TWELVE WEEK
FITNESS & NUTRITION
PROGRAMME
FOR WOMEN

Real results
No gimmicks
No airbrushing

GAVIN & ALISON MOREY

BLOOMSBURY
EY

Note
While every effort has been made to ensure that the content of this book is as technically accurate and as sound as possible, neither the author nor the publishers can accept responsibility for any injury or loss sustained as a result of the use of this material.

Published by Bloomsbury Publishing Plc
50 Bedford Square
London WC1B 3DP
www.bloomsbury.com

Bloomsbury is a trademark of Bloomsbury Publishing Plc

First edition 2014

Copyright © 2014 Gavin Morey and Alison Morey

ISBN (paperback): 978-1-4081-9639-7
ISBN (ePdf): 978-1-4081-9640-3
ISBN (EPUB): 978-1-4081-9641-0

A CIP catalogue record for this book is available from the British Library.

This book is produced using paper that is made from wood grown in managed, sustainable forests. It is natural, renewable and recyclable. The logging and manufacturing processes conform to the environmental regulations of the country of origin.

Typeset in URW Grotesk Light
Typesetting and page layouts by Susan McIntyre

Printed and bound in China by C&C Offset Printing Co

10 9 8 7 6 5 4 3 2 1

Acknowledgements
Cover photograph © Shutterstock
Inner photographs © the authors, except images of Alison in a black top © Grant Pritchard; images of food in chapter 6 and images before chapters 4 and 6 and pages 43, 55 and 110 © Shutterstock; and images in front of chapters: 1 © Wladimir Bulgar/Science Photo Library/Getty Images, 2 © Chris Gramly/Getty Images, 3 © Danita Delimont/Gallo Images/Getty Images, 5 © Joshua Hodge Photography/E+/ Getty Images, and 8 © webphotographeer/E+/Getty Images Illustrations by David Gardner, except the image before chapter 7 © Shutterstock
Commissioned by Kirsty Schaper

CONTENTS

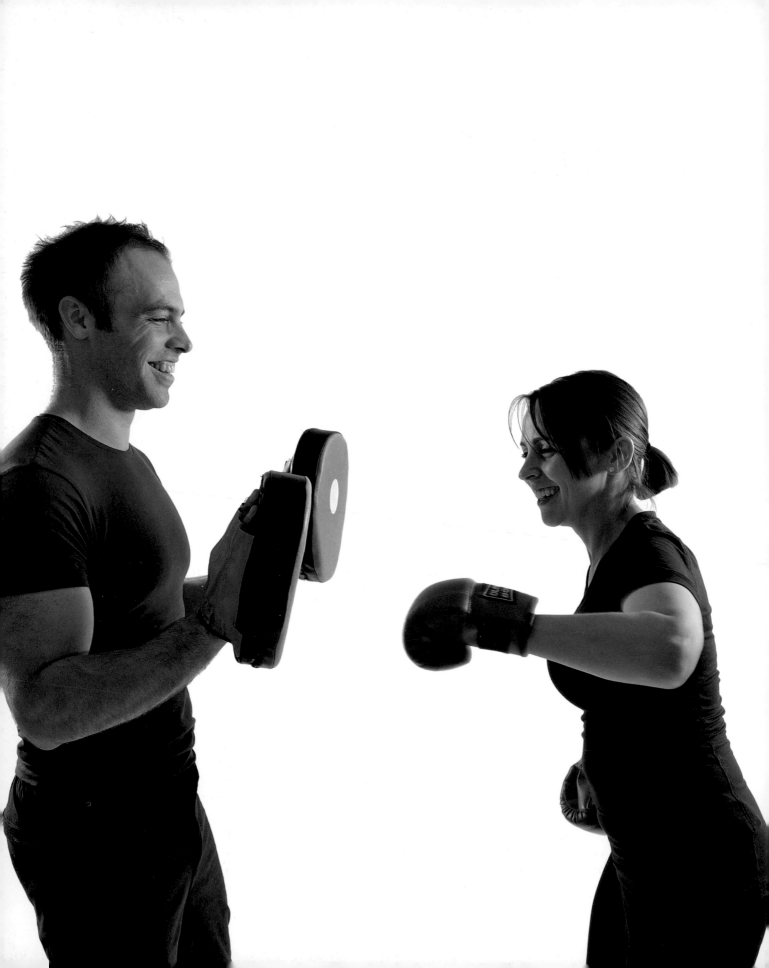

INTRODUCTION

My name is Gavin, and I am a personal trainer. I created the Twelve Week Fitness and Nutrition Programme, tailoring one for women and one for men – both with amazing results.

The Twelve Week Fitness and Nutrition Programme for Women has been designed to show you how to change your body and lifestyle for the better in just 12 weeks. This book is for those who want to change, and with this programme change will be inevitable. But how much you change is up to you.

How does the challenge work?

I noticed that most other 12-week programmes available on the market showed very unrealistic 'before' and 'after' shots, completely unachievable for the average person. I wanted to design a simple, achievable programme that anyone could follow in their own home, and that would be believable and possible for anyone willing to give it a try. It was important not to have any of the photos retouched, so what you see in this book is 100 per cent real. No gimmicks, no airbrushing, real results.

We used a home gym, bike, home health checks (glucose test, cholesterol test and blood pressure kit), other health tests readily available on the internet (fat percentage monitor, callipers, tape measure and peak flow meter), bleep tests, plumb line to check posture, and a home-made photo studio.

There are over 55 workouts in this book, with pictures of every aspect of the training, plus weekly pictures of Alison herself to show her progress throughout the programme. Over 80 of the exercises performed in this book are illustrated, each with a label explaining its purpose and how to perform it effectively.

Will the 12-week programme work for me?

The simple answer is it will work for anyone who wants to give it a go. Having done it herself, Alison is living proof that it works.

Let me now introduce you to Alison. I chose her to complete the programme as she is fairly typical of someone who wants to look and feel good, lose a bit of weight and become more toned. She works in a leading spa and knows how important it is to look after yourself. With irregular shift patterns and little spare time, however, she found going to the gym difficult, although she did play volleyball once or twice a week.

When I asked Alison if she would be my model for the 12-week challenge, her immediate reaction was a definite no. However, when I offered to give her the final say on the book after she'd completed the challenge, Alison finally agreed. And I'm delighted to say that she was over the moon with the results.

I needed to start Alison's training slowly and gradually build it up as, like most people, she'd had no previous experience of training. We began by introducing her to full body workouts with weights, and by gradually upping her walking to running. I then chose to incorporate weights to give Alison some shape and tone. The cardio training improved her fitness levels and decreased body fat. Finally, I introduced circuit training to reduce her body fat further, improve her cardio and increase her muscular endurance.

Although the training programme was a factor in getting Alison's body into shape, it was just as important for her to follow a sensible nutrition plan. Without following the nutrition plan, the results would not have been so impressive.

Injury and disclaimer

Muscles and injuries are my field of expertise, but before you begin any hard and strenuous exercise you should consult a GP. This is only to have reassurance from the medical field.

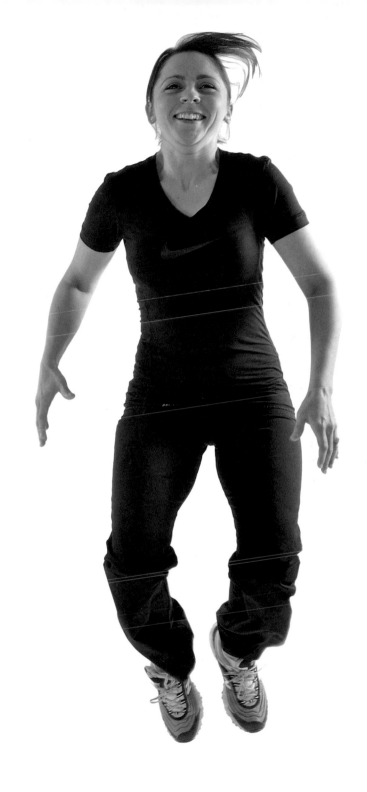

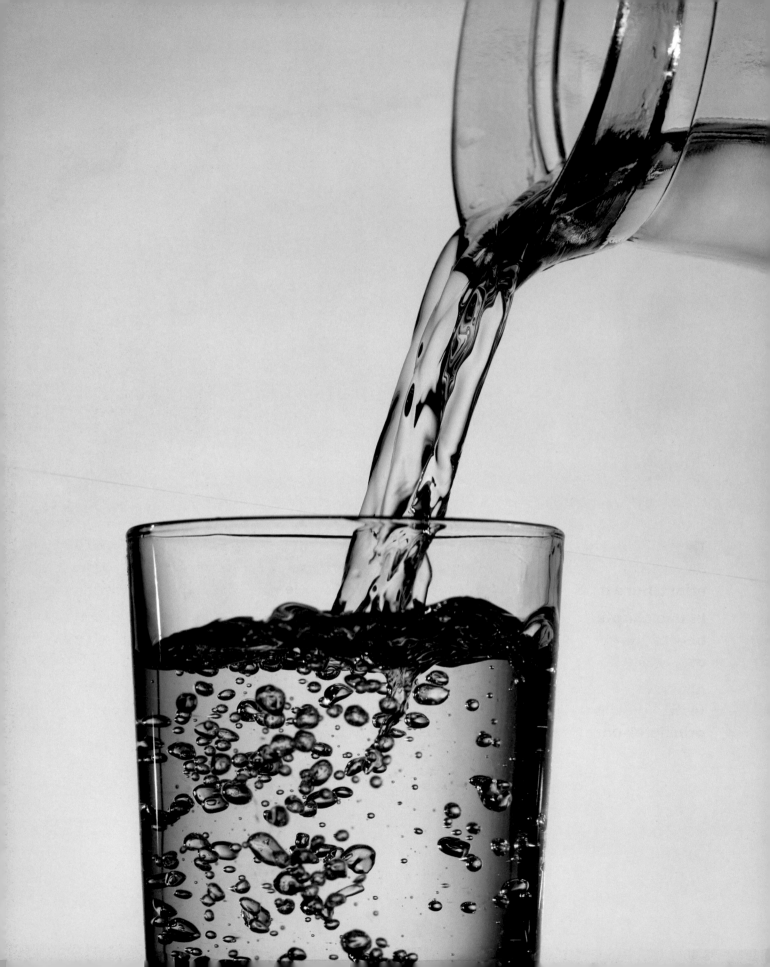

HEALTHY LIFESTYLE VERSUS UNHEALTHY LIFESTYLE

01

This book is here to show you the truth behind poor fitness programmes, faddy diets, fake photos and imagined results. To achieve your ultimate goal it takes effort, hard training, a healthy balanced diet, lifestyle changes and commitment.

In this chapter we look at how many times you will be training a week, and look behind the scenes at Alison's training plan. We shall also be taking a quick look at why Alison decided she wanted to change both her body and her lifestyle.

Alison's progress is shown through weekly photos, and weekly fitness and health tests. You will be guided step by step through all the training sessions, training principles and exercises in her personal diaries.

BEFORE THE CHALLENGE

What was Alison's lifestyle like before taking the challenge?

'Although I have quite a small body frame, at the age of 18 I gained weight by gorging on sweet things and tortilla chips. Combine this with eight years of sitting full time behind an office desk, and the result was a considerable amount of cellulite and chubbiness around my hips and thighs. Eventually this crept up to my waist too. I decided to join an outdoor pursuits club, eat fairly sensibly and work out playing volleyball a couple of times a week. However, I never really shifted much weight.

'I then decided to change my career path, which involved irregular shift work. This made it really hard to form regular eating and fitness routines. Eventually I had to give up my fitness club as it clashed with my work shifts. I would work most weekends, and never had quality time with friends and family. It wasn't long before I became very unhappy with myself.

'I suffer from asthma and it can be triggered by vigorous exercise, so I never really pushed my body past any pain barriers. My view was when I felt tired, I would stop. However, now I realise that the fitter I am, the less I'm held back by my asthma. Now I feel so much healthier, and it is all thanks to Gavin and the Twelve Week Fitness and Nutrition Programme for Women.'

How did Alison feel about the way she looked and felt?

'I felt so ashamed of myself and the damage I had done to my body – especially my thighs and general health. With excess weight and cellulite, I never felt confident wearing a bikini, and when Gavin asked me to wear one to show my progress in this book, I immediately said "NO!"

'I was self-conscious about my body and never liked the shape of it, particularly the flabby bits. I was often tired and exhausted, and always put this down to working too much and doing shifts with silly hours. I thought this was normal and that this was how everyone felt, but now I realise it was because I was unfit, unhealthy and stuck in a rut.

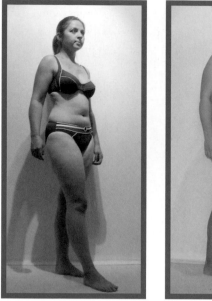 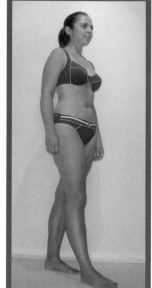

Week 1   Week 12

'I never gave my posture any consideration at all, I thought my body was the way it was because it was supposed to be like that. However, I did notice a considerable difference to my neck area after working for eight years at a desk with incorrect ergonomic desk settings – my neck curved, forming a slight hump. Also, I suffered from regular lower back pain.'

What did Alison used to eat?

'I didn't think I had that bad a diet before starting the 12-week programme. I like my sweet foods and would enjoy these as a comforter. I would always have breakfast, but either toast or cereals that are meant to be good for you. But I've since found out that they are high in sugar.

'As I am allergic to dairy I have never eaten any dairy products, so that was never too much of an issue with me. For lunch I would eat a sandwich or food provided for me at work. These meals tended to be high in carbohydrates, such as chips, jacket potatoes or pasta, and I would always finish with a sweet pudding of some sort.

'Again, I would snack during shifts with little cakes, sweets and crisps, and for dinner I enjoyed eating pasta and quite hearty and simple foods at home. However, when I was on shift work, I would eat pretty much the same as lunch. I love to bake and so if I had a sweet craving, I would bake something sweet and devour the lot. Again, I know that this is one of my biggest downfalls.

'I thought my diet was normal, but these foods eaten regularly over a period of 10 years or more made me overweight and extremely uncomfortable. Since doing my challenge, my diet has become much more balanced and varied thanks to Gavin's recipes.'

BEHIND THE SCENES

This is as real as it gets. By taking you into Alison's life, with real pictures and results, this book shows you that you can do anything you want if you put your mind to it.

I find it hard looking through the various health and fitness books and magazines that show these amazing results in just two weeks. These books promise you the earth, and to follow their diet normally consists of you following a bodybuilder's pre-contest diet. Of course this type of diet works, but trust me, I have trained a fair few amateur bodybuilders in my time and they do not follow this type of diet all year round.

Even now, you can see 'before' and 'after' pictures that are just unrealistic. They either look like they are completely different people, heavily airbrushed, or you can see that the photos have been taken after a far greater length of time than is claimed.

On a serious note, it is never good to lose weight too quickly as your body needs time to adapt to its new routine. Remember, with the yo-yo diet you will always end up putting on more body fat than you first started with.

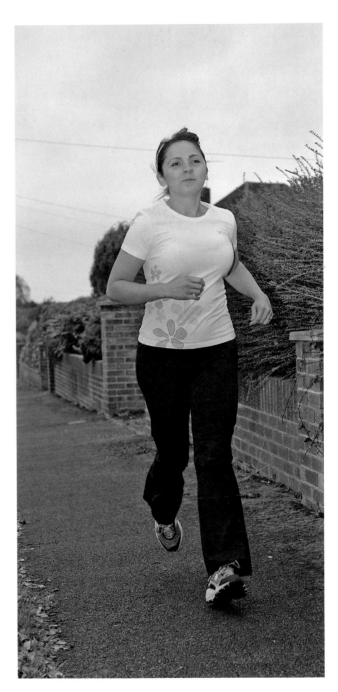

Fake tan or real tan?

I am against the use of fake tan in our photos as it goes completely against our ethos of no gimmicks. Alison has never used fake tan as she prefers the sun. The reason why you can see Alison becoming more tanned week by week was because we trained outdoors, where possible, during the summer months.

Remember, the sun is really vital for a healthy lifestyle and it gives our body lots of vitamin D. This is essential to help absorb and use calcium within our bodies, and it helps our immune system. Too much sun, however, can damage our skin and cause health concerns, so it is really important to use sun protection when you are outside for long periods or if UV levels are very high.

Real pictures or airbrushed pictures?

I need you, as the reader, to understand what it actually takes to get into shape, and if we ended up airbrushing any of the pictures we would be cheating not only ourselves but also you by showing something that cannot be sensibly achieved.

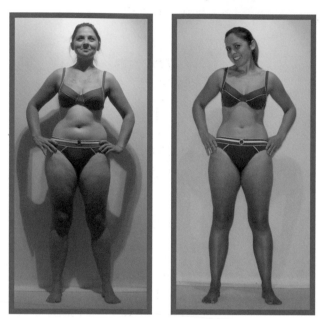

The style of these pictures is based on the photos you normally see in fitness magazines. The difference with these photos is that when you look closely, you will see Alison's flaws and blemishes – no airbrushing. These pictures are taken before and after Alison completed the 12-week challenge. What a difference.

Photographs

We chose to take photographs weekly to show you exactly what happened to Alison's body and what could happen to yours. Also, by taking weekly photos we can prove that the before and after photos were not separated by a longer period, so that you can follow Alison's progress with accuracy. Alison's photo was taken weekly and taken at approximately the same time of day to give you the truest results possible.

I decided not to use a professional photographer, but to take the photographs myself. This provides you with realistic view of Alison, as she has no special lighting or make-up to hide behind.

SUPPLEMENTS

I'm not sure why so many books say you have to drink meal replacement shakes and/or use supplements to reach your dream physique. That is a load of rubbish, and it angers me because this is not the case. You can achieve the body you want without any supplements, as Alison has in this book and I did in the men's book.

If you do choose to take supplements alongside your fitness and nutrition plan, please buy the best quality ones you can. I'm not against supplements, just the misuse of them. If you use them sensibly, they can aid in achieving your dream physique, but only if used alongside a balanced and healthy diet (or if you have a deficiency of some sort). Provided they are accredited, you should achieve excellent results.

In the next chapter, you will get to know your body inside and out, by recognising your body's health signs. You will start to understand how a poor diet or deficiency in vitamins or minerals can affect you. If you are suffering from a deficiency, then by all means either try eating the right foods or take supplements. However, following the 12-week programme should prove to you that you don't have to use supplements and protein/meal replacement shakes to get to where you want to be. It just takes the right training, nutrition, commitment, motivation and determination, all of which have to be fun.

FOLLOWING THE BOOK

Use this book and the training diaries as guidance and reference, to show you how hard you should train throughout the 12 weeks. You will be able to note down in your own training diary what you have been doing, the times you have been training, the weights you have been lifting, training RPE (rating perceived exertion), and so on. When following the workouts, please follow the exercises step by step to see what to do first. The training diary is your very own fitness programme, which you can take everywhere – even on holiday.

Alison used the training diary as a progress report showing what she was running or lifting, so the next time she attempted to do the same exercise she would always try to improve on it no matter how small the difference.

At the start of every week's training overview, you can jot down your feelings in your own personal diary next to Alison's. You will also notice the health tests you need to take in order to monitor your progress every week, and you can compare your results next to Alison's if you like. There are monthly tests for your glucose and cholesterol levels, postural analysis, etc., as well as the weekly tests of measurements, weight, body mass index (BMI), etc.

TRAINING

You will begin your training by exercising just three times for the first week. As the weeks go by, the number of training days will increase. I have done it this way to prevent overtraining, and to give you plenty of rest days so that your body can recover.

Near the middle, and towards the end of the programme, I have used shock tactics to try and get the most out of your muscles. You will also notice the mileage on the running and cycling picks up throughout the 12-week programme. This should enable you to comfortably run 10km (6.2 miles) at the end, as well as easily cycling over 15 miles.

How many times will you exercise?

In total, Alison exercised 57 times in the 12 weeks, exercising on average a little over four times a week, although it varied as the weeks went by. In the first week it was only three times, and by the end of the programme she was exercising up to seven times a week (which included dog walking).

On average, your training per week will be:
2 × cardio
1 × weight training
1 × circuit training

What exercises do I do?

You have a choice of over 80 exercises included in the book, with details of which specific muscles are being used. Although some of the exercises aren't utilised in the training, I have kept them in the book to give you as much choice and knowledge as possible on how to target specific muscles. Remember, variety is what we need.

How many rest days?

On average you will have at least two days off each week. Alison had about 28 rest days over the 12 weeks.

How long are the workout sessions?

The average time for the workout was 1 hour 2 minutes. Of course, this is an average. There were short training sessions of 20 minutes and long sessions of up to five hours (walking). Alison usually worked out either at 10.00 a.m. or 6.00 p.m., depending on her work shift patterns and days off.

Holiday and training

It is still possible to be good, eat well and train hard when you're on holiday. You can still exercise while you're away. Depending on the holiday, you can walk a lot, and most hotels have some sort of fitness suite you can use. Look at Chapter 3 on healthy eating to learn how to choose the right meals when you eat out.

Cheat days, training and nutrition

The purpose of the nutritional programme is not about dieting or dictating what you can and cannot eat. Its aim is not to reduce the amounts of food you eat, or even to deprive you of vital carbohydrates or fat, but to show that you can achieve a good physique by following a healthy plan that contains all your nutritional requirements.

When doing the fitness programme, Alison listened to whether her body was telling her if she was too stressed or overdoing things. You need to take these signs on board and change how you behave. This is why you have so many rest days at the beginning, to prepare your body for all the training you will undertake over the 12 weeks.

Training through all conditions

You may come up with all sorts of excuses why you can't train, but when you really want something badly enough, nothing should stand in your way.

Setting goals

I always tell my clients the importance of setting goals. This will motivate you all the way to the end, and push you to limits you might never have thought possible. When choosing your goals you should aim big, such as being able to run 10km. You should then have lots of little goals in between to keep you motivated and on track, like having mini markers every 2.5km.

Alison's big goal was to get the best results possible in the 12 weeks, and her little goals were all the training days during those 12 weeks.

You are reading this book because you have chosen your big goal. Use everything within this book to guide you to your goal and support you all the way.

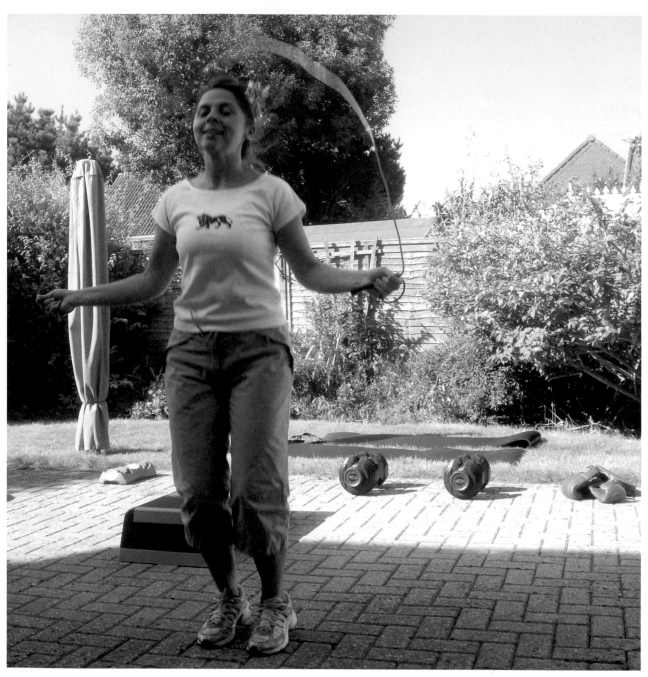

How do you get through the training on bad days?

The best ways to keep training through those tough days are never to lose your sense of humour, to train with a friend or a training partner, and to lift your spirits by remembering why you are doing this challenge in the first place. I advised Alison that she should train through rough days by thinking of the end result. It is also a good thing to train with other people as much as possible so you can motivate each other.

Never give up on the bad days. Having a training partner really does help you get through it.

DOMS – delayed onset muscle soreness

Often felt 24 to 72 hours after exercising, DOMS can cause pain, discomfort, stiffness and strength loss, which generally subsides within two to three days. Although the precise cause is still unknown, a theory recently developed states that DOMS is caused by the breakdown of muscular fibres. This is particularly apparent in strength/resistance programmes. The breakdown occurs due to stress and allows the muscles to grow stronger.

Try not to worry if you have DOMS. When you read through Alison's diary you will see she suffered from DOMS on a regular basis.

Remember these simple steps to help combat DOMS:

1. Stretch between sets while exercising.
2. Stretch at the end of the training session.
3. Stretch the muscles suffering from DOMS at least 6–12 times a day.
4. If you're really sore, do not exercise your muscles but take a day off to allow them to recover.

Overtraining

We start nice and slowly with the training to prevent overtraining. You don't want to exhaust your body so you won't be able to complete the 12-week programme. That is why the first three weeks are nice and easy, with the workouts gradually increasing in intensity over the 12 weeks.

Overtraining comes from training beyond the body's ability to recover. It can come from training too hard or too long without the adequate recovery and rest. If left too long this will backfire – it will decrease your performance in training and you will start to lose your physique.

The signs of overtraining:

- Feeling tired and drained.
- Lack of energy and the feeling of not wanting to train.
- Pain in your muscles and possibly joints.
- Drop in performance – diminished power, speed, strength, etc.
- Lack of concentration.

Treating overtraining

The only way to counteract overtraining is to stop all training and exercise, and rest for at least three days, or until you feel that your body and mind are functioning properly. When you rest, remember that it should be complete rest, and you should drink plenty of water and eat a little more food than normal. This will help your muscles recover back to their full capacity, and then you are ready to resume training. When you do go back into training, make sure that you take it easy for the first week and then gradually increase your performance.

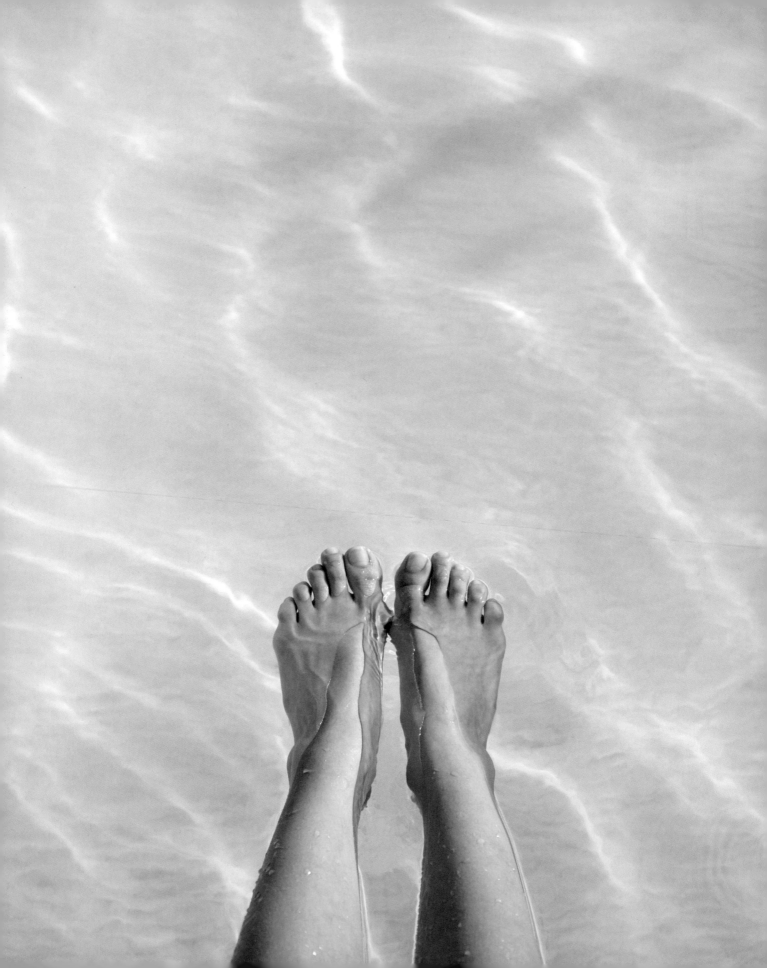

KNOWING YOUR BODY INSIDE AND OUT

02

It is important to know your body inside and out. What is normal for you may not be normal for someone else, and vice versa. Everyone can say they have noticed things about their body that were not normal for them at one time or another. Your body talks to you all the time, perhaps only in subtle measures, but by learning to read these signals it will enable you to act on anything that may be upsetting your well-being or disturbing your equilibrium.

The signs may be small, and you may feel that they are even unimportant, like having yellow fingers, for example. This could simply be a result of nicotine discolouration – however, it could also be a warning sign for a disorder in your liver or lungs. Try not to take anything for granted.

Knowing how to differentiate between these small signals before they turn into the actual symptoms of a disorder is a delicate matter, and should not be rushed. The following information is an easy reference guide to highlight some things that may be troubling you, and how you can watch out for signs of poor health in your own body.

TONGUE

We can detect a lot about the health of a person by looking at aspects of their tongue, such as changes to the shape, size, colour, texture and coating. In fact, the tongue is still used today in Chinese medicine to help diagnose various health concerns. The tongue is covered with several types of papillae or nodules that continually shed and grow like hair, making it a great source of information about our health.

This is a guide for a healthy tongue:

- **Size and shape** – normal and proportionate to the body
- **Colour** – salmon or pinky red shade
- **Texture** – smooth with no marks or cracks
- **Coating** – thin, white, moist coating across the whole tongue

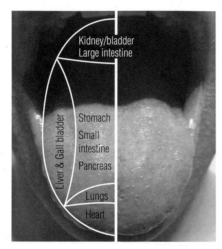

Week 1 – This is my own tongue at week 1 in the 'for men' 12-week programme. Please note the teeth marks on the side of the tongue and the slightly red tip. Both of these signs indicate poor nutrition, something that the 12-week programme can help alleviate by showing you how to eat a healthy balanced diet.

Here are some things to look out for when investigating your tongue. These could be caused by different conditions or could well be an indication of possible problems within certain body systems. Remember, this is just a guideline.

Size and shape

Big and unusually red – the protective papillae could be being damaged, for example, by teeth or dentures rubbing on the tongue.

Swollen – this could be due to poor digestion. For swollen sides of the tongue, it could be that the liver is being overworked, or there is a problem within the gallbladder.

Colour

Unusually red – possibly acute fever. If it is also smooth, it may indicate a vitamin B12 deficiency or an intestinal disorder where nutrients are not being adequately absorbed.

Red tip – indication of depression, a lack of sleep or stress.

Pale – possible lack of nutrients within the body such as vitamin B12 or folic acid. It may also be caused by a hormone imbalance.

Purple – poor circulation, poor nutrition or a lack of vitamin B-complex and minerals.

Texture

Peeling – dry mouth or a deficiency in vitamin B.

Teeth marks – normally occurs with a swollen tongue and could suggest digestion problems.

Scrotal tongue – an indication of an infection or poor nutrition.

Groovy tongue – something people are usually born with, and may not be noticed right away. It tends to become more noticeable as you age.

Coating

White – indication of the recovery from a recent fever or a poor diet lacking in fibre.

Black – possible reaction to antibiotics or to stomach medication. Poor oral hygiene, smoking, excessive use of mouthwash, infection, digestion or poorly managed diabetes may also cause this.

Brown and yellow – trapped bacteria and food or excessive smoking and coffee. Yellow coating is normally seen with a red tip.

TEETH AND GUMS

We all want those pearly white teeth and healthy gums to give the biggest and best smile imaginable. As a rule, I will usually brush my teeth twice a day, but please note that if you are following the information below, visit your dentist when it is next convenient.

Here are some things to look out for when investigating your teeth and gums. These could be caused by different conditions, or could well be an indication of possible future dental problems, so please consult your dentist if you have any concerns at all.

Teeth

Sensitive – caused by the thinning of your enamel layer (the outer layer that protects your inner dentine), which causes the dentine underneath to become exposed. Dental erosion, gum recession, gum disease, cracked tooth, tooth fillings and teeth bleaching can all lead to sensitive teeth.

Movement – there is a natural tooth movement that occurs throughout your life. It could be due to a tooth that is about to fall out, trauma, advanced gum disease or, if you are missing a tooth, the teeth on either side can move to fill in that space.

Discolouration – an indication of a poor diet, or caused by drinking coffee, soft drinks, tobacco, poor dental hygiene, disease, medication, trauma, advanced ageing, or choosing the wrong toothpaste.

Gums

Pain – this could be due to an injury, dental disease, tooth decay, scurvy, vitamin B deficiency, iron deficiency, Behçet's or Reiter's Syndrome.

Swelling – could be an indication of gum infection, monilia, oral fungal infection, gum disease, gingivitis, poorly fitted dentures, toothpaste or mouthwash allergies. It could also be a possible sign of malnutrition.

Bleeding – this could be due to trauma, disease, mouth sores, systemic conditions, pregnancy and hormonal changes, medication, and vitamin C and K deficiencies.

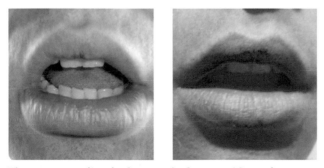

These are my lips before and after my 12-week programme. You can see on week 1 I had dry and slightly cracked lips but by week 12 I had supple and smooth lips.

LIPS

Dry and cracked lips could be caused by external factors such as cold weather, or may be a symptom of dehydration or a nutritional deficiency.

EYES

Your eyes are a big give-away and say a lot about you, how you are feeling, and ultimately how healthy you are. As an organ, the eyes are a great source of information for detecting those early signs of ill health. This is why your doctor will still occasionally examine your eyes when you visit.

Our eyes have more than two million working parts, which make them the second most complex organ in your body (the first is the brain), and while some say eyes are the windows to the soul, others have a more practical view.

Red and/or bloodshot – small blood vessels in the eyes become inflamed and dilated which causes bloodshot eyes. This may be caused by, or is an indication of, eye-strain, fatigue, colds, allergies, ocular rosacea, or a deficiency in vitamins B2 and B6 and amino acids commonly found in protein.

It is important to seek medical advice if you are suffering from bloodshot eyes along with any of these symptoms: severe headache, blurred vision, mental confusion, nausea/vomiting, or if you are seeing halos around lights. This may be an indication of an attack of acute glaucoma (a sudden increase in eye pressure).

Yellow eye – if the whites of your eyes turn yellow it could be a possible indication of a liver problem such as jaundice, gallbladder concerns, Gilbert's syndrome, sickle cell anaemia, pancreatic cancer or yellow fever.

Dry eyes – this condition occurs when the eyes don't produce enough tears to keep them moist. It is very common in women, especially after the menopause, due to the body's reduction of oestrogen.

This could also be environmental, for example, due to windy, dry or hot air, or air conditioning. A sluggish thyroid, constant contact lens usage, a deficiency in omega-3 and omega-6, or a reaction to prescriptive and non-prescriptive drugs can also cause dry eyes.

Watery eyes – too many tears being produced could

be linked to allergies, a deficiency in vitamin B2 or ocular rosacea.

Bags under the eyes – puffy pouches of skin under the eye. This is common as the skin around the eye ages and loses elasticity. Depression, insomnia or deprived sleep, crying, a high level of salt intake, a sluggish thyroid, fluid retention, kidney problems, or a bad reaction to medicine can encourage bags under the eye area.

Circles under the eyes – these could be indications of sleep deprivation, digestive problems, sluggish liver, eczema or allergies.

Bulging eyes – possibly due to an overactive thyroid. It is important to visit your doctor if you suspect this.

Yellowish lump/bump on the cornea – if you notice these small yellow lumps, don't worry, they tend to be age spots called pinguecula.

Spots on the eye – red spots on the whites of your eyes are usually blood vessels that have burst. It is normally caused by forceful sneezing or coughing, high blood pressure or injury.

NAILS

Your fingernails and toenails actually count as part of your skin, and are another great way of highlighting a number of medical and nutritional conditions. Nails are made of protein (keratin) and contain less water than skin, which makes them harder and protects the ends of the fingers and toes.

Fingernails take around four months to grow out, while toenails take at least six. If your nail growth is slower than average, it is possible that you have a fungal infection or a nutritional deficiency such as a lack of iron.

Healthy nails have the following characteristics:
- **Texture** – smooth, no ridges, thickness or cracks
- **Shape** – no exaggerated curving up or down at the ends
- **Nail bed colour** – pink
- **Colour of nails** – white

Here are some things to look out for when investigating your nails.

Texture

Horizontal ridges – these go from side to side across your nail and can be an indication of a thyroid concern, stress, vitamin B deficiency, or the result of a nail injury that has stunted nail growth.

Vertical ridges – these go from the nail bed up to the tip. They may be due to nutritional disorders, a lack of iron, or a kidney disorder.

Pitted nails – this could be caused by lack of vitamin C, psoriasis or deficiency in protein, and is a common sign for autoimmune disorders.

Thick nails – this could be a result of poor circulation, injury, fungal infection, poor diet or diabetes.

Rough nails – if they have a sandpaper-like texture, rough nails could indicate a skin or hair disorder such as psoriasis or eczema.

Brittle or cracked nails – often this is due to the use of harsh cleaning products, a thyroid disease, iron deficiency, vitamin A deficiency, or a lack of calcium.

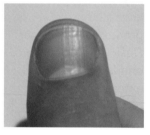

Looking at my thumbnail from week 1, you will notice that I have vertical ridges across the nail and a horizontal ridge at the top. This indicates nutritional deficiency.

Shape

Nails curve upwards (resembles a spoon) – could be a possible nutritional deficiency, a lack of iron, or a vitamin B12 deficiency.

Nails curve downwards (clubbed nails) – could be an indication of bowel disease, liver disease or a lack of oxygen in the body. Once this condition occurs, it is normally permanent.

Nail bed colour

Blue – may be caused by a lung disorder.

Yellow – sign of a heavy smoker, jaundice or yellow nail syndrome (this is a rare condition however).

Pale – possible sign of anaemia.

White spots – may be due to nail separation from the nail bed, nail warts, zinc or calcium deficiency, or systematic conditions that affect the skin, lungs and other organs.

HAIR AND SCALP

The hair defines the overall health of a person like no other part of the body. You could say that our luscious locks are a barometer of our general health. Hair condition is a true reflection of the nutrition it receives from the scalp – so the better the diet, the better the hair condition.

Hair is made up from protein (keratin) and minerals, which go through the hair growth cycle. The hair has a growth phase, followed by a resting phase, and then a shedding phase. It then repeats the cycle.

When we look at hair, we are looking at its condition, texture and volume to gauge how well our bodies are nourished.

Here are some things to look out for when investigating your hair.

Condition

Dry scalp – this could be due to the environment, hard water, poor diet, or the improper use of hair products.

Flaky scalp/dandruff – dandruff is not contagious and is not usually a serious problem. Some cases of excessive dandruff with intense itching and patches of flaky skin elsewhere on your body are most likely to be a form of eczema.

A flaky scalp may be caused by, or is an indication of, a fungus (malassezia), hormone changes, stress, neurological disorders, infrequent shampooing, skin ailments (psoriasis or infections), or the improper use of hair products.

Brittle and split ends – could be due to the environment, a poor diet, lack of protein and essential fatty acids, thyroid disease, menopause, excessive washing and drying, using bleaching and dying products, iodine deficiency, pregnancy, or the improper use of hair products.

Volume

Thinning hair/hair loss – this is normally determined by our genes and the ageing process, but may also be caused by a poor diet, lack of iron, or possible thyroid disease.

Texture

Dry – this can be an indication of a poor diet, the environment, lack of protein and essential fatty acids, thyroid disease, menopause, excessive washing and drying, using bleaching and dye products, iodine deficiency, pregnancy, or the improper use of hair products.

Greasy/oily – occurs due to an overproduction of sebum, a waxy substance from the sebaceous glands, which keeps the hair supple, soft and waterproof. Fine hair tends to be greasier due to having more sebaceous glands. It may also be caused by genetics, the improper use of hair products or a lack of regular hair cleaning.

SKIN

Our skin is a reliable indicator for assessing general health as it is quite obvious when a person is run down, tired or ill by simply looking at their skin. Just think of all those skin creams and serums produced and marketed to millions of people across the world, claiming to dispel aged or tired looking skin. A good routine and a healthy, balanced diet are the basis for picture-perfect skin.

Our skin protects us from the environment, provides a unique barrier to infection, and helps excrete waste and toxins from within the body. It regulates and maintains a healthy balance of fluids and minerals, and is of course the source of our sensory receptors for touch. It is the largest organ of the body, and is indirectly linked to almost every part of your body, except the eyes and teeth.

Here are some things to look out for when investigating your skin.

Colour

Pale – could be an indication of anaemia or iron deficiency.

Blue tone – may be caused by oxygen deficiency in the blood, exposure to cold temperature, lung disease or heart disease.

Yellow tone – could be jaundice, the consumption of too much beta-carotene (foods such as carrots), or too much vitamin A.

Grey tone – can be caused by smoking, a sluggish liver, cardiovascular disease or feeling unwell.

Red tone – rosacea, over-exertion, inflammation or burns can contribute to a red skin tone. Caught in the early stages, rosacea may cause flushing or blushing, but can progress to permanent redness. The rash consists of tiny pimples as well as dilated blood vessels under the skin and may be found on the face and body, which can cause an itching and burning sensation.

Texture

Dark patches on the skin – possible indication of diabetes and insulin resistance, a hormonal disorder, or an adrenal gland concern.

Scaly rash – can be an indication of psoriasis, an infection or emotional stress.

It is common to find random lumps and bumps either on top of or beneath the skin surface from time to time, and most of these are harmless. Some, however, are not. If you notice a change in the size or shape of a lump or bump do not hesitate to see your doctor. Early detection of any pre-cancerous or cancerous cells will help treatment. Listen to your body.

Facial skin

We get oily and dry skin on both our body and face. Here are some things to look out for when investigating your facial skin more closely.

Colour

Rosy cheeks – these can be due to a hot flush, over exertion, rosacea, sun damage, or an autoimmune inflammation disease.

Dark patches – these can result from pregnancy, sun damage, a reaction to medication or contraceptive pills, or indicate high levels of oestrogen.

Texture

Oily/greasy – caused by overproduction of sebum, a waxy substance from the sebaceous glands. This could be an indication of stress, pregnancy, hormone imbalance, medication, genetics, or poor diet (high intake of sodium, sugar and saturated fat). The improper use of cosmetic products or a deficiency in vitamin B2 could also cause an outbreak. It is not all bad news, however; your natural sebum slows down the signs of ageing.

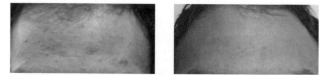

Look at the amazing difference 12 weeks can make to your skin with the right nutrition, cosmetics and advice.

It is important to highlight the difference between dry skin and dehydrated skin.

Dry skin – this lacks the oils and moisture to keep skin supple and regulated. If your face never shows an oily shine and you've never even had a pimple (let alone acne), you are most likely to have normal to dry skin. Dry skin may be caused by genetics, or you may be deficient in essential fatty acids (omega-3, omega-6 and omega-9) and/or vitamins A and B. Hormones, skin disorders such as eczema, the environment, and the improper use of cosmetic products could also dry your skin.

Dehydrated skin – this is caused by a lack of water within the cells of the skin. If you have had visible pores, especially around your chin, nose or eyebrows and are prone to spots, but your skin has a dry and scaly appearance, you probably have dehydrated skin. It could be due to dehydration throughout your body, skin disorders (eczema), the improper use of cosmetic products or the environment.

Combination skin – this is characterised by oily patches in certain areas and dry/dehydrated areas in other parts of your face. The normal areas for the oily patch are known as the T-zone: the forehead, nose, cheeks and chin. This is due to these areas having more sebaceous glands than other areas of the face, like the eyes and jaw line. With this combination skin type, awareness must be given to the cosmetic products that you use so that you do not aggravate the problem areas further.

Sensitive skin – thin or fine-textured skin reacts quickly to hot and cold temperatures, and so is easily affected by the environment (sun burn and wind chills). This skin type is usually dry and delicate, and prone to allergic reactions. Again, awareness must be given to the cosmetic products you use so as to not irritate the skin.

Skin care routine

There are a lot of things you can do to keep your skin healthy, feeling fresh and soft, and looking young. Maintaining a healthy diet, getting enough exercise, staying hydrated, avoiding any sun damage to the skin, and having low stress levels are all things that aid in keeping skin healthy. Following a skin care routine can also help. The skin care cycle has three main steps that should be followed daily to ensure a truly glowing complexion.

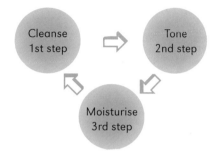

What is cleansing?

Throughout the day your skin is exposed to all kinds of things that clog up your pores, such as exhaust fumes, pollution, bacteria and dirt. Your skin naturally loses dead cells, excretes sweat (laced with toxins that your body is pushing out) and excess sebum.

By the end of the day, all this grime lies on the top of the skin and needs removing. When you cleanse, you remove this build-up. Oil-based, clay and scrub cleansers will also remove the top layer of dead skin.

What is toning?

This step is so simple and so often overlooked. Ultimately it is crucial to balance the skin, add nutrients and increase hydration. Toning removes any remaining grime left by the cleanser (which is especially important with oil-based cleansers), and will balance the pH of the skin. It will also aid in the tightening of pores, and helps the skin absorb oils more effectively.

What is moisturising?

This is the most important step in the cycle, and helps keep skin young and soft. Think about a piece of leather, for example. Adding oil keeps it from drying out, losing vibrancy and wrinkling. Cleansing removes the skin's natural oils on dry skin; on oily skin it signals to the skin to stimulate more oil production often causing overproduction. By not replacing these oils, the skin must work harder to balance itself.

A moisturiser is not just oil, though – it should be a blend of good quality ingredients, as it sinks into the skin. Using a cheaper alternative often means cheaper ingredients that will have a long-term negative effect on the skin's appearance.

CELLULITE

What is cellulite?

Cellulite is subcutaneous fat within fibrous connective tissue, but the term 'cellulite' is often used to describe the dimpling appearance of the skin that can represent an orange-peel texture. This is caused by fatty deposits that sit just below the skin. Cellulite generally appears in the thighs, buttocks and abdomen, and can affect both men and women.

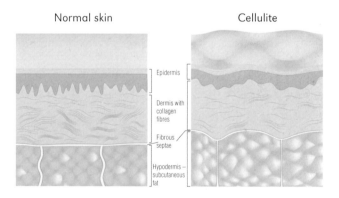

What causes cellulite?

There are a number of theories, but the cause is not fully understood. Here is a list of common causes:

- *Diet* – a poor and unbalanced diet, generally high in fats and carbs.
- *Lifestyle* – an inactive/sedentary lifestyle.
- *Genetics* – we inherit our parents' genes.
- *Hormones* – hormones regulate our body.

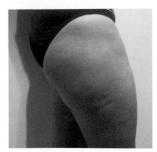
Week 1

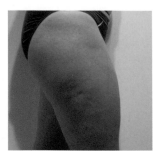
Week 4

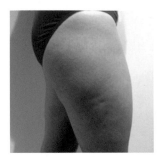
Week 8

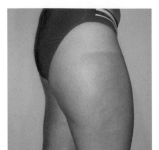
Week 12

See the reduction in cellulite from following the 12-week programme, and with a little help from the cellulite and lymphatic massages (see pages 339–340).

How did Alison get rid of her cellulite?

In addition to massage, Alison used an exercise programme that accelerates the breakdown of cellulite. Below are some methods for achieving the best results:

- *Skin:* regularly scrub the area of cellulite then moisturise your body. Rub and massage area.
- *Diet:* healthy and balanced; large variety of foods, herbs and spices; drink at least eight glasses of water a day.
- *Exercise:* any form of fat-burning exercises; become more active; use the myo stretch routine (see page 340) weekly.
- *Massage:* cellulite massage; lymphatic massage; muscular massage.

You need to break down the cellulite (with your hands), eat healthily to lose weight, and then exercise to increase your blood flow, all of which will get rid of the unwanted cellulite. If you can combine these together as Alison did, then you will achieve similar results.

LOOKING AFTER YOUR BODY

With all of the information you have just gained, you may now be wondering what you can do to help yourself.

One thing you may have noticed is that poor nutrition – lacking in vitamins and minerals – plays an important role in giving signs of poor health. By changing the way you eat, and by choosing a rounded diet that is nutritious and high in vitamins and minerals, your body will return to full health.

For any health concerns that you may have, you can help yourself in many ways, ranging from homeopathic remedies and supplements to holistic therapies. Whatever concerns you may have, remember there is nothing too big or too small for your GP. They are there to help you.

TAKE CONTROL OF THE BASICS

When we look at the basics for health, we are looking at the situations that we face every day of our lives. How we handle stress, how we overcome tiredness, and how we get the most out of ourselves.

It is these situations that change the way we look at life and make us into who we are. If we can take hold of these basics, we will be able to get more out of ourselves and others.

STRESS

We feel stress when pressure is placed upon us, whether actual or imagined. It can be harmful, but a certain amount can be good for us to help motivation, performance and productivity. Too much stress, however, can prompt depression, so please keep a close eye on yourself and others.

People react differently to stress; some have a higher threshold than others. Reasons for stress are very broad and unpredictable. It is a common fact that stress can be caused by demanding deadlines at work, the loss of a loved one, relationship concerns, financial pressures or illness. These and many more concerns can cause anxiety and stress, which can lead to physical, emotional and mental health problems. When we are faced with circumstances that are stressful to our mind and body, the body releases hormones (chemicals like cortisol and adrenaline), which help regulate our responses internally.

Adrenaline, for instance, is released to help us cope with dangerous or unexpected conditions. These invoke the flight or fight impulse – the biological response to acute stress. It is interesting, however, that when faced with a situation in which you are prevented from either fleeing or fighting, such as being in a crowded underground station, these chemicals are not released. If you have a build-up of these chemicals due to them not being used the consequences are felt throughout the body, such as an increase in blood pressure, heart rate and sweat production.

Stress can cause single or multiple conditions. The list below is not meant to scare you, it is simply to emphasise the need to try to control and minimise any stress you may feel in your life.

- Heart disease
- Muscular tension
- Pain
- Diet
- Depression
- Weight gain/loss/obesity
- Digestive problems
- Sleep problems
- Autoimmune diseases
- Lower immunity causing more colds, feeling run down, etc.
- Raised cholesterol
- Skin complaints

Stress responses

Stress affects our bodies in many ways and on many levels. Have a look below to understand your stress responses.

Physiological – tension from posture or overuse.
Emotional – anger, fear and hate are all reflected in our postures.
Behavioural – posture imbalance from habit.
Structural – the body and posture will change to meet any stress imposed upon it.

You can follow these steps to help control your own stress levels.

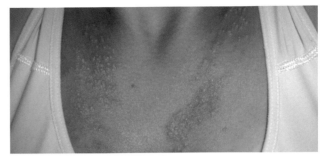

Week 1

Week 4

As you can see from these pictures, Alison was suffering from stress due to her work and lifestyle. We managed to beat the stress and calm down the skin dramatically within a short period by following the steps in this chapter.

Step 1 – your stress levels

These are influenced by numerous things. The key is to have the knowledge and power to monitor your own responses, and to seek help or advice when something gets a little too much for you to cope with. How you take control is up to you.

Step 2 – your sense of control

Have confidence in yourself and your ability to perform. Support from friends and family will encourage you to look on the positive side and to share some of your concerns, and will act as a buffer for life's stresses, resulting in you feeling less vulnerable.

Step 3 – your attitude

Try to have a more optimistic outlook. The ability to manage your emotions and bring them back into balance will enable you to become more calm and relaxed.

Step 4 – *your understanding and preparation*
Learn from past stresses and try to be prepared for similar future stresses.

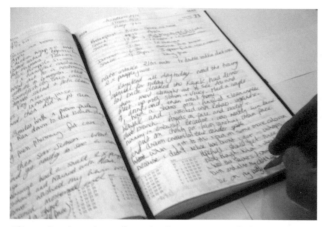

Alison jotting down her day's events and thoughts in her health diary.

Keeping track of stress
During the 12-week programme we used the RPE scale to track stress levels. As you can see from the graphs opposite, Alison's stress levels were fairly high at the start, but gradually decreased by eating healthily, exercising and taking control of your body's condition and lifestyle.

RPE (rating perceived exertion)
The RPE scale is a simple method of measuring how a person handles stress on their body. The original scale was introduced by Gunnar Borg, who rated exertion on a scale of 6–20, although many health practitioners now use a revised scale of 0–10, developed by the American College of Sports Medicine. RPE can be applied to absolutely anything.

0   Not stressed at all
1   Very, very light stress
2   Very light stress
3   Fairly light stress
4   Light amount of stress
5   Moderately stressed
6   Fairly stressed
7   Stressed
8   Very stressed
9   Very, very stressed
10 Stress is severely affecting life

Energy levels
It's a fact: having more energy in the body fights fatigue and reduces stress levels. We have all felt tired and lacking in energy from time to time, especially during busy or stressful periods. But if you know the cause then the solution is often easy. More often than not, the reasons are found in our everyday life and habits.

Energy levels can be affected by your diet, how much sleep you get and even your emotional state. There are many contributing factors that affect the balance of our emotional and physical state, which ultimately affect our energy levels. You should ask yourself how many of the following items you are managing to help keep your batteries charged:

• Having regular exercise
• Drinking plenty of water
• Eating a balanced diet
• Sleeping well
• Controlling stress levels
• Managing your emotional state

Keeping track of tiredness levels
During the 12-week programme, use the RPE scale to track your progress in overcoming tiredness. We changed the stress levels for a tiredness rating:

0   Not tired at all
1   Very, very little amount of tiredness
2   Very little amount of tiredness
3   Fairly little amount of tiredness
4   Small amount of tiredness
5   Moderately tired
6   Fairly tired
7   Tired
8   Very tired
9   Very, very tired
10 Too tired to stay awake

The results show how Alison was handling her energy level on a daily basis. As you can see, her tiredness was fairly high at the start of the 12 weeks, but gradually decreased as she started to eat healthily, exercise, and basically gain control of her body and its condition. Although she did suffer from a fair amount of tiredness, she was able to manage it by following the steps above.

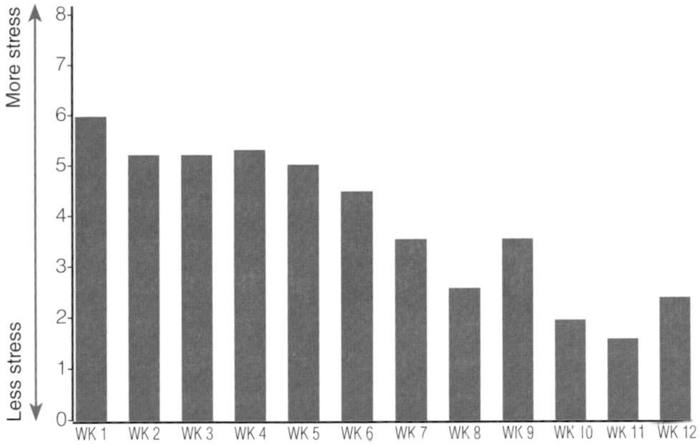

Stress level results

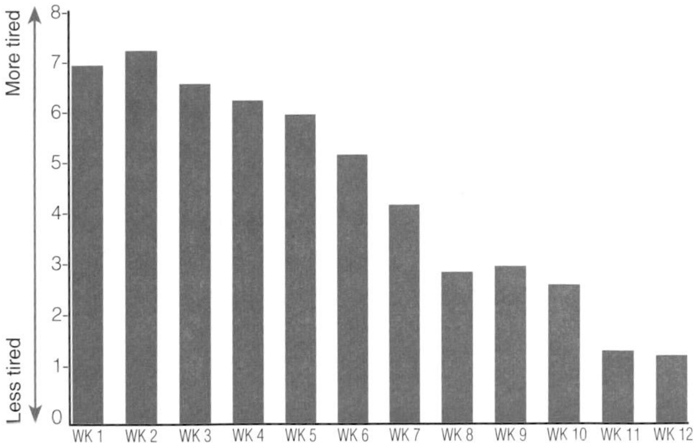

Tiredness level results

SLEEP

Sleep is as important as eating and drinking, which is why we spend one third of our lives doing it. It is absolutely vital for maintaining normal levels of cognitive skills including speech, memory, innovative and flexible thinking, and it gives the body a chance to recuperate and recover from all of the day's activities.

We all become agitated and stressed when we are tired. The most simple and mundane tasks may become a source of stress due to sleep deprivation. Most adults need around eight hours of sleep on a regular basis to function well, although some require more than others. It is believed the likes of Napoleon, Florence Nightingale and Margaret Thatcher all survived on just four hours sleep a night.

Sleep is triggered by hormones that are active in the brain, and respond to cues from the body and the environment. Some of our growth hormones trigger the release of proteins throughout the body to build and repair cells during sleep. Sleep deprivation can prevent this and affect the immune system.

Sleep occurs in a recurrent series of 90–110 minute bursts, and is divided into two categories relating to eye movement levels: REM (rapid eye movement) sleep, and non-REM sleep, which is about 80 per cent of all sleep.

During non-REM sleep, your breathing and heart rate slow and blood pressure will be low. This type of sleep is divided into four stages:

Level 1 – transition between wakefulness to sleep
Level 2 – makes up 50 per cent of sleep, slowing breathing and heartbeat
Level 3 – very low respiration and heartbeat
Level 4 – leads to rapid eye movement sleep known as REM, or Level 5

My average amount of sleep per night was 6 hours, 36 minutes, while Alison slept on average 7 hours and 5 minutes per night.

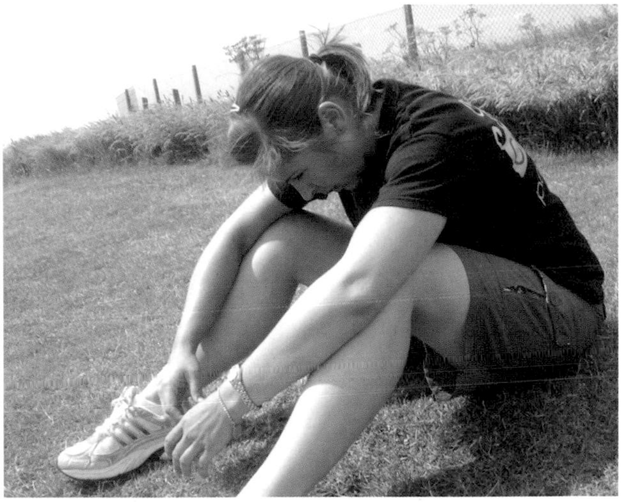

The first week of training was hard both mentally and physically. Alison was tired and looking forward to resting and sleeping. Sleep helps our bodies recover for the next day's activities.

HYDRATION

Water makes up more than two thirds of the weight of the human body, around 60–70 per cent depending on size, shape and the amount of lean tissue (muscle). Muscle consists of approximately 75 per cent water, fat is around 14 per cent, blood has around 82 per cent, and lungs have 90 per cent. Astonishingly, the human brain is made up of 95 per cent water. A mere 2 per cent drop in our body's water supply can trigger signs of dehydration, and without water we would die within days.

Water is the most important nutrient for the body. It helps keep your cells, tissues and organs running smoothly, efficiently and effectively. Some of the ways water keeps your body working is by helping to keep it at a constant internal temperature, preventing constipation, and cushioning your joints and protecting your organs. Fluids are vitally important when you are ill, particularly when you lose more water due to fever, diarrhoea or vomiting.

Your body needs a continuous supply of water to stay hydrated. By maintaining an adequate hydration level, your body will feel all the more healthy.

Reasons why water is special:
- Helps to fight fatigue and tiredness
- Allows you to exercise, train harder and maintain your strength
- Is the best detoxing agent available
- Helps digestion
- Regulates your metabolism
- Serves as a lubricant
- Forms the base for saliva
- Forms fluids that surround and protect joints
- Regulates the body temperature as cooling and heating is distributed through perspiration
- Helps get rid of waste

If you always wait until your mouth is dry to drink water, then you are probably waiting too long and are likely to be dehydrated. Dehydration causes a fuzzy short-term memory, trouble with basic cognitive skills and difficulty focusing on smaller print. Are you having trouble reading this? If so, drink up.

Water comes packaged in different forms, so you can have a little variety throughout your day. Did you know that a glass of milk or a serving of juice is actually about 90 per cent water? Some foods have high water content too, such as fruits, vegetables, yoghurts and soups. Enjoying these foods regularly can contribute to your water intake, and also provide you with many of the vitamins and minerals your body needs.

Here's something to think about: a common mistake is confusing thirst for hunger, so why not drink water if you feel hungry between meals?

How much water is enough? It is recommended that we consume between 1.5 and 3 litres a day. During the 12-week programme Alison drank 1.5 litres a day (eight glasses) on average, and that's excluding the fruit drinks, herbal teas and food she consumed. Don't be put off by plain water. Add cordial to it to make it a little tastier.

POSTURE

Posture plays such an important role in the health of your body, but more often than not it is simply overlooked. The ideal skeletal alignment and consequent good posture involves teaching your body to stand, lie, walk and sit in positions that require the least amount of strain on supporting ligaments during any bodily movement. Having good posture keeps bones and joints in the correct alignment so that muscles are used correctly. It prevents fatigue because muscles are being used more effectively (and therefore using less energy), and even contributes to a good appearance – more supermodel, less hunchback.

Analysing your posture

Your posture provides a lot of information about the state of your body. Postural analysis allows you to see which areas of the body are under more stress than others, which could result in backache.

The easiest way to see if you have a good posture is to stand next to a plumb line to see if any body parts are out of sync. You can use this method to identify any postural faults and to help to distinguish which areas you need to strengthen or release. The side view posture test hypothetically divides the body into front and back sections of equal weight.

During the 12-week programme, you should take photos of your posture from the side and front to see the improvements in your posture. This method

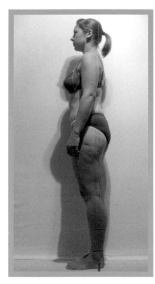 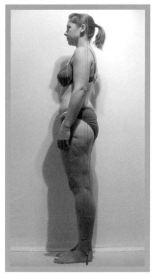 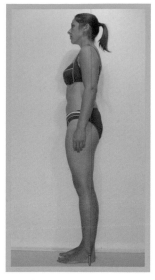 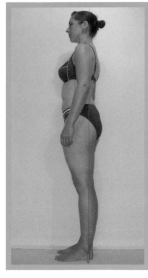

Week 1   Week 4   Week 8   Week 12

Again, the results speak for themselves, but you may also notice the weight loss as well. This plays just as important a role as everything else mentioned.

is not as accurate as if you were to visit a health professional, but it is something that can be done at home. Please note, you will need someone to help you with this test.

Set-up
Postural alignment equipment:
- Plain wall
- Plumb bob and line (coloured string if possible, available from most DIY stores)
- Picture hook
- Tape measure
- Camera

Tie the plumb line string to a picture hook in the ceiling in front of the wall you are going to stand in front of.

Standing barefoot, ensure the plumb line passes slightly forward of the ankle and approximately through the apex of the arch of the foot.

Then measure the distance between the wall and your feet, as well as between your feet themselves, and use these measurements to ensure you are positioned in the same way every four weeks when you take photos of your posture.

Analyse, compare and diagnose your own posture

against that of a neutral posture using the following guidelines and pictures. If you have a misaligned posture then use the relevant information given to strengthen or stretch your muscles to realign yourself.

Neutral posture

In the neutral position, all the muscles are working in harmony with each other, and there are no elongated, weak, or short and strong muscles.

■ Strong muscles
▢ Elongated muscles

Common misaligned posture types

	Elongated or weak muscles	Exercises to strengthen muscles	Short or strong muscles	Exercises to stretch muscles
▓ Strong muscles ▒ Elongated muscles				
Kyphotic posture	Neck flexors, upper back, external obliques, and hamstrings (slightly elongated but may or may not be weak)	• Reverse shrugs • Bent-over lat raises • T-bar row	Neck extensors and possibly your pectorals	• Static stretch for the chest on a wall trapezius stretch • Static stretch for the trapezius muscles
Lordotic posture	Abdominals and hamstrings may or may not be elongated	• Reverse curl • Reverse crunch • Stiff leg deadlifts	Lower back and hip flexor/rectus femoris	• PNF stretch for quad lying face down • Developmental stretch for the lower back while lying down • Developmental stretch for hip flexor stretch
Flat back posture	Hip flexors and the back may seem elongated with a flat back, but they may not be weak	• Reverse crunch • Deadlifts • Dorsal raises	Hamstrings and the abdominals are frequently strong	• PNF stretch for hamstring muscles • Developmental stretch for sitting hamstring muscles • Static stretch for the abdominal muscles
Sway back posture	Hip joint flexors, external oblique, upper back extensors and neck extensors	• Bent-over row • Single arm cable row	Hamstrings and the upper part of the internal oblique; lower back is normally strong but not short	• Developmental stretch for sitting hamstring muscles • PNF stretch for hamstring muscles
C-shape posture	Lateral trunk muscles, the hip adductors (inside thigh), inside of calf muscles, and on the opposite side the hip abductors (gluteus medius muscle), and also TFL (front of hip) – side where pelvis tilts lower is weak side		Hamstrings and abdominals are often strong. For instance, the hip/pelvis that is raised/tilted up has tight lateral muscles, hip adductors (inside thigh), inside calf muscles and on the opposite side the abductors (gluteus medius muscle). Also look at the TFL (front of hip). Strong muscles are opposite side to weak muscles.	

If a person with a neutral posture stands side on, the plumb line should pass through the following areas:

- *Head:* lobe of the ear.
- *Cervical spine:* the neck presents a normal anterior curve.
- *Thoracic:* the thoracic spine should curve slightly in a posterior direction and the plumb line should pass midway through the shoulder joint.
- *Lumbar:* the lumbar should curve slightly anterior.
- *Pelvis:* the front (anterior) and the back (posterior) of your hip should be at the same angle.
- *Hip joint:* slightly posterior to the centre of the hip.
- *Knee:* slightly anterior through the axis of the knee joint. The knee should be neither flexed nor extended.
- *Ankle:* past the ankle and through the apex of the arch of the foot.
- *Feet:* Your feet should be in a neutral position, with your toes angled outward slightly at approximately 8 to 10°, and your heels together.

There are five common misaligned posture types, detailed in the table opposite.

Scoliosis

An S-shape posture, where the shoulder is raised higher on the same side as a raised hip, could be scoliosis. Scoliosis is the abnormal curvature of the spine to the sides, which should be diagnosed by a doctor observing the movement in your back.

Help to realign your posture

Now you can identify which category your posture falls into, you can take the correct steps to amend it by strengthening and shortening the weak muscles with exercise, and by elongating the short, strong muscles by stretching them. Exercises and stretches found within the 12-week programme can help with realigning posture, and massage can also help to alleviate muscular tension.

UNDERSTANDING AND TESTING YOUR BODY'S HEALTH

In order to monitor your progress and to demonstrate your eventual results, you should take health tests before, during and after the 12-week fitness and nutrition programme. We've opted for home testing instead of visiting a GP every week. These tests are not as accurate as those you may receive from your doctor, so perhaps visit your GP before and after your 12-week programme. This will ensure both sets of your results are accurate, and if you do have any health concerns before you start the programme, your doctor will be able to advise you.

Most of the home health-testing kits are easily available at a pharmacy or online.

Equipment needed for the health tests:
- Accurate scales
- Tape measure
- Glucose home test
- Cholesterol home test
- Callipers
- Body fat percentage reader
- Peak flow meter
- Watch
- Blood pressure monitor

Each of the following tests was taken at the start of the programme, with some repeated on the last day of each week, and all taken every four weeks.

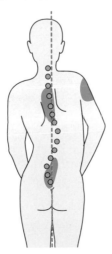

■ Strong muscles
□ Elongated muscles

Tests	Every week	Every 4 weeks
Height and weight	×	×
BMI	×	×
Resting heart rate (RHR)	×	×
Blood pressure (BP)	×	×
Body fat percentage	×	×
Measurements	×	×
Glucose		×
Cholesterol		×
Lung function		×
Calliper tests		×

Height and weight

Although your height will give you no relevant information on its own, you will need it in order to work out your BMI.

Jumping on the scales every day is not the most accurate way to follow your progress, and try not to put too much pressure on yourself to lose a specific amount of weight each week. Don't weigh yourself every day, as this can be very disheartening, but do it every Sunday on test day. You will need to weigh yourself to work out your BMI.

Body mass index (BMI)

There is no average weight or size that a person should be, but there is a method to discover if we fit into the general health practitioners' recommendations. Using height and weight measurements we can use the BMI to determine a healthy weight for your height.

For the 12-week programme, we used a body fat percentage monitor for calculating BMI, but you can use the BMI equation below to calculate it if you don't have one.

$$\text{Weight (kg)} \div \text{height (m)} = x$$
$$x \div \text{height (m)} = \text{BMI}$$

For example, if you weigh 80kg and you are 1.75m tall, your BMI would be 26.1 (80 ÷ 1.75 = 45.7, then 45.7 ÷ 1.75 = 26.1). Using the chart below, you can see that the end figure would mean that the person

is overweight. Please note, however, that BMI should not be relied upon by bodybuilders or athletes as they have a higher than normal amount of muscle mass.

The BMI chart	
Underweight	13–18
Normal weight	19–24
Overweight	25–29
Obese/seriously overweight	30–40
Dangerously overweight/morbidly obese	40+

Resting heart rate (RHR)

This test measures your heart's efficiency in pumping blood around the body when you are in a resting state. The RHR is able to tell you how fit you are, and by following the 12-week programme you should see a steady decrease in your heart rate as your heart becomes more efficient. Try and take your RHR readings as soon as you wake up in the morning, to get your best record.

You can find your RHR by simply finding your pulse on the thumb side of the wrist and counting your heartbeat for one minute with your index and middle finger to see what result you have.

Alison's resting heart rate at the beginning of her fitness plan was 77 beats per minute, and by the end of week 12 it had decreased to 50 beats per minute.

The table opposite shows the average RHR for a female. Mark where you are on the table to see how fit you are right now, and then mark it again in 12 weeks' time.

Blood pressure

Checking blood pressure is essential, as it directly affects your health. Blood pressure testing measures the strength of your heartbeat and the pressure of the circulating blood against the walls of your blood vessels. An ideal, healthy blood pressure is 120 over 80. The first number is your systolic blood pressure (the highest pressure when your heart beats), and the second number is your diastolic blood pressure (the lowest pressure when your heart relaxes between beats).

Women RHR						
Age	18–25	26–35	36–45	46–55	56–65	65+
Athlete	<60	<59	<59	<60	<59	<59
Excellent	61–65	60–64	60–64	61–65	60–64	60–64
Good	66–69	65–68	65–69	66–69	65–68	65–68
Fair	70–73	69–72	70–73	70–73	69–73	69–72
Average	74–78	73–76	74–78	74–77	74–77	73–76
Poor	79–84	77–82	79–84	78–83	78–83	77–84
Very poor	85+	83+	85+	84+	84+	84+

Blood pressure	Systolic	Diastolic
Low	70–90	40–60
Ideal	90–120	60–80
Pre-high	120–140	80–90
High	140–190+	90–100+

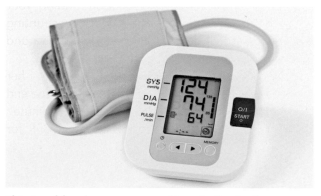

This is a blood pressure monitor similar to the one used in the 12-week programme.

Alison's blood pressure was at 112/68 in week 1, and after completing the 12-week programme it was 110/61.

Body fat percentage test

This is a quicker and more convenient version of the calliper test. However, the results are not quite as accurate. If you do this test every week it will allow you to see the change and will keep you on track.

There are a number of body fat monitor models available; some are similar to normal bathroom scales that you stand on with bare feet, others are hand-held. The monitor passes a low-level, imperceptible electric current through your body. Fat contains limited water and is not a good conductor, so it impedes the current. As lean body tissue contains mainly water and electrolytes, this conducts the current throughout the body, giving you a reading. By measuring your lean body mass, the monitor can predict your fat mass.

For best results, the monitors should be used at the same time of day, once a week, with minimal clothing being worn. You will also need to empty your bladder before use, as this will affect the results. Also, avoid alcohol and use the device straight after exercising.

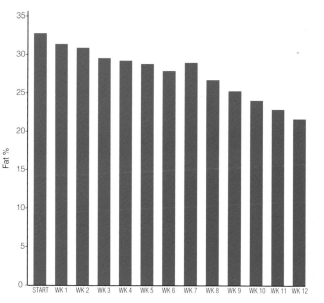

Alison's body fat percentage results for the 12-week programme.

Measurements

Measurements are a great way of showing how the body is reacting to exercise and nutrition on the 12-week programme. With the results of your measurements and your fat percentage, you will be able to see if you are losing body fat rather than just losing weight (which may well just be fluid).

To take measurements accurately, you will need someone else to take them for you so your body can relax in a standing position. Take measurements while cold and relaxed, and at the same time every week throughout the 12-week programme. Please take careful note of exactly where you are taking your measurements from, and ensure that you measure from exactly the same place every time, in order to keep your results as precise as possible.

Neck: measure down from where the ear lobe and jaw connect. The measurement will be down to the largest part of the neck. Take a note of the measurement, and then measure around the neck for the result.

Chest: place the tape measure around the upper torso, measuring from the nipples and keeping the tape in the same alignment all of the way around.

Upper arm: look at the arm and mark out the largest circumference. Measure up from the lateral epicondyle of the humerus (the bony bit on the outside of the elbow). Take note of the measurement, and then measure around the circumference for the result. Repeat for the opposite arm.

Waist/naval: place the tape measure around your abdomen, measuring from the belly button and keeping the tape in alignment all the way around.

Hips: place the tape measure around the hips over the anterior superior iliac spine (or the bony parts either side of your hip). Make sure the tape goes all of the way around and is in alignment with the front.

Upper thigh: look at the widest part on the upper thigh and mark. Measure up from the head of the fibula (or the bony part on the outside of the top of the lower leg). Take note of the measurement, and then measure around the circumference for the result. Repeat for the opposite thigh.

Calf: look at the largest part on the calf and measure around its circumference. Repeat for the opposite calf.

Glucose test

This test measures the amount of glucose in the blood, and is used to detect hyperglycaemia (higher than normal glucose levels in the blood) and hypoglycaemia (lower than normal glucose levels in the blood). It also helps identify diabetes.

For the tests, we used a fasting blood glucose test for ease, which required eating no later than 10.00 p.m. the night before, and taking the test at around 8.00 a.m. the following morning. Keeping the test criteria the same provides the best results. Please make sure that you read and follow the instructions on the specific test kit that you use.

The result guidelines for the fasting blood glucose test are in the table below, measured in millimoles per litre (mmol/l).

From 3.6 to 6.0 mmol/l	Normal fasting glucose
From 6.1 to 6.9 mmol/l	Impaired fasting glucose
7.0 mmol/l and above	Probable diabetes

Cholesterol test

Our bodies need a certain amount of cholesterol to make cell membranes, insulate nerves and produce hormones. Cholesterol is a waxy substance produced in the liver and other organs. We can also absorb cholesterol from foods such as eggs, red meat, cheese and more. Too much or too high a cholesterol level can affect your heart.

There are two forms of cholesterol, one of which is good for you while the other is bad.

Good cholesterol

High-density lipoprotein (HDL) picks up and transports surplus cholesterol from the body tissues back to the liver, where it is broken down and passed out of the body.

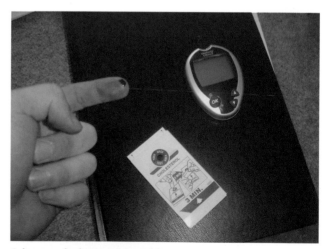

A home cholesterol test kit.

Bad cholesterol

Low-density lipoprotein (LDL) transports cholesterol from the liver around the rest of the body. When there is more LDL in the blood than the body needs, the cholesterol accumulates in the body tissues, such as the walls of the coronary arteries. Here it can build up and affect the heart function.

A home test kit simply measures the total amount of cholesterol. Please remember to read and follow the instructions. The levels of total cholesterol fall into the following categories:

Ideal level	3.9–5.2 mmol/l
Mildly high level	5.0–6.4 mmol/l
High level	6.5–7.8 mmol/l
Very high level	7.8+ mmol/l

Lung function test

The lung function test is measured by a peak flow meter, a small hand-held device used to measure how fast a person can exhale. The peak expiratory flow rate (PEFR) shows how well your airways are performing.

Even though Alison suffers from asthma, you can see her lung performance increases quite considerably due to improvements in her health and fitness levels.

To measure PEFR

- Breathe in as deeply as possible
- Blow out into the meter as hard and fast as possible

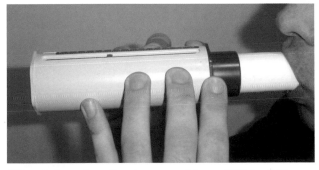

Alison's lung function increased from 370 to 450 as her fitness improved over the course of the programme.

- Take note of its result, repeat three times and record your highest rate

Average female lung function results								
Age	Height (m)							
	1.45	1.50	1.55	1.60	1.65	1.70	1.75	1.80
25	365	383	400	416	433	449	466	482
30	357	374	390	407	423	440	456	473
35	348	365	381	398	414	431	447	464
40	339	356	372	389	405	422	438	455
45	330	347	363	380	397	413	429	446
50	321	338	354	371	388	404	420	437
55	312	329	345	362	379	395	411	428
60	303	320	336	353	370	386	402	419
65	294	311	327	344	361	377	393	410
70	285	302	318	335	352	368	384	401

Calliper test

This test measures skin folds to calculate your body's fat percentage. You will need to have another person available to help take the measurements for this test, but again this can be done at home.

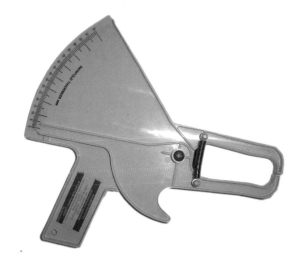

Calliper

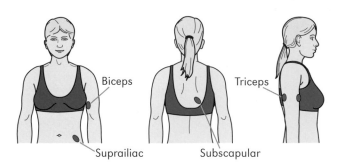

Biceps

Triceps

Suprailiac

Subscapular

Areas to measure

To take the calliper test:
- Use the left-hand side for all of your measurements with your arms hanging freely.
- Pinch 1cm above the area being measured with the calliper.
- Measure all your calliper positions so that the next reading will be taken in the same place.
- The pinch should be maintained throughout the reading for a specific area before moving on towards the next area.
- Take the measurement a couple of times to gain the most accurate reading, allowing the skin to return to normal between readings.

Areas to measure
- *Biceps* – vertical fold for the pinch. Measure half way between the shoulder and the elbow directly on to the biceps to take the reading.
- *Triceps* – vertical fold for the pinch. Measure half-way between the shoulder and the elbow directly on the triceps to take the reading.
- *Suprailiac (waist)* – diagonal fold for the pinch. Measure directly above the hip.
- *Subscapular* – diagonal fold for the pinch. Measure 1–2cm down at 45° directly from the bottom of the shoulder blade.

Now add all four of your calliper measurements (biceps, triceps, superiliac and subscapular) together to get your total skin folds measurement.

Apply your total skin folds measurement to the appropriate tables below:

Average female calliper test results			
Total measurements for all four skin folds (mm)	Age 16–29 (fat %)	Age 30–49 (fat %)	Age 50 (fat %)
14	9.4	14.1	17.0
16	11.2	15.7	18.6
18	12.7	17.1	20.1
20	14.1	18.4	21.4
22	15.4	19.5	22.6
24	16.5	20.6	23.7
26	17.6	21.5	24.8
28	18.6	22.4	25.7
30	19.5	23.3	26.6
35	21.6	25.2	28.6
40	23.4	26.8	30.3
45	25	28.3	31.9
50	26.5	29.6	33.2
55	27.8	30.8	34.6
60	29.1	31.9	35.7
65	30.2	32.9	36.7
70	31.2	33.9	37.7
75	32.2	34.7	38.6
80	33.1	35.6	39.5
85	34	36.3	40.4
90	34.8	37.1	41.1
95	35.6	37.8	41.9
100	36.3	38.5	42.6
120	39	40.8	45.1
130	40.2	41.9	46.2
140	41.3	42.9	47.3
150	42.3	43.8	48.2
Lean	<14	<14	<16
Optimal	15–21	15–21	17–21
Slightly overweight	22–25	22–26	22–26
Overweight	26–32	27–32	27–32
Obese	>33	>33	>33

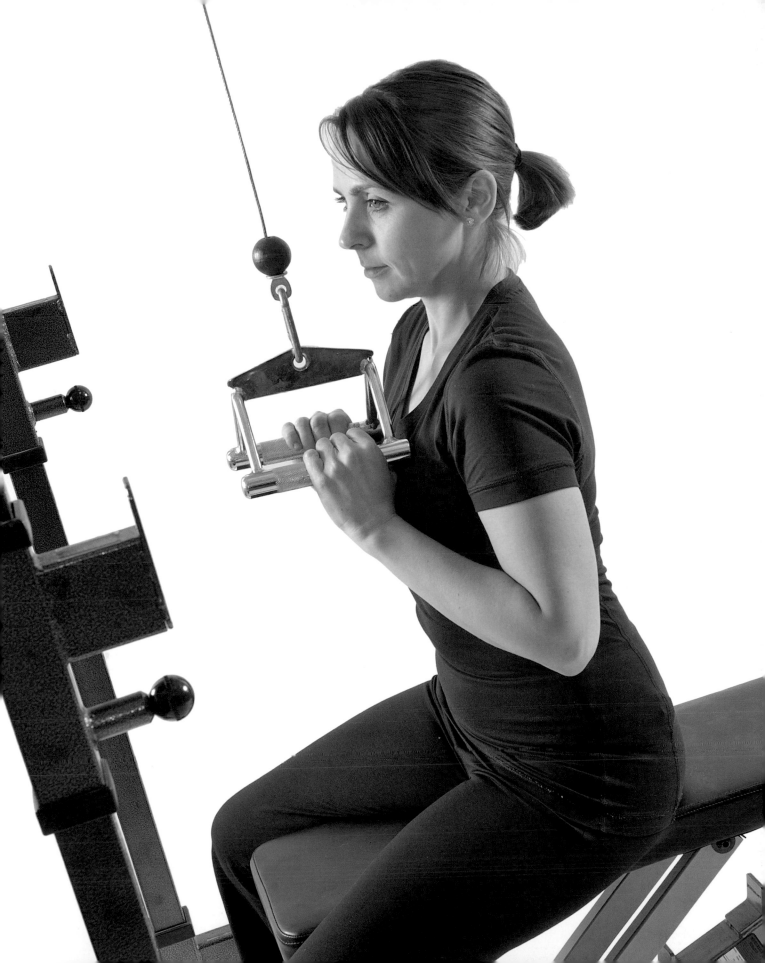

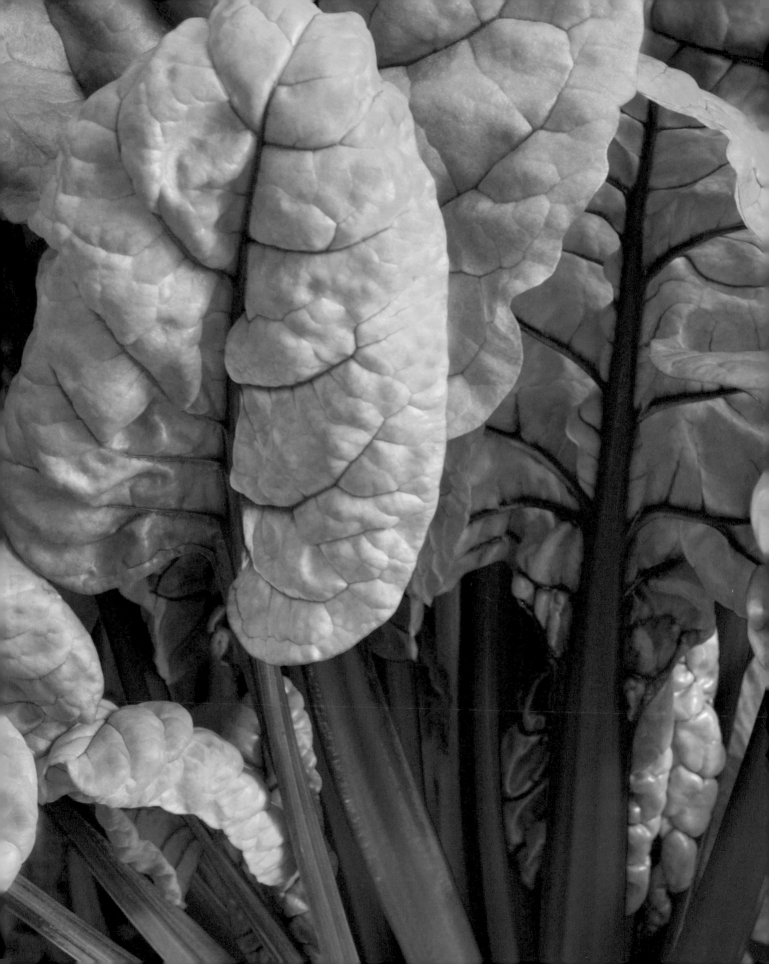

HEALTHY EATING

03

KNOWING YOUR FOODS AND FOLLOWING THE PLAN

The meals and recipes in this book are easy to follow and have been created with a family of four in mind (but do feel free to make smaller amounts for individual portions). It is important to show that following a healthy and balanced nutritional diet will improve you and your family's health, fitness and well-being. The recipe section will guide you through the number of meals that you should consume each day, when and how to prepare them, and even supplies you with detailed weekly shopping lists to save you time.

The shopping lists include all of the ingredients that you will need for each week's recipes, and you can find printable versions online (www.bloomsbury. com/9781408196397), which you can print off and take with you with you when you go shopping. The lists are divided into sections, from carbohydrates through to meat, fish, fruit and vegetables, and you will find shopping much quicker and easier with them. Please feel free to amend the lists to incorporate your existing cupboard contents.

Vegetarians and vegans can substitute tofu, soya or Quorn products for meat and fish in recipes. Non-dairy alternatives are suggested throughout the recipes (Alison is allergic to dairy products).

HEALTHY EATING VERSUS UNHEALTHY EATING

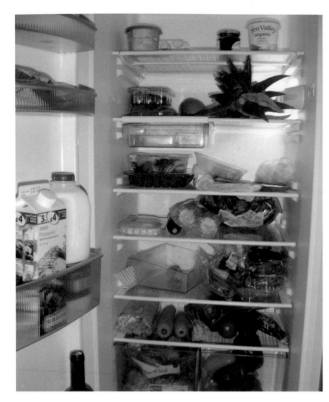

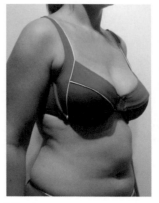

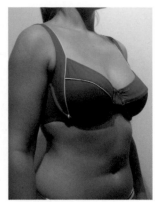

Week 1   Week 12

It is never too late to make a difference, and with some changes to your fitness, nutrition and lifestyle you can make big changes, with great results.

Starting your weight loss

You may be wondering if the nutrition programme is going to work for you. Well, Alison followed it and look at the great results she got.

By eating a healthy balanced diet, Alison's skin cleared up, her attitude was extremely positive and her health results increased, as did her fitness results. When you get the right nutrition it contributes to around 60–70 per cent of how you look and feel.

If you have mistreated your body, you have the ability to change your health and well-being for the better, as our bodies are great at adapting to new lifestyles and diets.

The best way to start this plan is by emptying the contents of your fridge and cupboards – get rid of all the junk and unhealthy foods. Not only will

this give you a fresh start, but it will also stop any temptations further down the line.

KNOWING YOUR FOODS

Foods come in various forms, and have a variety of benefits for our bodies. We have natural foods and processed foods, and here we find out why natural foods are so much more important for us.

Here is a quick rundown of every important type of food group/property that you are likely to come across:

- *Carbohydrates* – our main source of energy.
- *Proteins* – essential for growth and repair of muscle and other body tissues.
- *Fats* – a source of energy and important in relation to fat-soluble vitamins.
- *Minerals* – these are inorganic elements that occur in our bodies, and which are critical to its normal function.
- *Vitamins* – water- and fat-soluble vitamins play important roles in many chemical processes in the body.
- *Water* – essential for our body's healthy functioning. It makes up 60–70 per cent of the human body, and is used to carry nutrients around.

Carbohydrates (carbs)

Carbohydrate (meaning 'carbon plus water') is the most widely eaten food type in the world. Along with fat and protein, carbohydrate is an essential nutrient, but what makes carbs different is that they are easily converted into energy by the body.

Carbohydrates come in two forms – simple and complex.

Simple carbohydrates – various forms of sugar, such as glucose and sucrose (table sugar). These simple carbs have smaller molecules, making it easier for them to be absorbed into the body and used as energy. Fruit, dairy products and honey contain large amounts of simple carbohydrates.

Complex carbohydrates – composed of long-string simple carbs. This means the body absorbs the large molecules at a slower rate than the simpler molecules, which gives us energy at a slower rate than simple carbs, but faster than fats and protein. Complex carbs consist of rice, bread, beans and root vegetables (e.g. potatoes).

Carbohydrates can also be classed as refined or unrefined.

Refined carbohydrates – highly processed products, with all of the goodness such as fibre, bran, vitamins and minerals stripped away, but still giving the same amount of calories.

Refined products often include vitamins and minerals that have been added in an unnatural way, giving the food little nutritional value.

You should reduce or eliminate these types of refined products, such as white bread, white rice, cakes, commercial cereals, biscuits, crisps, bagels and croissants from your diet. If you tend to get most of your carbs from these refined products, you run a higher risk of getting type-2 diabetes and becoming obese.

Unrefined carbohydrates – untouched products still retaining their original nutritional value. Brown rice, wholegrain bread, muesli and yams are all unrefined carbs.

If you consume more carbohydrates than your body needs at any one time, your body stores some of these within cells as glycogen and converts the rest into fat. So remember, only eat what you need to remain satisfied.

Protein

The body needs proteins to maintain and replace tissues, and to function and grow. If the body is getting enough calories, it does not use protein for energy. If more protein is consumed than is needed, the body breaks the protein down and stores its components as fat.

Protein is the main building block in the body, and is the primary component of most cells: muscle, connective tissues, hair and skin are all built from protein.

Protein consists of units called amino acids, strung together in complex formations. Because proteins are complex molecules the body takes longer to break them down. As a result, they are a longer-lasting source of energy than carbohydrates.

Amino acids – the 20 amino acids found in proteins convey a vast array of chemical versatility. The body synthesises some of them from components within the body, but there are nine amino acids that the body cannot synthesise. These are called essential amino acids, and they must be consumed within your diet.

Essential amino acids – adults need eight of these nine amino acids: isoleucine, leucine, lysine, methioninie, phenylalanine, threonine, tryptophan and valine. Infants also need a ninth one – histidine.

The percentage of protein the body can use to synthesise essential amino acids varies from protein to protein. The body can use 100 per cent of the protein in an egg, and a high percentage of the proteins in milk and meats.

Fats

Fats are complex molecules composed of fatty acids and glycerol. The body needs fats for growth and energy, and the body also uses them to synthesise hormones and other substances (such as prostaglandins) needed for the body's activities.

Fats are the slowest source of energy, but the most energy efficient form of food. Each gram of fat supplies the body with about nine calories – more than twice that supplied by proteins or carbohydrates.

As fats are such an efficient form of energy, the body stores any excess energy as body fat. The body deposits excess fat in the abdomen (omental fat) and under the skin (subcutaneous fat) to use when it needs more energy. The body may also deposit excess fat in blood vessels and within organs, where it can block blood flow and damage organs, often causing serious disorders. The different types of fats are listed below.

Saturated fats – these are more likely to increase cholesterol levels and increase the risk of atherosclerosis. Products containing saturated fats include: meat products (especially beef), coconut and palm oil, as well as artificial hydrogenated fat.

Monounsaturated fats – normally lowers LDL cholesterol (the 'bad' cholesterol), and is found in both plant and animal products, such as olive oil, canola oil and peanut oil, and in some plant foods such as avocado.

Polyunsaturated fats – these tend to lower blood cholesterol levels, and are found in plant sources such as safflower, sunflower, corn and cottonseed, and oils like olive oil and walnut oil.

Essential fatty acids (EFAs) – these are necessary fats that the human body cannot synthesise, and must be obtained through diet. EFAs are long-chain polyunsaturated fatty acids derived from linolenic, linoleic and oleic acids. There are two types of EFAs: omega-3 and omega-6 (omega-9 is necessary yet 'non-essential' because the body can manufacture a modest amount on its own, provided essential EFAs are present). EFAs are found in products such as oily fish, nuts and seeds.

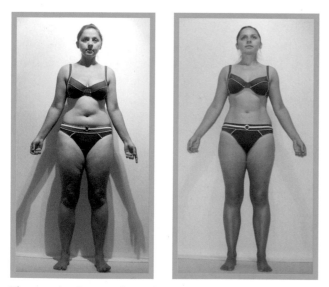

The results from reducing fat and sugar intake and eating healthily speak for themselves – this is week 1 compared with week 12.

Vitamins and minerals

Vitamins and minerals make our bodies work properly, and although you get vitamins and minerals from the foods you eat every day, some foods contain more vitamins and minerals than others.

Vitamins

Vitamins fall into two categories: fat soluble and water soluble.

Fat soluble – vitamins A, D, E and K dissolve in fat and can be stored in your body. Some of these stay for a few days, some for up to six months. Then, when it's time for them to be used, your body utilises them.

Water soluble – vitamin C and the B-complex vitamins such as vitamins B6, B12, niacin, riboflavin, thiamin, pantothenic acid, biotin, folic acid and folate acid, all need to dissolve in water before your body can absorb them. Because of this, your body cannot store these vitamins. Any vitamin C or B that your body does not use as it passes through your system is lost as waste. So you need a fresh supply of these vitamins every day.

Minerals

Minerals are necessary for three main reasons:
1. Building strong bones and teeth
2. Controlling our cells and body fluids
3. Turning the food we eat into energy

Whereas vitamins are organic substances (made by plants or animals), minerals are inorganic elements that come from the soil and water, and are absorbed by plants or eaten by animals.

Your body needs larger amounts of some minerals, such as calcium, to grow and stay healthy. Other minerals like chromium, copper, iodine, iron, selenium and zinc are called trace minerals, because you only need very small amounts of them each day.

Salt (sodium)

Most of our dietary salt comes from the foods we eat, and other salt comes from the drinks we consume.

Both sodium and chloride are essential not only to life, but to good health – it has always been that way. The body's salt/water ratio is critical to a healthy metabolism. The human blood contains 0.9 per cent salt (sodium chloride), and salt maintains the electrolyte balance inside and outside its cells.

Salts are found naturally in food and drink as well as coming in the form of sea salt, table salt, rock salt etc. There is a good side and a bad side to salt.

The bad side of salt – unnatural/processed salt has been stripped of all the goodness that sea salt provides, such as minerals. Salt makes your body hold on to water, and the extra water stored in your body raises your blood pressure. So the more salt you eat, the higher your blood pressure. The higher your blood pressure, the greater the risk and strain on your heart, arteries, kidneys and brain. This can lead to heart attacks, strokes, dementia and kidney disease.

The good side of salt – sea salt is actually good for you when it is natural and has not been refined. It comes directly from the sea, and not only is it full of minerals, but it can also enhance flavours to make our food taste even better.

Salt is essential to our health and development. We need the vital electrolytes in salt (sodium and potassium) to control water levels in the blood and tissue.

A healthy intake of sea salt aids in balancing:
- Blood sugar levels
- The absorption of food in the intestines
- Acts as a strong and natural anti-histamine
- Can help clear mucus and phlegm from the lungs

We chose not to add any extra salt to any of the recipes in this book, and will leave it up to you whether you add salt to your food for that extra bit of taste. If you do choose to use salt for seasoning, please use sea salt.

Herbs and spices

Herbs and spices add flavour and nutrients to dishes without fat or calories, and are derived from the roots, buds, bark, leaves and fruit of plants.

Herbs are usually the leaves of certain plants, and have been used to treat diseases for thousands of years. Herbs such as basil, chilli, oregano, fenugreek and rosemary are very beneficial to our health.

Many spices contain antioxidants that protect against cancer and heart disease, and can even help with controlling blood sugar. There are other spices with properties that fight *E. coli*, listeria, *Staphylococcus* and fungus. This is why most of the meals within the 12-week programme have herbs and spices in them.

The nitty gritty

Rest assured, the nutrition programme is very easy to follow. Whether you are going to commit to the 12-week programme, or if you just want to try the recipes, they are all simple and straightforward to follow. The recipes are not fixed, and you are free to swap the meals around. Even pick a different week entirely if you wish – the choice is yours.

FOLLOWING THE PROGRAMME

The recipes are very easy to follow, and are presented as simple step-by-step instructions. All recipes are designed to feed four people, so remember to halve all quantities if cooking for two or divide by four if it's just for yourself. To help you manage your time, you will find advice about preparing items in advance for the following day's lunch or dinner (such as when split peas need to be soaked overnight). You may also consider keeping a nutritional diary, similar to the training diaries that appear for each of the 12 weeks in Chapter 6 (or combine the two into a single diary). This kind of record can be useful for keeping track of which recipes work best for you.

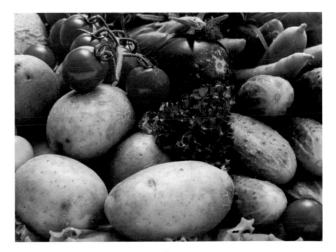

Choosing the foods for you

When looking through the recipes you may wonder what to do if you don't like one of the key ingredients, such as sweet potato or fish.

The recipes have been designed to be versatile, so that you can swap and change the ingredients to suit you and your taste buds.

Major ingredient alternatives

- Specified fruit → any fruit (not too many grapes, though)
- Sweet potato → potato, yam, butternut squash
- Baked potato → sweet potato, yam, butternut squash
- Fish → white meat
- Pork → beef
- Chicken → turkey

Choice of foods

When following the 12-week nutritional programme, Alison would always choose turkey over chicken. Also, she always chose rice milk/soya milk over skimmed milk.

For the following ingredients I would recommend that you use the same, as they are more beneficial for the body:

- Cold-pressed extra virgin olive oil
- Organic rice milk, unsweetened soya milk and skimmed milk
- Low fat bio live yoghurt
- Organic balsamic vinegar
- Natural organic or nut and seed muesli
- Make all of your own sauces and dressings
- Brown sugar
- Free range organic eggs
- Free range poultry and meat from the local butchers
- Fruit juices

The main point to remember when choosing a fruit juice drink is to buy one that is not made from concentrate and is 100 per cent natural, with no added sweeteners or preservatives.

Bad day? Bad week? Don't panic!

This is not an eating plan that denies you any naughty foods or treats. Alison still had the odd off-day. When you do get a bad day, sit back for a moment, analyse what you are doing, and ask yourself:

- Are you eating for the sake of eating?
- Are you eating because you're hungry?
- Have your treat foods got out of hand?
- Are you depriving yourself of snacks/treats?
- Are you missing meals?
- Are you drinking enough water?
- Are you eating or drinking more sugary foods than normal?

Just ask why you are having your bad day, and perhaps you will stop and think before you reach for the bad food.

If you do have a bad day – or an entire bad week – try not to panic. Limit these days as much as possible, but remember this: don't give up. If you hang in there and turn your food back around to being good, you can actually lose more weight than you put on with unhealthy eating. Your body will get a shock but it will always adapt to its current circumstances.

If you find this hard to believe, look at the progress Alison made over the 12 weeks:

Week 5 fat %: 28.4
Week 6 fat %: 27.4
Week 7 fat %: 28.4
Week 8 fat %: 26.3
Week 12 fat %: 21.3

You will notice that during week 7, the weight started to creep up due to a series of bad days (OK, a bad week). However, from week 7, in just five weeks, Alison managed to lose 7.1 per cent body fat by turning around the way she was eating.

The increase was due to having too many treat foods and starting to have a taste for sugar. Having analysed what was being eaten, she counteracted it by following the nutritional programme precisely, with sensible snacks just like the ones listed later in this chapter.

There is a noticeable change around Alison's midriff, especially in the last four weeks.

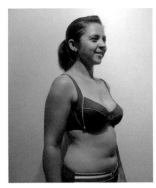
Week 5

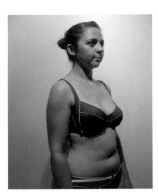
Week 8

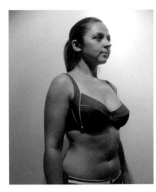
Week 12

Eating out

Don't panic if you're going to eat out. Look at it as a treat that you deserve from time to time, but of course that doesn't mean run wild and eat what you want. On average Alison ate out once every three weeks, and all you need to remember is the basics of food.

Perhaps lean towards fish or protein dishes with fresh food, less sauce, and not so many starchy carbohydrates.

Foods to avoid when eating out are as follows:
- Creamy dishes
- Starchy carbohydrates
- Deep fried food
- Pan fried food
- Battered food
- Bread
- Chips
- Desserts

Don't be afraid to state how you want your food cooked when ordering. For instance, you may ask for a jacket potato instead of chips or dressing on the side rather than over your meal. If you do need something sweet after dinner go for fresh fruit, or if you find that too boring share a dessert with someone.

I also recommend that you try to stay clear of take-aways and convenience foods if you can.

Treat foods

You will notice that from time to time I would have foods that would be classed as bad foods or 'treat foods'.

Think of it this way: you are not a robot, and you are not on a diet – you are on a healthy eating plan. This 12-week nutrition programme consists of 80–90 per cent healthy eating, with the rest being considered naughty.

The treat days will act as motivation too, and help keep you on track towards your potential end goal. If, however, you are the sort of person who cannot just have a little treat (you have to finish the entire tub of ice cream), then resist and don't have any treats at all. You know your body – just don't starve it of the nutrients it needs.

I suggest that you don't buy treats on your main shopping trips, and don't leave them out on display. You won't be so tempted to eat them if they're sitting in the cupboard.

Desserts and snacks

During the 12-week programme Alison had two healthy desserts a week, which would normally be yoghurt and fruit, fruit salad with seeds, or just a fruit salad. However, for the first two weeks of the programme she had no desserts at all, and kept to the recipes exactly.

Snacks are just that: snacks. They are not mini meals, so don't treat them as such. Don't purchase snacks that are high in sugar or fat (carbohydrate sugar over 5g or saturated fat over 5g). Surprisingly, this discounts all of the cereal bars on offer at your local supermarket. Try to stay clear of them, as these bars will tend you to give you a sugar craving, which in turn makes you hungry.

Listed below is a suggested list of snacks to eat

per week. The quantities listed are what Alison had on average each week.

Snack list

- Melon, mango or coconut – 1 to share
- Peach, plum, or kiwi – 1
- Pineapple – 1 to share
- Orange or nectarine – 1
- Berries (blackberries, goji, blueberries, raspberries or strawberries) – 2 portions
- Pear – 1
- Banana – 5
- Apple – 5
- Wholegrain crispbread – 3
- Crackers/flat breads – 1
- Small bowl of muesli (if really hungry) – 2
- Yoghurt/soya yoghurt (four dessert spoons) – 1
- Nuts (cashew, pine or occasionally mixed nuts) – 2 to 3 handfuls
- Soya nuts – 3 to 4 handfuls after training sessions
- Seeds (pumpkin or sunflower) – 2 to 3 handfuls
- Pitta bread/wrap with salad and protein filling – 1

You can snack four to five times a day at random intervals – or just when you need to.

Caffeine and alcohol

As part of the 12-week fitness and nutrition programme, Alison chose to live a healthy lifestyle that did not cut out any essential dietary needs, but also not to completely remove the sociable side of her lifestyle, which included drinking alcohol, tea and coffee. She simply chose the healthier option when doing so. For example, when she had a choice between teas or coffees, she chose green tea, herbal tea or decaffeinated tea and coffee. When she was drinking alcohol, she avoided beer and opted for a spirit like vodka with a fruit or diet mixer.

During the 12-week programme you may have parties to go to, or you might meet up with friends at your local pub. Here is a little advice as to what to choose:

- Spirit with fruit or diet mixer over ales/lager/beer
- Red wine over white wine
- Guinness or ale over beer/lager
- Cider over beer/lager

On average Alison consumed a little over one alcoholic drink per week. The average alcohol unit consumption was 2.4 per week, which is the equivalent of having one pint of beer or two single spirits with a diet mixer a week.

Relishes and dressings

Here are some great healthy dressings that you can make easily at home and are used in the weekly recipes:

Houmous

1 large can chickpeas, drained
2 cloves garlic
2–3 tablespoons olive oil
1 dessertspoon tahini (sesame seed spread)
Tzatziki
1 clove garlic, crushed
200g yoghurt
¼ cucumber, finely grated
½ red onion, finely chopped
1 tablespoon parsley, chopped
1 tablespoon mint, chopped

Avocado relish

2 avocados, peeled and chopped
1 tablespoon lime juice
½ small red onion, finely cut
2 tomatoes, chopped

Relish

1 bunch fresh parsley
6 anchovy fillets
Zest of 2 lemons, grated
115ml lemon juice
60ml olive oil

Mint dressing

150g yoghurt
2 tablespoons mint, chopped
½ tablespoon olive oil
2 tablespoons lemon juice

Basil dressing

1 tablespoon olive oil
1 clove garlic, crushed

1 tablespoon lemon juice
1 tablespoon basil leaves, shredded

Salad dressing
4 tablespoons yoghurt
¼ cucumber, grated
1 tablespoon olive oil
1 tablespoon balsamic vinegar
2 teaspoons black pepper
2 teaspoons dried dill

Nutty delight dressing
3 tablespoons olive oil
3 tablespoons yoghurt
Sprinkle of pine nuts
½ tablespoon balsamic vinegar
Black pepper

Mustard dressing
1 tablespoon Dijon mustard
1 tablespoon olive oil
2 teaspoons cider vinegar
1 teaspoon water

Dill dressing
1 tablespoon fresh dill, chopped
250g yoghurt
1 clove garlic, crushed
1 teaspoon balsamic vinegar

All-purpose dressing
2 tablespoons olive oil
1 tablespoon balsamic vinegar
1 clove garlic, crushed
1 teaspoon Dijon mustard
Black pepper

Ginger dressing for the wok
2 tablespoons light soy sauce
2 teaspoons lime juice
1 teaspoon ginger, grated

Spicy dressing 1
2 tablespoons lime juice
1 tablespoon fish sauce
1 tablespoon light soy sauce

1 clove garlic, crushed
1 red chilli, de-seeded and chopped

Spicy dressing 2
1 red chilli, finely sliced
½ teaspoon ground cumin
1 tablespoon lime juice

Coriander and yoghurt dressing
500g yoghurt
2 tablespoons coriander, chopped
1 clove garlic, finely chopped
4 teaspoons lemon juice
1 teaspoon ground cumin

Food portions and presentation
Within each recipe and shopping list, all the ingredients that you will need for breakfast, lunch and dinner are listed. This is just a guideline, as sometimes (for example, during the week) you might eat two turkey breasts instead of the one recommended, or increase the muesli recommended for breakfast to give you the energy you need for the day ahead. Bear in mind that all recipes are designed for four people, so adjust quantities according to how many people you are cooking for.

Surprisingly, the presentation of your food is almost as important as how it tastes. It has been proven that good food presentation can make your food taste better due to your brain perceiving that the food looks delicious and smells delectable before even tasting it. So take your time with all your meal presentations.

Shopping lists
Items in the shopping lists are organised in alphabetical order under categories of fish, meat, dairy, carbohydrates, fruit, vegetables, herbs and spices, and other. This will help you be in and out of the supermarket with more ease and efficiency. All the lists have been designed to cover every meal, but you do need to add healthy snacks to your list.

When you start, you will notice that the amounts are very precise, but these are just recommendations. For instance, if you cannot find 12 tomatoes, only a pack of eight, don't worry because the recipes are adaptable.

If, for example, you don't like to eat sweet potatoes or butternut squash, you can eat yam instead. If you would rather eat turkey instead of chicken because it is leaner and healthier, you can. You are the boss, just be good to yourself.

It is important when you are shopping to not worry so much about the calories, but look carefully at the carbohydrates (sugars), and the fats (saturated) that you are popping into your supermarket trolley.

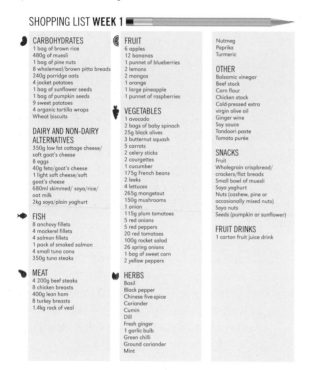

WHEN TO EAT

There is a lot of stipulation on what time you should eat. We all have different lifestyles and routines, but sometimes it is just physically impossible to eat at a certain time. All you have to remember is that you need to eat breakfast, lunch and dinner – do not worry too much about the timings. If you are eating later in the day keep your food portions smaller than normal, increase the protein and decrease your carbohydrate intake.

When to eat on training days

The food we eat before and after exercise is important both for comfort and for performance.

The major source of fuel for active muscles is carbohydrate, which is stored in the muscles as glycogen. It takes time to fill glycogen stores completely, and what you eat following exercise either helps or hinders this process.

You should aim to eat 1.5 hours before or after exercise. Again, in reality this is just a rough timing to help as a guide. Sometimes you might eat breakfast and be cycling to work within 40 minutes, so just listen to your body and decide what's right for you. When you finish exercise, try to eat protein within 30 minutes to fuel your muscles and help them repair. I use soya nuts as my post-exercise snack.

Foods that normally help with performance before exercise

As glucose is the preferred energy source for most exercises, the meal before should contain carbohydrates that are easy to digest, plus protein and a small amount fat. For example, a turkey salad wrap or soya nuts with a piece of fruit or a fruit smoothie.

Foods to avoid before exercise

Foods that are high in fat and/or fibre are digested slowly and remain in the stomach longer, so try to avoid these. These foods include meat, chips, chocolate bars and cakes.

Exercising on a full stomach

This is not ideal, as any food remaining on your stomach can cause cramp, stitches, nausea or even diarrhoea. To make sure you have enough energy while exercising you should eat between one and four hours beforehand, depending on the type and quantity of food you are eating. Remember, everyone's different so we recommend experimenting to find out what works best for you.

Exercising in the morning

If you are the sort of person who exercises early in the morning, or you have a big race that day, then it's best to wake up a little bit early to ensure you have your pre-exercise meal (breakfast) and enough energy to perform to the best of your ability. The closer you are to performing your exercise, the less you should be eating.

Exercising in the evening

You can either choose to train before or after your evening meal. It is completely up to you. If you prefer to train straight after work, ensure you eat a healthy snack at least one hour before you exercise, and then eat within an hour – or preferably half an hour – of finishing.

However, if you choose to train after dinner, take into account what we've already mentioned about exercising on a full stomach – work out what is going to be best for you.

The most important thing to remember is to hydrate before and after exercise.

What you eat after exercise

The first thing to do after any exercise is to drink water, replacing any fluids you will have lost.

It is then very important that you replace your glycogen stores and consume carbohydrates (such as a piece of fruit) within 15 minutes. The reason for this is that carbohydrate consumption stimulates insulin production, which aids muscle glycogen production (repairing your body faster).

If within half an hour you can also consume protein with the carbohydrates, the insulin response almost doubles. The protein provides the amino acids necessary to rebuild muscle tissue that will have been damaged during training.

In short, to give your body the best possible chance of recovery and repair after strenuous exercise you should aim to eat a 4 to 1 ratio of carbohydrate and protein within half an hour of finishing.

FREQUENTLY ASKED QUESTIONS

Will I get bored with the 12-week nutrition plan?
The recipes have been created so that you don't eat the same meals each week and you have a different dinner recipe every day for the whole 12 weeks. With this wide variety and varied cooking, your taste buds should not be feeling neglected.

Will I be able to feed the whole family?
This is a plan based around a family of four.

Will I get hungry?
To be honest, there will be times when you will feel hungrier than usual, but there will also be days where you feel full. When you first start the programme your body and eating habits will change, so you will probably find that the first two weeks are the most demanding. The programme has been particularly devised to fulfil your appetite with tantalising meals that will keep hunger at bay.

On some days of the fitness programme you may require more food for certain days. Follow the plan and use my diary as a guide, and you should end up getting where you want to be.

Are the shopping lists easy to follow?
Items on the shopping lists have been organised according to common categories, as well as being in alphabetical order. This will enable you to shop quickly and easily. You can access them online and print them off to take to the supermarket.

Did you use supplements?
No. This is mainly to show that if you are on the right healthy eating plan, then you don't need any supplements. Having said that, I am not against supplements as some of them are beneficial for the body

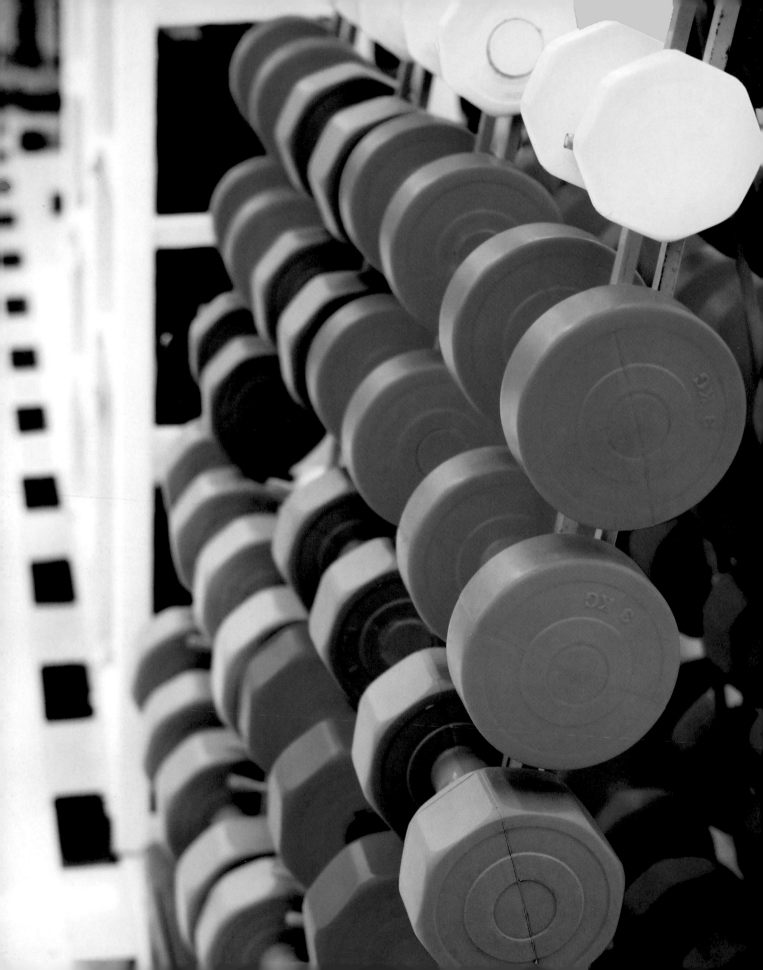

TRAINING BASICS AND SET-UP

04

The 12-week programme will be very challenging, both mentally and physically. It will change your fitness levels, physical shape, confidence, posture, skin and eating habits – and hopefully change you into what you want to become.

This chapter looks at the basics of weight training, running and cycling, and then the set-up and equipment needed to complete the programme.

WEIGHT TRAINING

Repetitions (reps)

A rep is a contraction of the muscle followed by the extension – for example, arm-curling the dumbbell up and back down to the start.

The general rule:
Upper body: 10+ reps
Lower body: 15+ reps
Strength training: 1–8 reps
Toning: 10–15 reps
Muscular endurance: 15+ reps

When you start your reps you should be pushing about 60–80 per cent of your maximum effort, and by the end of the last set you should be at 80–100 per cent of your maximum effort.

When you are training, do not worry about getting bigger muscles. It will take you a lot longer to put on muscle mass, and within the 12-week

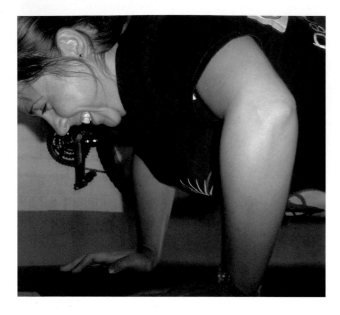

programme we are using rep ranges of 12+ for the majority of the time. We do use lower reps between 6–12, but this is to strengthen and stabilise your posture, joints and muscles.

Sets

A set is a specific number of repetitions performed for different exercises.

The general rule is the larger muscle groups (e.g. thighs, back and chest), the more sets. Normally you would aim for around 10 sets per large muscle group. For smaller muscle groups (e.g. biceps and triceps), you need to do fewer sets, usually around 6–9 sets. These are just average recommendations.

Full range of motion

Full range of motion enables the entire muscle to be contracted with up to 90–100 per cent instead of, say, only 50 per cent with a partial rep. There are some exceptions if you are doing specific advanced training which involves partial or half reps.

When Alison performed her exercises, it was important to note how many repetitions and sets per exercise she completed, plus the technique and full range of motion.

Technique

Technique is the most fundamental part of training. When you perform with a good technique you ensure maximum muscle contraction and minimum injury to your muscles.

It is important to choose the appropriate weight for the exercise to maintain quality of technique. If you are trying to isolate a muscle group and you're lifting too heavy a weight, your technique will be altered, so that other muscles will become involved in helping you perform that exercise.

Remember – it is the quality of the movement, not the quantity.

Resting between sets

Choosing how much time you rest between your sets depends on how you are training. Either way, you do not want your muscles to recover too much, but just enough to continue your workout, unless you are after strength training.

Alison tended to rest between one and three minutes on the weight training sessions. During circuits and endurance-type exercises, Alison tried not to rest at all between any sets. This is to keep both the heart rate up and the muscles full of blood and lactic acid.

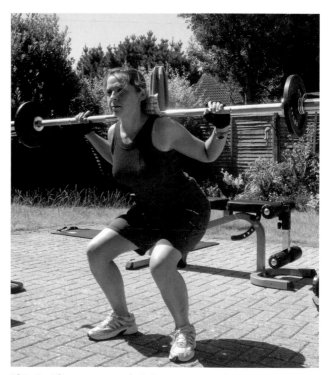

This is Alison on week 5. You can see her focus on the technique.

Breathing

When people are training, they seem always to worry about how they breathe when lifting weights. The general rule when breathing should be:

- Exhale on the way out for effort.
- Inhale after effort.

Rating perceived exertion (RPE)

This scale is handy to describe the intensity of training sessions. Alison used the RPE throughout her training sessions, to show you how hard she felt her body was working. Use the same scale for your own training to monitor your progress.

0 Nothing at all
1 Very, very light
2 Very light
3 Fairly light
4 Light
5 Moderate
6 Fairly hard
7 Hard
8 Very hard
9 Very, very hard
10 Maximum effort possible

The RPE for cardiovascular (CV) sessions shows you the intensity of how hard and fast to run. For instance, if it was 7/10 for running, that would convert to running at 70 per cent effort.

Training average RPE

7.5/10 = 75 per cent of rate of exertion per training session.

Energy average RPE

You can apply the RPE scale to anything, such as your energy levels: 0 = not much energy at all and 10 = maximum energy.

Stress average RPE

In the training diary the RPE scale is used for recording stress: 0 = not much stress at all and 10 = maximum stress.

GYM SET-UP

We set up a home gym in my garage that Alison used. Most people have gym memberships, but if you are not able to access a fully equipped gym, we recommend the purchase of dumbbells and a bench. You will need somewhere to do pull-ups and a floor mat for the floor exercises.

Equipment

The equipment listed below should give you everything you require.

Weights

You don't need to buy both adjustable weights, just buy the appropriate ones for you.

- Adjustable dumbbells 5lbs (2.25kg) to 52.5lbs (24kg)
- Adjustable dumbbells 10lbs (4.5kg) to 90lbs (41kg)
- 150kg Olympic weights and 7 foot Olympic bar
- Bench
- Rack and cable

Attachments

- Single handle
- Rope
- Lat pull-down bar with rack and cable bar
- Close grip handle
- If required, Olympic adjustment, from standard size bar diameter to Olympic size diameter

Other

- Bosu
- 4kg or 8kg kettle bell
- Abs mat
- Step box
- Full-length mirror (for correcting your technique)

RUNNING

Technique

The type of surface will determine how you run. For example, when running on soft surfaces like sand you should run in other people's tracks or by shuffling and digging your toes into the sand. This will use your calves more than when running on hard surfaces.

When running on hard surfaces, the general rule is a heel to toe contact. As your heel comes into contact with the ground it rolls along the foot and you then push off using the toes. Keeping your stride open keeps the stress off your knees and hips and sends it through your body.

Relax your whole upper body to enable your heart, lungs and legs to work more effectively. If you run with your hands clenched, for instance, blood will be taken from your legs and other areas needed for running and be pumped into your clenched hands. In turn, this results in decreasing your effectiveness in running. Your arms should be relaxed and in rhythm with your feet.

Breathing

The most important part of running is finding your rhythm, whether this is from breathing or by your strides. Either way, this enables you to relax so that your breathing becomes deeper in inhalation and exhalation. What we are trying to prevent here is shortness of breath. This results in oxygen being deprived from your muscles, which can cause cramp.

RUNNING SET-UP
Gait

It is very important to wear the correct footwear when training, and especially when running. You can go to a specialist running shop, where they will look at your feet and running style and prescribe trainers

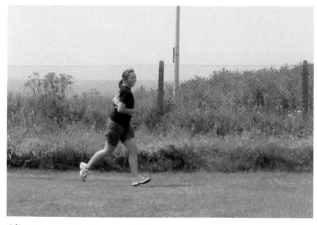

Alison running in week 1.

especially for you. Or, you can do a simple home test and prescribe your own trainers. Once you know your feet, it is easier for you to look for a pair of trainers to suit you. You need to look to see if you pronate, supinate, or neither.

Knowing your foot type – home test

To establish your foot type at home, the quickest way is to wet your feet and then stand on a dry area, so you can clearly see an imprint of your feet.

From the pictures below you can determine what foot type you have.

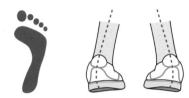

Supinated foot – high arch: foot doesn't roll over before toe-off, foot strike

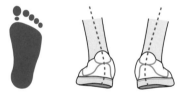

Over pronated foot – flat foot: foot rolls in excessively during foot strike but rolls to the inside

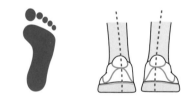

Neutral foot: ideal biomechanics

Trainers

What to look for in trainers: comfort, durability, performance, weight, style and price.

Types of trainers:

- Neutral/cushioning – neutral biomechanics
- Anti-pronation – over-pronators
- Motion control – biomechanical disorders and pronation control
- Racers – light, neutral and flexible

Clothing

- Running socks
- Cycling shorts
- Running shorts
- Breathable sports top
- Trainers
- Speed and distance watch

CYCLING

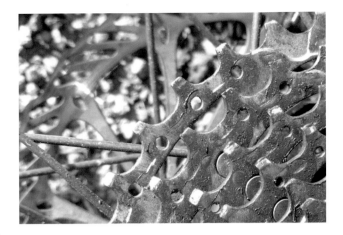

Technique

After setting up the bike, the correct cycling technique will require you to push through the ball of your foot on the way down while pulling the pedal up with your hip flexors – push and pull. When attempting a hill, you will need either to shuffle back on to the seat to push and pull with more power, or to stand.

Comfort and efficiency in cycling must go hand in hand. You need to find a relaxed and comfortable position. You should never sacrifice comfort for speed. You need to concentrate on maintaining a still upper body – by relaxing your shoulders you can help conserve your energy.

Breathing

You need to find your own rhythm, which will enable you to relax into your cycle.

Cadence

Learning to cycle at a high cadence is going to be the best fundamental skill you can learn. You should be aiming for a cadence between 80rpm and 90rpm, or if you're strong in cycling try to reach 100rpm.

To count your cadence all you need to do is count the number of revolutions you pedal over 15 seconds, then multiply it by four.

Bike set-up

Type of bike

It is important to get the best bike to suit your pocket, and one that meets your cycling needs, depending on the type of cycling you do.

The type of bike you require depends on the surface on which you will be cycling and what you want to use it for. Use the list below to understand what factors you need to consider:

- Type – off-road, road or hybrid
- Performance
- Maintenance
- Weight
- Comfort
- Style

Alison's bike is a mountain bike, as she prefers to cycle off-road or on cycle tracks. Her bike cost £350. As we started to increase the miles and Alison cycled more, she realised that she would have preferred to invest a little more money in a hybrid bike so it would be easier to ride on-road too.

Bike frame – to get the correct frame size for you should go to a specialist bike shop and allow them to fit you out with the correct size.

Saddle height – prop yourself up against a wall or get a friend to hold your bike. Place one heel on the pedal at the lowest point of the revolution – that leg should be straight but not locked out. This incorporates the use of the quadriceps muscles.

Saddle position – at 3 o'clock, the anterior aspect of the patella (front of the kneecap) should line up with the centre of the pedal axle. To achieve this you can move the saddle forwards or backwards, as well as tilting the saddle up and down.

Tyre pressure – for a road bike with 700c high-pressure wheels, the correct pressure will be around 100–120psi. For a mountain bike being ridden off-road the tyre pressure will be anywhere from 35 to 60psi.

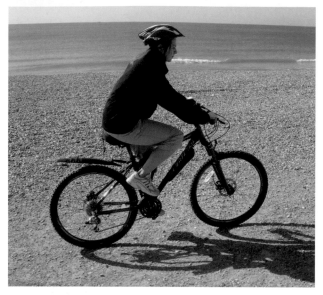

Alison trained mostly on her own mountain bike, which proved a lot harder for her than if she had ridden a lighter bike.

The psi varies with each manufacturer, so please check the recommendations on the sidewall of the tyre first.

CYCLING EQUIPMENT
Clothing
- Windproof T-shirt
- Windproof jacket
- Lightweight waterproof jacket
- Cycling gloves
- Cycling shorts
- Cycling shoes

Other
- Bike bag
- Waterproof dry bag
- Water bottle/hydration pack
- Speed and distance bike computer
- Pedals with/without clips
- Pump
- Bell
- Adjustable allen keys
- Spare inner tube
- Puncture repair kit
- First aid kit

WHEN TO TRAIN
You can train at any time throughout the 12-week programme. You just have to choose what time suits you to get the most out of your workouts, whether it is first thing in the morning or last thing at night. Alison worked out at various times throughout the 12-week programme, although she preferred working out in the evenings.

REST AND RECOVERY
Rest days are almost as important as training days. It's during sleep and rest that your body recuperates from all its hard work, repairing and building your muscles to become more toned, stronger and fitter. You should have total rest on the specified rest days.

Our bodies don't respond well to extremes. For example, if you eat too much you gain weight. However, if you eat too few calories, your body shuts down and your weight loss screeches to a halt. The same goes for exercise. You need to find a happy medium to coax your body to change in the way you want it to.

Why should you rest and recover after training?
Your body doesn't become stronger when you work out, but when you rest. For example, when you lift weights, you create little tears within your muscle fibres (which is good so don't worry). When you rest, the muscle fibres begin to repair themselves, growing back stronger than before. So, as your muscles grow and become stronger, you are able to lift more weight. If you don't allow those muscles adequate rest, however, the fibres won't have a chance to heal, and may even weaken, until eventually you could even injure yourself with a pull or a tear.

Recovery is influenced by many factors, including healthy eating, hydration and sleep. There are also more complex factors such as work and family stress. You need to be aware of the influence your personal lifestyle can have on your recovery.

If it is clear you are not overtraining, then consider if your lifestyle could be the cause of your deterioration. If you are experiencing stress at work or at home, try reducing the number, duration and intensity of your training sessions. Below are some tips on how to achieve this.

Active rest – you can help flush out lactic acid and other waste products that build in your muscles by doing very gentle exercise, such as walking or a very light swim or cycle. The key is to enjoy the activity and not to work your muscles too hard.

Passive rest – do no activities at all. Enjoy a day off seeing family or friends, or just lazing around at home. The choice is yours.

Stretching – stretching can help increase the range of movement and efficiency of muscles, reduce the likelihood and seriousness of injury, extend your training life, and reduce muscle fatigue and soreness. Stretching can easily be incorporated into your day – for example, when at your desk, or even while watching television.

Spa benefits – soak in a spa or use the sauna to help your muscles recover faster. You can try to stretch while in the spa. Alternating hot and cold water in the shower helps flush out waste products and bring oxygen to tired muscles.

Refuel – the body is most efficient at absorbing nutrients straight after training. Eating immediately after your workout supports the body's need to repair itself.

Sleep – it is during sleep that the growth hormone sets to work, protein production occurs, and our mind and body are recharged. The amount of sleep required varies from person to person, but most people fully recover after between seven and nine hours sleep.

Rehydrate – the harder you train, the more water you need to drink. Drinking enough before and immediately after your workout is your key to success.

FITNESS TESTS

You should take fitness tests at the start of your training programme, and every four weeks, to monitor your progress and your eventual results. Ongoing testing acts as a morale booster, and highlights areas in which you are not performing to the best of your abilities. By taking the following fitness tests every four weeks, it gives your body the time and opportunity to adapt and get fitter and stronger.

Bleep test

The bleep test measures your aerobic fitness level over a 20-metre distance. It involves you running continuously between two lines measured 20 metres apart, in time with the audio bleeps.

Scoring on the bleep test

Use the table below to assess your individual scores taken during the bleep test.

Level	Speed (km/h)	Shuttles	Distance (m)	Cumulative distance (m)
1	8.5	8	160	160
2	9.0	8	160	320
3	9.5	8	160	480
4	10.0	9	180	660
5	10.5	9	180	840
6	11.0	10	200	1040
7	11.5	10	200	1240
8	12.0	10	200	1440
9	12.5	11	220	1660
10	13.0	11	220	1880
11	13.5	12	240	2120
12	14.0	12	240	2360
13	14.5	13	260	2620
14	15.0	13	260	2880
15	15.5	13	260	3140
16	16.0	14	280	3420
17	16.5	14	280	3700
18	17.0	15	300	4000
19	17.5	15	300	4300
20	18.0	15	300	4600
21	18.5	16	320	4920
22	19.0	16	320	5240
23	19.5	17	340	5580

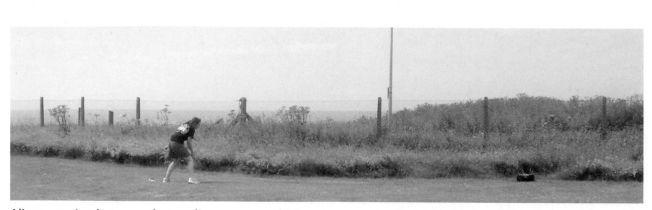

Alison running between the two lines measured 20 metres apart – the bleep test

You will start off with a slow speed, which will gradually increase as the levels increase. At the end of each level you will hear the bleeps getting closer together, which continues each minute.

If you have reached the line before the bleep, you must wait until you hear the bleep before running again.

Note: if the line is not reached in time with the bleep you have a chance to turn and catch up the pace for two more bleeps. The test is stopped if you are unable to reach the line in two consecutive ends, or if you fail to reach the line with a 2m gap.

Bleep test equipment
- Tape measure to measure the distance
- Cones or some type of markers
- Bleep test audio track

The bleep test audio track is commercially available at very low cost (or even free) as a CD or as a download to play on laptop, iPad, etc. Enter 'bleep test' in a search engine to find the many options.

The results below are not predictions for maximal oxygen uptake, but are indicators for aerobic fitness.

Age	Excellent	Good	Average	Fair	Poor
14–16	10/9	9/1	6/7	5/1	4/7
17–20	10/11	9/3	6/8	5/2	4/9
21–30	10/8	9/2	6/6	5/1	4/9
31–41	10/4	8/7	6/3	4/6	4/5
41–50	9/9	7/2	5/7	4/2	4/1

Each score shows the test level and the number of shuttles completed successfully (e.g. 4/6 = level 4 and 6 shuttles completed).

Muscular endurance tests
In the following tests you have one minute to perform as many repetitions as you can. This will be a good guide to your muscular endurance, as well as being a great way of motivating yourself to do better.

The results shown are from my years in the fitness industry, and represent an average of what I have recorded and seen. See Chapter 7 for guidance on how to perform these exercises.

Press-ups
Do full press-ups if you can, otherwise ¾ press-ups.

Age	17–19	20–29	30–39	40–49	50–59	60–65
Excellent	> 35	> 36	> 37	> 31	> 25	> 23
Good	27–35	30–36	30–37	25–31	21–25	19–23
Above average	21–27	23–29	22–30	18–24	15–20	13–18
Average	11–20	12–22	10–21	8–17	7–14	5–12
Below average	6–10	7–11	5–9	4–7	3–6	2–4
Poor	2–5	2–6	1–4	1–3	1–2	1
Very poor	0–1	0–1	0	0	0	0

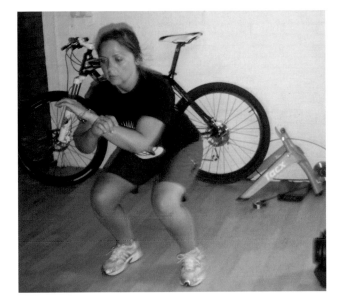

Squats

Do full squats to test your leg endurance.

Age	18–25	26–35	36–45	46–55	56–65	65+
Excellent	> 43	> 39	> 33	> 27	> 24	> 23
Good	37–43	33–39	27–33	22–27	18–24	17–23
Above average	33–36	29–32	23–26	18–21	13–17	14–16
Average	29–32	25–28	19–22	14–17	10–12	11–13
Below average	25–28	21–24	15–18	10–13	7–9	5–10
Poor	18–24	13–20	7–14	5–9	3–6	2–4
Very poor	< 18	< 20	< 7	< 5	< 3	< 2

Half sit-ups

To test your abdominal endurance, do half sit-ups and not full ones.

Age	Under 35	35–45	Over 45
Excellent	50	40	30
Good	40	25	15
Average	25	15	10
Below average	10	6	4

Dips

Completed as a bench dip.

Excellent	75+
Good	55–74
Average	35–54
Below average	35 and under

Pull-ups

There is no time limit, but you must keep hanging from your hands and keep your feet off the floor at all times.

The average result for pull-ups for women is 3–5. Initially Alison could hardly do half a pull-up, but after the 12 weeks she managed to do just over four of them, which she was really pleased with.

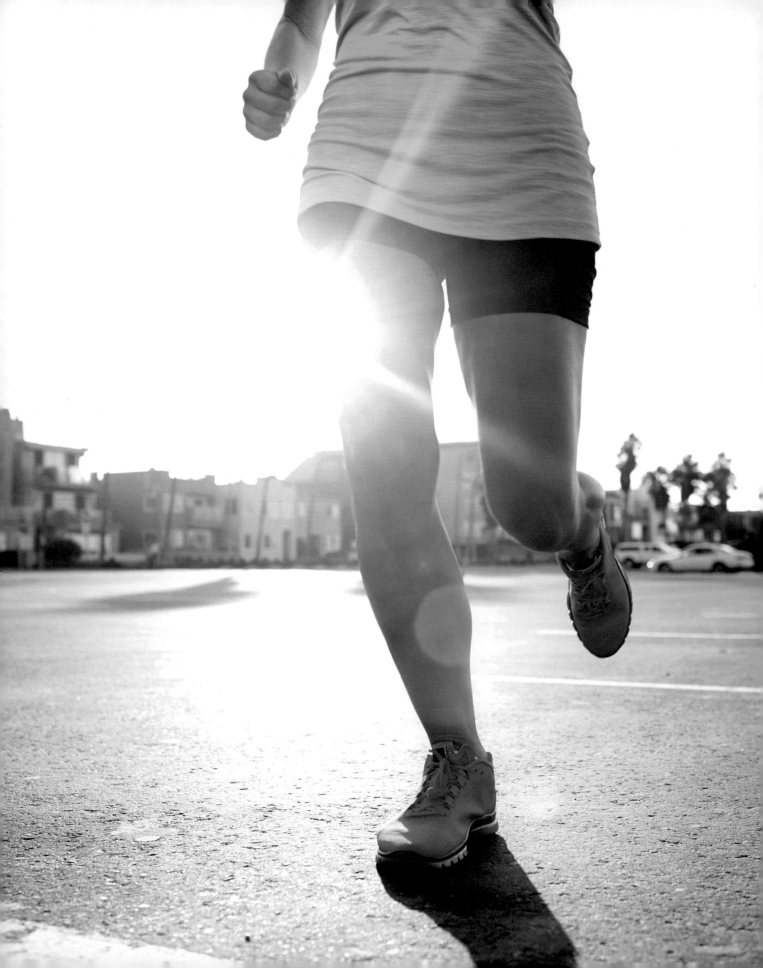

LET'S GET STARTED

05

Within the 12-week fitness programme you will do 57 different workouts and use over 80 different exercises to get the body you want. We will look at the basic training methods, warm-ups, cool-downs and quick stretches to get the most out of your muscles.

WEIGHT TRAINING

I am sure you have seen those people who use the gym regularly but have bodies that never change shape. This is due to several different reasons, but the main ones are:

- Lack of knowledge and technique
- No variety – using the same routine continuously
- Never increasing their performance (e.g. not increasing the weights when lifting)

We need to use as many different methods while training to get the most out of our bodies. This will encourage our bodies to get bigger and stronger, as our bodies won't become accustomed to the same routine.

Have a look through the different types of training methods I used, and take note so that you can use it to do your best.

Supersets
These are two exercises performed in a row without stopping. For example, perform squats followed by lunges.

Superset

	Static lunges (bosu)			Squat thrusts		
Sets	1.	2.	3.	1.	2.	3.
Reps	15	15	15	15	15	15

For example, this superset means completing three sets of 15 reps of static lunges and three sets of 15 reps of squats. Perform the first of three sets of static lunges, followed by the first set of three squats without stopping. After performing the first set of both exercises you can rest, then repeat until you have completed three sets of both exercises.

Drop sets

Perform an exercise with a heavy weight to reach failure (see below). Lower the weight and reach failure again. Keep lowering the weight until specified.

Pyramid training

This has a warm-up, a maximum and a cool-down all in one. Begin at the bottom of the left side of the pyramid and climb up until you are all the way at the top and then come back down on the right hand side to the base. The numbers represent the repetitions.

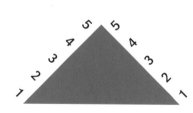

Set 1 = 1 pull-up,
set 2 = 2 pull-ups ...
set 5 = 5 pull-ups,
set 6 = 5 pull-ups,
set 7 = 4 pull-ups ...
set 10 = 1 pull-up.
Total pull-ups = 30.

Negative pull-ups

Use negative pull-ups if you are unable to perform more than three repetitions in a row. If you find that you cannot perform negative pull-ups, do lat pull-downs (see page 305). Negative pull-ups will strengthen your back quickly, so eventually you will be able to perform more than three reps in a row.

Start with your chin at bar level, either by stepping on a step box or object or by getting your training partner to lift you up to the top (with a little help from yourself). Slowly lower yourself in a count

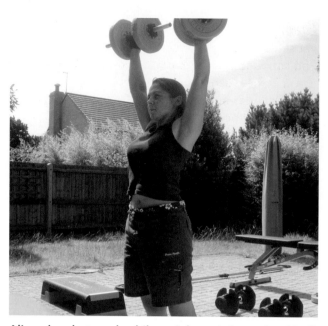

Alison hard at work while weight training – dumbbell press.

of five seconds back down to the bottom, until your arms are straight. This counts as one negative rep. Then repeat the number of reps specified.

Press-ups

With all of the press-ups you will be performing over the next 12 weeks, you must be able to perform at least 20 in a minute. If you are unable to perform 20 regular press-ups, you should be looking to perform ¾ press-ups. As soon as you can perform 60+ ¾ press-ups in a row, you should then be able to perform 30 regular press-ups.

If you find you prefer the ¾ press-ups, you can do them throughout the 12 weeks, like Alison, but of course you will get better results from doing full press-ups.

If you find ¾ press-ups difficult then you can try box press-ups. This is when you position yourself on all fours with your hands in line with your chest and do the press-ups from this position.

FAILURE

To train to failure, you continue a set until you can't do any more repetitions with that weight without stopping or losing technique.

Example:

1st set: warm-up set, 20 reps.

2nd set: add weight that allows your muscles to fail between 15 and 20 reps.

3rd set: add more weight to allow your muscles to fail between 10 and 15 reps.

4th set: using the same weight, allow your muscles to fail between 10 and 15 reps.

Forced rep

Get your training partner to spot you, to force extra reps to complete your set.

Weights

Heavy weights

We use heavy weights within this programme to strengthen your muscles, joints and posture. When using heavy weights follow the failure guide above. The rep range you are aiming for with heavy weights is 6–10 reps. If this is your first time with heavy weights, you should train with someone and take your time.

When you see heavy weights within the workouts please remember to increase the weight as much as comfortably possible, so that you get the most out of your workout.

Endurance weights

Most of the time we use endurance training in circuits, but we also introduce it into your weight training sessions. This will help tone your muscles while lifting a weight that pushes your limits. You will find this workout harder than most due to feeling the lactic acid burn. But remember, keep going.

Every time you see endurance weights written in the training diary, please choose a weight that pushes your boundaries. If the weight you choose was not hard enough just increase it, or if it was too heavy then lower it.

CARDIOVASCULAR TRAINING

Run PT (physical training)

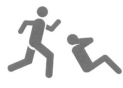

Alison enjoyed running and exercising outside, so if you can, try to perform the running and exercises outside instead of in a gym.

Run for the specified distance, and then perform the exercise with the number of sets and repetitions required, before moving on to the next exercise or run with no rest in between.

The running should be at 75 per cent of your maximum effort (RPE 7.5/10), and the exercises should be with good technique and as fast as you can to keep your heart rate up.

Cycle PT

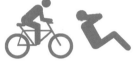

This is to be done in the same fashion as the run PT.

Running

We start the running nice and slow, as we want to have a steady build-up phase for your fitness. It is all about getting outside and running.

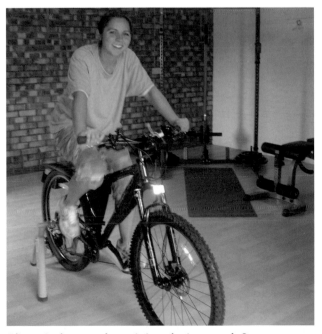

Alison indoor cycle training during week 8.

What if I can't run?

If you are unable to run through personal or health reasons, please do not give up straight away. You can match the running time or distance specified and swap it with another cardiovascular (CV) exercise.

What alternative exercises do you recommend?

Walking, swimming, rowing, using a cross trainer machine and cycling on your bike or on a spin bike.

On the longer runs, just try to keep in your aerobic zone most of the way. This should be at a comfortable pace, so you are able to hold a brief conversation with your training partner. If, however, you find it hard to talk, you are probably running too hard and you are out of your aerobic zone, so slow down.

Depending on your fitness levels and ability to run, beginners should use the timed runs and the more advanced should run the distance and time it.

Fartlek training

Fartlek (Swedish for 'speed play') is a training method that blends continuous training with interval training. This means running for as long as you can comfortably (note the time), walking to recover (note the time), and repeating the time patterns. Alison used fartlek training due to her not being able to run comfortably for more than five minutes. Alison's time pattern was four minute run and one minute walk, until she completed the time specified.

It does not matter if you walk for longer than you run, if this is what best suits you and your body at the beginning. As long as you push yourself each time you run, you will steadily progress by walking less and jogging more.

Cycling

I recommend you time a certain route and distance, and on subsequent rides try and match the time or, if possible, beat it.

Circuits

When exercising in circuit training, the most important thing is to push yourself as hard as you can and never rest in between any exercise or CV-based exercise.

WARM-UP

The warm-up is to prime your muscles, heart and lungs in preparation for your training session. You should slowly increase your intensity as you go through your workout, which will increase your heart rate and blood pressure.

Cardiovascular (CV) training sessions

Use five minutes before you start your CV session to perform the same exercise, but gradually build up the intensity until you feel that your body is thoroughly warmed up.

Weight and circuit training sessions

The following routine warms up all your muscles and systems and takes about five minutes.

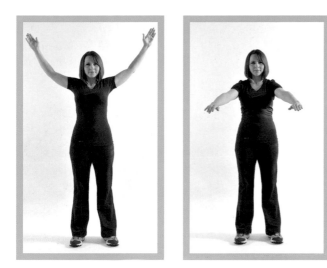

Arm circle forwards and backwards

Start with a small circle forwards about the size of a golf ball and gradually increase the circle size until you are rotating them to the maximum. For the arm circle backwards repeat by going in reverse.

Breast stroke and reverse breast stroke

Perform the breast stroke technique used for swimming. As you are going through the technique make sure you are really stretching forwards, and on the way back try to open up your chest to feel a stretch in your pectorals.

For reverse breast stroke, repeat by going in reverse.

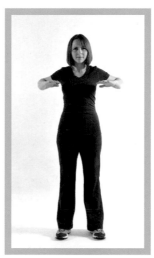
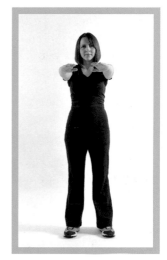

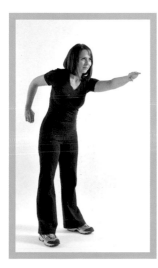
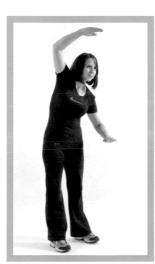

Front crawl and back stroke

The front crawl is the same as the swimming technique. When performing, make sure you're really trying to rotate each arm forwards and allow your hips to move with the movement. Reverse the direction in the same way for the back stroke.

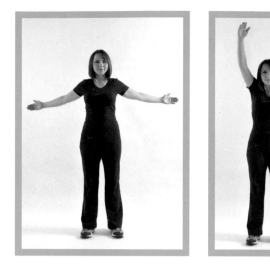

Butterfly stroke forwards and backwards

The butterfly stroke is the same as the swimming technique. As you are performing the stroke gradually increase the speed of the rotations forwards and then backwards.

Military press

Perform the military press movement, trying to feel a little burn in your shoulders.

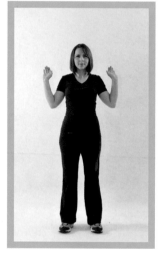

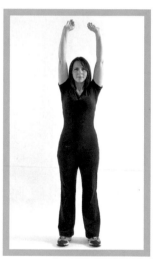

Roll hips in circles

Place your hands on to your hips, with your feet a shoulder-width apart, roll your hips in one direction and then in the other. As you roll your hips around in a circle, try to make sure the movement is coming from your hips and not from your legs.

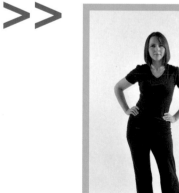

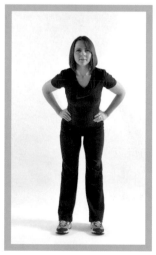

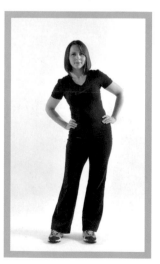

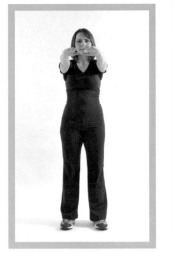
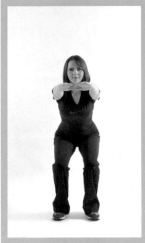

Squats

Perform 10–30 squats to feel your whole body loosen up. As you start off with the squats, you can start with half squats and gradually increase into full deep squats.

<<

Calf raises

Perform the calf raises as normal, and really try to stand on your tip-toes to feel your calves.

>>

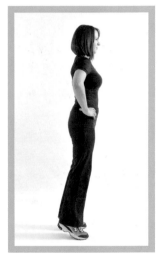

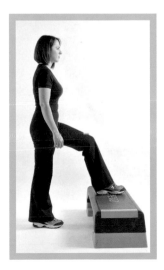

Step-ups

Perform any type of step-ups until you feel your heart rate increase. This should take no longer than three minutes.

<<

You can now add in stretches if you feel you need to release some muscles, or, if your muscles are ready, you can now start your training session.

When beginning your weight training sessions, do the first exercise with no weight and perform the motion with strict control, normally around 20 reps. Then use the first set with a light weight. After that, you will be ready to lift heavy weights and get stuck in.

Try to stretch in between all of your sets and exercises. Make sure you're stretching the muscle that you're exercising as this helps to open up the muscles and to incorporate more of the muscle fibres into the next set. This in turn helps you gain more tone, strength and definition.

COOL-DOWN

The cool-down phase is to make a transition for your muscles, heart and lungs to a resting or near resting state. You should slowly decrease your intensity as you go through your cool-down, which will decrease your heart rate and blood pressure.

CV training sessions

Once you have finished your training session, slow the pace down gradually until you are either spinning your legs out with no resistance if you are cycling or gradually slow to a walk if you are running. Keep moving at the slower pace until you feel your body relax and your heart rate decrease. Once you feel nice and relaxed, you can perform the stretches.

Weight and circuit training sessions

Complete the cool-down in the same manner as the CV cool-down. Normally when I finish circuit training or weight training, I go for a walk and try to relax my body. I might use some of the warm-up movements to make sure my muscles feel free of lactic acid, such as arm circles.

Once your heart rate has come down, perform the stretches.

WARM-UP AND COOL-DOWN STRETCHES

Try to stretch after the cool-down to make sure you don't ache too much the next day, and to help release the tension from within the muscles.

Alison used the myo stretch (meaning the muscle stretch) throughout the 12-week programme on a weekly basis to work on specific muscles that felt tight. It is an hour-long stretching routine that encompasses the majority of the muscles within your body.

You can follow this routine (see page 340), or below are a few basic stretches that I would include in my training routine. Do these between sets and at the end of training sessions.

How to stretch

When you stretch, there is no specific time to hold each stretch. Remember one thing, though: the smaller the stretch the better, so listen to your body. You need to find a stretch that gives you no burning sensation, shaking within the muscle or pain, but instead a stretch that is small enough so you can just feel it.

THE **STRETCHES**

Calf (gastrocnemius) stretch

Place both hands on a wall in front of you. Extend one leg backwards as far as comfortable, keeping it straight and your front leg bent. Make sure your feet are parallel with each other, and push up diagonally into the wall while pressing your heel down into the floor. You should feel a stretch in the back of your lower leg.

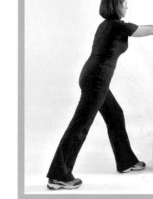

>>

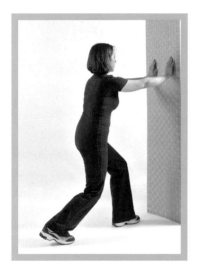

Soleus stretch

Place both hands on a wall in front of you. Extend one leg backwards, and maintain a bend in it. Make sure your feet are parallel with each other, and push up diagonally into the wall while pressing your heel down into the floor. You should feel a stretch deep in the back of your lower leg.

<<

Hamstring stretch

Stand with one foot on a chair or raised object. Keep your leg slightly bent and your foot flat on the chair. While keeping your back straight, lean forwards from your hip and tilt your bum upwards. You should be able to feel a stretch in the back of your thigh.

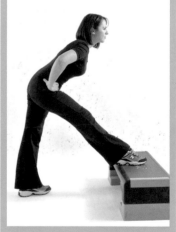

>>

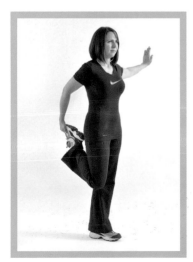

Quad stretch

Stand on one leg either balancing or holding on to a wall or object. Keep your whole body straight and your legs in line with each other. Your knees should be together and, holding your foot behind your buttock, tilt your hip forwards. This enhances the stretch on the front of your thigh.

<<

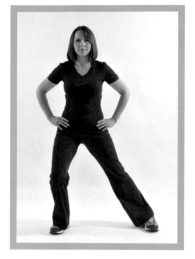

Adductor stretch

Stand with your feet wide apart. Keep one leg straight with the toes pointing forwards. Bend the other leg and allow your foot to turn outwards to balance you. While in this position, lower your groin towards the ground – to get more of a stretch you can lean your body towards your straight leg.

Hip flexor stretch

Extend one leg backwards as far as is comfortable, and keep it bent. Place both feet parallel with each other. Push your pelvis forwards, and lean slightly backwards towards your back leg. If you require, you can support yourself next to a wall or object to balance yourself.

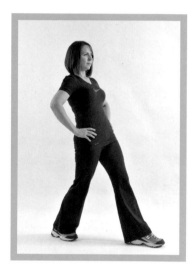

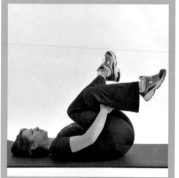

Glute stretch

Lie on your back on the floor face up. Cross one leg over the other leg, and rest your foot on the thigh. Start to bring your foot towards your buttock. Grasp the thigh just under the knee. Pull the leg up and towards your chest.

Abdominal stretch

Lie face down on the floor, keeping your hands in front of you about a shoulder-width apart. Keep your hips, legs and feet flat on the ground. Raise your torso off the ground until your arms are almost straight.

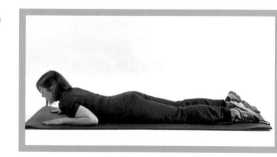

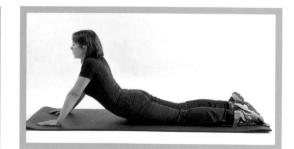

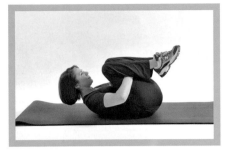

Lower back stretch

Lie on your back, face up. Hold on to the back of your thighs just underneath the knees. Pull your knees towards your chest, allowing your buttocks to rise off the ground.

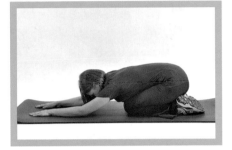

If you cannot feel the stretch there is an alternative method. Kneel on the ground, with your weight on your heels. Reach forwards with your hands, and let your head relax between your arms.

Lat stretch

Place your feet shoulder-width apart, and extend one arm across your body in front of you. Reach across as far as possible with your hands while leaning slightly forwards. The key is to try and arch the side of your back. You can vary this by holding on to an object or doorway. This will give you a deeper stretch into the lats.

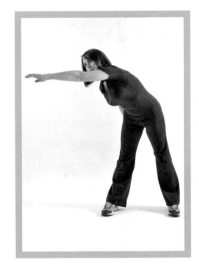

\>\>

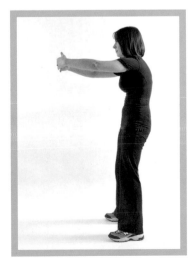

Rhomboid stretch

Place your hands together in front of you at about shoulder height. Reach forwards as far as is comfortable with your hands, trying to round the middle/upper part of your back.

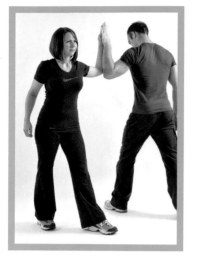

Pectoral stretch

Stand alongside a wall, with your feet shoulder-width apart. Bend your arm to a 90° angle at the elbow, and rest your forearm on to the wall or door frame. At the same time place the same-sided leg forwards. Turn your body and shoulders away from the bent arm until you feel a stretch. The same can be achieved with a workout buddy, as pictured here.

Anterior deltoid stretch

Place your hands into the base of your back. Drop your shoulders forwards and raise your chest up just like you're taking a deep breath. You should feel a stretch at the front of your shoulders.

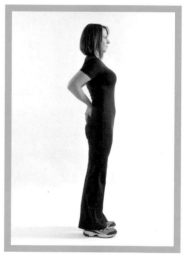

Deltoid stretch

Place one arm across the front of your body. You can either keep that arm straight or you can bend it to a 90° angle. Pull your arm in and towards the opposite arm until you feel a stretch.

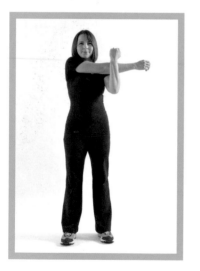

Triceps stretch

Place one hand up and behind your head with your elbow pointing upwards. With your other hand (depending on your flexibility) either pull the elbow down from the top or push the elbow from the front.

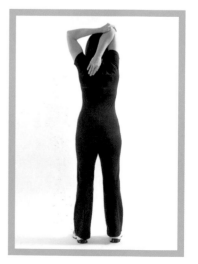

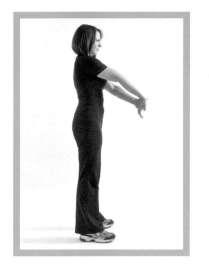

Biceps stretch

Hold on to a bench with your hands facing towards your body and your forearms facing away from your body. Keep your arms straight and lean backwards and down until you feel a stretch.

Forearm flexor stretches

With one hand, hold on to the opposite fingers and straighten your arm so your forearm is facing upwards. Then pull your fingers towards your body.

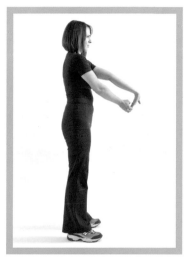

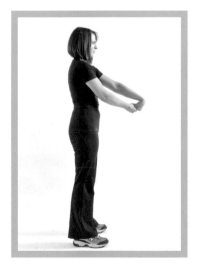

Forearm extensor stretches

With one hand, hold on to the opposite fingers and straighten your arm so your forearm is facing down. Then pull your fingers towards your body.

Trapezius and neck stretch

While looking straight ahead and keeping your head up, allow your head (ear) to drop towards one of your shoulders. Once in this position, pull the opposite shoulder down with your other hand to feel a stretch in your upper trapezius.

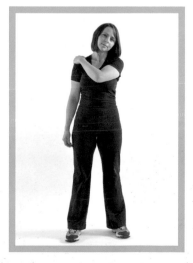

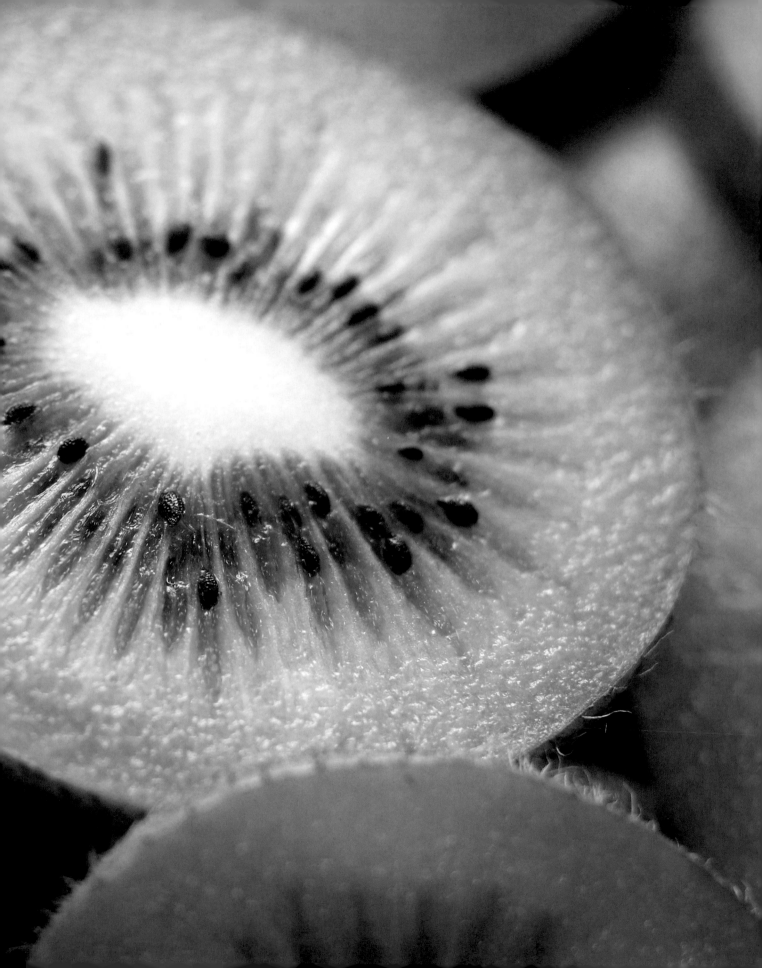

NUTRITION PLANS AND TRAINING SESSIONS

06

THE BEGINNING

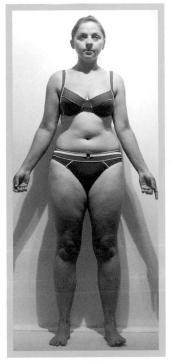
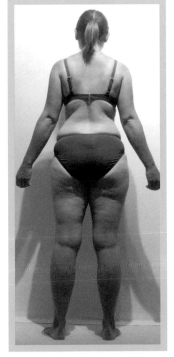

Front view of Alison at the beginning of week 1.

Back view of Alison at the beginning of week 1.

HEALTH CHECK **AT THE BEGINNING**

ALISON'S RESULTS

Statistics

Weight (kg)	57
Height (cm)	157.3

Health tests

BMI	23
RHR	77
BP	112/68
Fat (%)	32.1
Glucose	6.2
Cholesterol	5.2
Lung function	370

Measurements (cm)

Neck	31.75	
Chest	90.17	
Arms	R: 29.85	L: 29.21
Navel	81.28	
Hips	91.44	
Thighs	R: 60.33	L: 59.06
Calves	R: 35.56	L: 35.56

Calliper test (mm)

Biceps	8
Triceps	18
Waist	15
Subscapularis	19
Total	60
Calliper fat (%)	31.9

Fitness tests

Bleep test (20m) level	4.5

Maximum reps in one minute

¾ push-ups	15
½ sit-ups	35
Squats	39
Dips	23
Max pull-ups	½

YOUR RESULTS

Statistics

Weight (kg)	
Height (cm)	

Health tests

BMI	
RHR	
BP	
Fat (%)	
Glucose	
Cholesterol	
Lung function	

Measurements (cm)

Neck		
Chest		
Arms	R:	L:
Navel		
Hips		
Thighs	R:	L:
Calves	R:	L:

Calliper test (mm)

Biceps	
Triceps	
Waist	
Subscapularis	
Total	
Calliper fat (%)	

Fitness tests

Bleep test (20m) level	

Maximum reps in one minute

¾ push-ups	
½ sit-ups	
Squats	
Dips	
Max pull-ups	

WEEK ONE NUTRITION PLAN WEEK 1

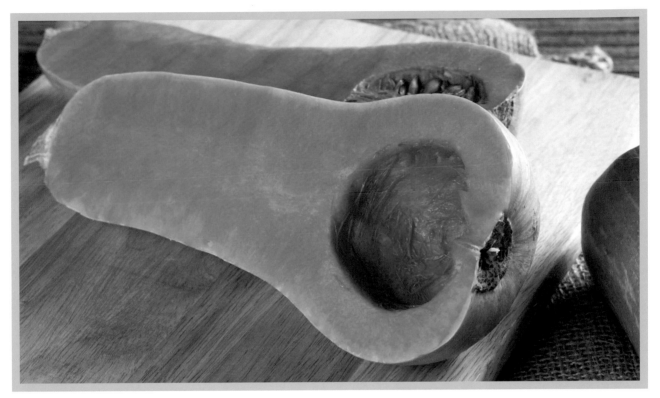

WEEK 1 OVERVIEW

Day	Breakfast	Lunch	Dinner
1	Muesli with fresh fruit	Smoked salmon pitta	Beef stir fry
2	Fruit porridge	Tuna and olive salad	Chicken with roasted sweet potatoes
3	Fresh fruit and seeds	Tuna salad with sweet potato	Slow roasted orange veal
4	Wheat biscuits or muesli with fruit	Turkey wrap	Jacket potatoes with cheese
5	Fruit salad	Butternut squash and vegetables	Spicy salmon
6	Fruit smoothie 1	Pitta turkey salad	Grilled tandoori chicken
7	Omelette	Butternut squash and coriander soup	Mackerel salad

SHOPPING LIST **WEEK 1**

CARBOHYDRATES
1 bag of brown rice
480g of muesli
1 bag of pine nuts
8 wholemeal/brown pitta breads
240g porridge oats
4 jacket potatoes
1 bag of sunflower seeds
1 bag of pumpkin seeds
9 sweet potatoes
4 organic tortilla wraps
Wheat biscuits

DAIRY AND NON-DAIRY ALTERNATIVES
350g low fat cottage cheese/
soft goat's cheese
8 eggs
40g feta/goat's cheese
1 light soft cheese/soft
goat's cheese
680ml skimmed/ soya/rice/
oat milk
2kg soya/plain yoghurt

FISH
8 anchovy fillets
4 mackerel fillets
4 salmon fillets
1 pack of smoked salmon
4 small tuna cans
350g tuna steaks

MEAT
4 200g beef steaks
8 chicken breasts
400g lean ham
8 turkey breasts
1.4kg rack of veal

FRUIT
6 apples
12 bananas
1 punnet of blueberries
2 lemons
2 mangos
1 orange
1 large pineapple
1 punnet of raspberries

VEGETABLES
1 avocado
2 bags of baby spinach
25g black olives
3 butternut squash
5 carrots
2 celery sticks
2 courgettes
1 cucumber
175g French beans
2 leeks
4 lettuces
265g mangetout
150g mushrooms
1 onion
115g plum tomatoes
5 red onions
5 red peppers
20 red tomatoes
100g rocket salad
26 spring onions
1 bag of sweet corn
2 yellow peppers

HERBS
Basil
Black pepper
Chinese five-spice
Coriander
Cumin
Dill
Fresh ginger
1 garlic bulb
Green chilli
Ground coriander
Mint
Nutmeg
Paprika
Turmeric

OTHER
Balsamic vinegar
Beef stock
Corn flour
Chicken stock
Cold-pressed extra
virgin olive oil
Ginger wine
Soy sauce
Tandoori paste
Tomato purée

SNACKS
Fruit
Wholegrain crispbread/
crackers/flat breads
Small bowl of muesli
Soya yoghurt
Nuts (cashew, pine or
occasionally mixed nuts)
Soya nuts
Seeds (pumpkin or sunflower)

FRUIT DRINKS
1 carton fruit juice drink

RECIPES **WEEK 1** DAY 1

BREAKFAST MUESLI WITH FRESH FRUIT

240g muesli (60g per person)

Serving of milk (soya/rice/oat or skimmed milk)

Fruit of your choice, cut into chunks (1 piece of fruit per person)

1 Pour muesli into a bowl, add milk.
2 Serve with fruit.

LUNCH SMOKED SALMON PITTA

4 wholemeal pitta breads (hot or cold)

Smoked salmon

Soft goat's cheese/low fat soft cheese (small serving per person)

2 spring onions, finely sliced

200g baby spinach

4 large tomatoes, sliced into quarters

1 red pepper, finely sliced

1 Cut open the pitta bread and spread the goat's cheese thinly across one side.
2 Add the smoked salmon and sprinkle on the spring onions.
3 Serve with spinach, tomatoes and red pepper.

DINNER BEEF STIR FRY

2 teaspoons corn flour

115ml beef stock

2 tablespoons soy sauce

800g of lean steak

1 tablespoon olive oil

1 garlic clove, finely chopped

2cm piece ginger

150g mushrooms

100g of mangetout

4 spring onions, chopped

Brown rice

1 Blend together the stock, corn flour and soy sauce.
2 Mix the beef, olive oil, garlic and ginger in a large bowl.
3 Heat a large frying pan or wok, and when hot add beef mixture and heat until meat is brown, then set aside.
4 Add the spring onions, mangetout and mushrooms to the hot pan, and fry until slightly crunchy.
5 Add the stock and corn flour mixture to the pan, stir over high heat until sauce has thickened.
6 Add the meat back into the pan, heat and stir well. Serve with brown rice.

RECIPES **WEEK 1** DAY 2

BREAKFAST FRUIT PORRIDGE

240g of porridge oats (60g per person)

2–3 apples, chopped

120ml of water or milk (soya/rice/oat or skimmed milk) – enough to cover the oats and apples

1 Slowly bring the water and/or milk to the boil in a saucepan. Add the oats and chopped apples.
2 Cook for 10 minutes, stirring continuously until thickened. If the mixture becomes too thick, add more water or milk. Serve immediately.

LUNCH TUNA AND OLIVE SALAD

175g French beans, topped and tailed

350g fresh tuna steaks

115g baby plum tomatoes, halved

8 anchovy fillets, drained on kitchen paper

25g stoned black olives in brine, drained

Fresh basil leaves to garnish

For the dressing:

1 tablespoon olive oil

1 garlic clove, crushed

1 tablespoon lemon juice

1 tablespoon basil leaves, shredded

1 Boil the French beans in a small saucepan for 5 minutes, or until slightly tender. Drain and keep warm.
2 Season the tuna steaks with black pepper, and place tuna on grill rack and cook for 4–5 minutes on each side, or until cooked through.
3 Drain the tuna on kitchen paper, and flake the tuna into bite-size pieces using a knife and fork.
4 Mix the tuna, French beans, tomatoes, anchovies and olives in a bowl and keep warm.
5 Mix all of the dressing ingredients together and pour over the tuna salad. Garnish with basil and serve.

DINNER CHICKEN WITH ROASTED SWEET POTATOES

3 sweet potatoes, chopped

1 butternut squash, peeled and chopped

1 red onion, peeled and chopped

6 spring onions, finely sliced

40g feta/goat's cheese, cut into small chunks

4 chicken breasts, sliced

2 tablespoons olive oil

1 teaspoon dried basil

3 tomatoes, roughly chopped

Handful of lettuce per person

1 Preheat oven to 190°C (375°F). Place the sweet potatoes and butternut squash into an ovenproof dish and drizzle half of the extra virgin olive oil over the top, mix well. Place into the oven and cook for 35–45 minutes.
2 Meanwhile, heat the rest of the olive oil over a medium heat and cook the chicken breasts for 8–12 minutes, until golden brown and thoroughly cooked.
3 Add the red onion, spring onions, dried basil and tomatoes to the sweet potatoes and butternut squash dish, stir well and cook for a further 5 minutes.

4 Sprinkle the cheese over the top and cook for another 3–4 minutes.

5 Serve the sweet potatoes and butternut squash topped with cheese with the chicken on a bed of lettuce leaves. Decorate with spring onions.

Lunch for tomorrow:
TUNA SALAD WITH SWEET POTATO
Consider preparing extra sweet potatoes for your lunch in advance.

RECIPES **WEEK 1** DAY 3

BREAKFAST FRESH FRUIT AND SEEDS

8 tablespoons soya/plain yoghurt

Sprinkle of sunflower or pumpkin seeds

2 pieces of fruit of your choice per person

1 Mix together the soya/plain yoghurt, seeds and fruit.
2 Divide into four portions.

LUNCH TUNA SALAD WITH SWEET POTATO

4 sweet potatoes, cooked (1 per person)

4 small tinned tuna (1 per person)

100g rocket leaves

4 tomatoes, roughly chopped

¼ cucumber, roughly chopped

50g mangetout

1 red pepper, sliced

1 tablespoon balsamic vinegar

1 tablespoon olive oil

1 Preheat oven to 190°C (375°F).
2 Cut the sweet potatoes into small chunks and drizzle with a tablespoon of extra virgin olive oil. Cook in the oven for 30–40 minutes.
3 Place rocket leaves, mangetout, tomatoes, cucumber and red pepper into a salad bowl.
4 Add balsamic vinegar and olive oil and mix well.
5 Serve with tuna, sweet potatoes and salad.

DINNER SLOW ROASTED ORANGE VEAL

1.4kg rack of veal, trim fat

2 carrots, sliced lengthways

2 courgettes, chopped

2 red onions, chopped

2 tablespoons olive oil

4 spring onions, finely chopped

Orange zest, finely grated

60ml of orange juice

For the dressing:

1 butternut squash, peeled and chopped into small pieces

150g low fat natural/soya yoghurt

2 tablespoons fresh mint

½ tablespoon olive oil

2 tablespoons lemon juice

1 Preheat oven to 200°C (400°F). Put butternut squash, carrots, courgettes and onions into a large baking dish. Drizzle over half of the olive oil and mix well.

2 Mix the spring onions, orange zest, orange juice and the rest of the olive oil to make a mixture.

3 Place veal on a wire rack set over vegetables and coat meat with mixture.

4 Roast veal for 40 minutes, or until cooked throughout.

5 Remove meat from oven, cover with foil and rest for 10 minutes.

6 Mix all of the dressing ingredients in a bowl, and serve vegetables and meat with a drizzle of dressing over the top.

Lunch for tomorrow: TURKEY WRAP

Consider preparing the turkey in advance for tomorrow's lunch.

RECIPES WEEK 1 DAY 4

BREAKFAST WHEAT BISCUITS OR MUESLI WITH FRUIT

560ml milk (soya/rice/oat or skimmed milk)

2–3 wheat biscuits or 240g of muesli (60g per person)

1 piece of fruit of your choice

1 Place your choice of cereal in a bowl and add milk.

2 Serve with fruit.

LUNCH TURKEY WRAP

4 turkey breasts, cooked and sliced

4 organic wholewheat wraps, serve hot or cold

200g mixed salad

4–5 tomatoes, sliced

1 red onion, finely chopped

1 yellow pepper, sliced

4 tablespoons of soya/plain yoghurt

1 Heat some extra virgin olive oil (½ tablespoon) in a frying pan over a medium heat.
2 Slice and cook 4 turkey breasts (1 per person) until golden.
3 Place the salad, red onion, tomatoes, yellow pepper and cooked turkey breasts into a salad bowl and mix well.
4 Drizzle over the yoghurt and add the salad to the wrap and roll up.

DINNER JACKET POTATOES WITH COTTAGE OR GOAT'S CHEESE

4 large baking potatoes (cut a cross in the centre of each potato and prick the skins with a fork)

3 teaspoons sun-dried tomato purée

½ teaspoon ground coriander

1 tablespoon olive oil

4 spring onions, finely chopped

1 fresh green chilli, deseeded and finely chopped

1 tablespoon fresh coriander

350g low fat cottage cheese/ soft goat's cheese

Handful of pine nuts

Side salad:

Generous amounts of mixed salad leaves

4 large tomatoes, chopped

1 red pepper, chopped

¼ cucumber, chopped

1 Preheat oven to 200°C (400°F). Bake the potatoes for one hour, or until soft and cooked. Meanwhile prepare the salad.
2 Mix the sun-dried tomato purée and ground coriander together in a bowl.
3 Just before the potatoes are ready, heat the olive oil in a small saucepan. Add the spring onions and chopped chillies, and cook for 2–3 minutes, stirring occasionally until soft.
4 Stir in the sun-dried tomato paste and cook for a further 1 minute. Remove from heat and stir in the chopped coriander.
5 Place the cheese in a bowl and stir in the tomato mixture.
6 Divide the cheese mixture equally among the potatoes.
7 Serve with salad and add a sprinkle of pine nuts over the top.

Lunch for tomorrow:
BUTTERNUT SQUASH AND VEGETABLES
See the following page and consider preparing your lunch in advance.

RECIPES **WEEK 1** DAY 5

BREAKFAST FRUIT SALAD

8 tablespoons soya/plain yoghurt
(2 tablespoons per person)

80g oats

60g sunflower seeds or pumpkin seeds

4–5 pieces of fruit (preferably ones in season)

1 Dice fruit into chunks and divide into four portions.
2 Add 2 tablespoons of soya/plain yoghurt to each portion and sprinkle with oats and seeds

LUNCH BUTTERNUT SQUASH AND VEGETABLES

1 butternut squash, peeled and chopped

2 sweet potatoes, peeled, and diced into cubes

1 leek, chopped

1 red onion, quartered

1 tablespoon, olive oil

Handful of coriander, chopped

Handful of rocket leaves per person

For the dressing:

¼ grated cucumber

4 tablespoons soya/plain yoghurt

1 tablespoon olive oil

1 teaspoon balsamic vinegar

2 teaspoons black pepper

2 teaspoons dried dill

1 Preheat the oven to 190°C (375°F). Place the butternut squash, sweet potatoes, onion and leek into a large baking dish. Drizzle with olive oil and season with black pepper and coriander.
2 Cook for 30–40 minutes, or until vegetables are cooked. Stir if necessary.
3 Meanwhile, place all dressing ingredients into a small bowl and mix well.
4 Remove from the oven and serve with rocket leaves, and drizzle the dressing over the top.

DINNER SPICY SALMON

4 salmon fillets

2 teaspoons Chinese five-spice powder

2.5cm ginger, cut into thin strips

2 tablespoons ginger wine

2 tablespoons soy sauce

1 Rub Chinese five-spice powder into both sides of the salmon fillets.
2 Place vegetables into a bowl, and add ginger wine and soy sauce.
3 Preheat the grill to a medium heat. Boil water and add the rice.

1 tablespoon olive oil

Brown rice

Side vegetables:

1 leek, finely shredded

1 carrot, sliced lengthways

115g mangetout, cut into thin strips

4 Place the salmon fillets on the grill and brush with some soy sauce. Cook for a few minutes on each side.

5 Meanwhile, heat the olive oil in wok or frying pan and stir fry vegetables for 3–5 minutes.

6 When the vegetables and salmon are cooked, transfer to plates and serve with brown rice.

Marinade for tomorrow's dinner *GRILLED TANDOORI CHICKEN*

Consider prepearing for tomorrow's dinner in advance (marinate in fridge overnight).

RECIPES **WEEK 1** DAY 6

BREAKFAST FRUIT SMOOTHIE 1

2 large mangos, peeled and chopped

4 bananas, chopped

2 handfuls of raspberries

Blend mangos, bananas and raspberries, and serve.

LUNCH PITTA TURKEY SALAD

4 wholemeal pitta breads

4 turkey breasts, cooked and sliced

Generous amount of salad leaves

1 avocado, sliced

1 red pepper, sliced

1 yellow pepper, sliced

2 spring onions, finely chopped

½ tablespoon olive oil

4 tablespoons of soya/plain yoghurt

1 Place the salad leaves, avocado, peppers and chopped spring onions in a salad bowl and mix.

2 Slice open the pitta bread and fill with turkey, salad and a dollop of soya/plain yoghurt.

3 Serve immediately.

DINNER GRILLED TANDOORI CHICKEN

100g natural soya/plain yoghurt

4 chicken breasts, diced

300g spinach

1 handful of coriander, chopped

8–10 tablespoons of sweetcorn

Brown rice

For the marinade:

1 tablespoon tandoori paste

1 teaspoon cumin

300g natural soya/plain yoghurt

1 tablespoon lemon juice

1 garlic glove, crushed

1 In a bowl, add the marinade ingredients together and mix well.
2 Add the diced chicken and coat with marinade. Leave in the fridge for at least 2–3 hours.
3 Preheat grill to a medium heat and cover a baking tray with baking paper.
4 Skewer the chicken and place on to a baking tray. Grill for 8–12 minutes, or until chicken is cooked (keep turning).
5 Boil the rice and add the sweetcorn for the last 2 minutes.
6 Serve the chicken, spinach, sweetcorn and rice. Pour the remaining yoghurt over the top and garnish with coriander.

RECIPES WEEK 1 DAY 7

BREAKFAST OMELETTE

8 eggs (2 eggs per person)

4 tablespoons of cold water

8 teaspoons of extra virgin olive oil

400g lean ham

1 courgette, finely sliced

4 spring onions, finely chopped

1 Cook one omelette at a time, beat the eggs with some water in a bowl.
2 Heat the extra virgin olive oil in a non-stick pan over a high heat and pour in the eggs. Cook for 2 minutes, or until the mixture just begins to set.
3 Place ham and courgette on top of the egg mixture and cook until the omelette has set.
4 Sprinkle on the spring onions, fold omelette in half, and serve.

LUNCH BUTTERNUT SQUASH AND CORIANDER SOUP

900ml of chicken stock

1kg butternut squash, peeled and chopped

1 onion, roughly chopped

2 carrots, roughly chopped

2 celery sticks, roughly chopped

1 garlic clove, crushed

1 teaspoon paprika

½ teaspoon turmeric

½ teaspoon ground coriander

½ teaspoon ground nutmeg

1 In a large saucepan bring chicken stock to the boil. Add the vegetables and spices and bring back to the boil.
2 Reduce heat and simmer for 20 minutes, or until vegetables are soft.
3 Allow to cool and serve.

DINNER MACKEREL SALAD

4 cooked mackerel, skin removed

Generous amount of mixed salad leaves

1 red pepper, sliced and deseeded

4–5 tomatoes, sliced

¼ cucumber, sliced

For the dressing:

3 tablespoons of soya/plain yoghurt

Pine nuts, small sprinkle

½ tablespoon balsamic vinegar

Black pepper

1 Place mixed salad leaves, peppers, tomatoes and cucumber on a plate.
2 Cut the mackerel into pieces and place on top of salad.
3 To make the dressing, mix the yoghurt, pine nuts and balsamic vinegar in a small bowl and add black pepper to taste. Add dressing to salad.

Lunch for tomorrow
BEETROOT SALAD
See page 96 and consider preparing rice and shallots for your lunch in advance.

TRAINING DIARY **WEEK 1**

WEEK 1 OVERVIEW
Day 1: Weights – whole body
Day 2: Rest
Day 3: CV – run
Day 4: Rest; cellulite massage
Day 5: Circuits
Day 6: Rest
Day 7: Rest; myo stretch

ALISON'S DIARY

Day 1 (Monday)
Today is the first day of my 12-week programme and I'm really looking forward to seeing how my body changes. I'm quite stressed at the moment so it's possibly not the best time to start, and I have some stress blisters on the top of my chest to prove it.
Tiredness 6
Stress 6
Sleep 7 hours

Day 2 (Tuesday)
Playing volleyball tonight, hopefully I can remember how to play as it's been a while. I was a bit stiff (DOMS) from yesterday's workout and today's volleyball session. I'm going for a run in the morning so hopefully I can move when I wake up.
Tiredness 6
Stress 7
Sleep 6 hours 30 minutes

Day 3 (Wednesday)
I went for my first run in ages. It took me a while to find a comfortable breathing pattern and to settle my breathing. I had to stop to get my breath back regularly but I did improve by the end of the session.
Tiredness 7
Stress 6
Sleep 7 hours

Day 4 (Thursday)
The stress blisters are ready to pop and the soreness has subsided. I needed some extra brain food as I had an exam to take (which I passed). I also had a cellulite leg massage from myo Clinic. One word, ouch! I was told the first will always be the most painful as all the cellulite needs to be broken down.
Tiredness 8
Stress 6
Sleep 8 hours

Day 5 (Friday)
Feeling good today. I had a comment at work saying that I had lost some weight but it might have been because I wore a different style uniform top to work that was more flattering.
Tiredness 8
Stress 6
Sleep 5 hours 45 minutes

Day 6 (Saturday)
Feeling a bit low and hormonal today and ended up missing lunch due to work. Not happy. I did catch up on sleep though, which was brilliant.
Tiredness 7
Stress 6
Sleep 9 hours 30 minutes

Day 7 (Sunday)
Tests today, a bit scared about my results but also nervous about having my photos taken in my bikini. Had an emotional moment this morning after the tests, but the results were very positive and so were the photos, so all good.
Tiredness 8
Stress 6
Sleep 8 hours 30 minutes

TRAINING SESSION **WEEK 1** DAY 1

ALISON'S SESSION

AM Rest

PM Training session Weights – Whole body

Time trained 3.30–4.20 p.m.

Session time 50 minutes

RPE 7/10

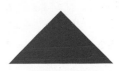

WORKOUT

Regular pull-ups
Negatives: 1–3 and 3–1
Total: 12

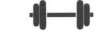

Dumbbell press
Set and Rep: 1. 15　2. 15
Weight (lb):　　5　　10

Squats bosu (upside down)
Set and Rep: 1. 13　2. 13　3. 13
Weight:　　　–　　　–　　　–

Lunges
Set and Rep: 1. 12　2. 12
Weight:　　　–　　　–

¾ Regular press-ups
1–4 and 4–1
Total: 20

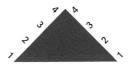

Half sit-ups: 2 × 15

Single side leg levers: 2 × 10 each side

Pelvic tilts: 3 × 15

YOUR SESSION

AM

PM　Training session Weights – Whole body

Time trained

Session time　　hour(s)　　minutes

RPE　/10

WORKOUT

Regular pull-ups
Negatives:　　　and
Total:

Dumbbell press
Set and Rep: 1.　　2.　　3.
Weight (kg):

Squats bosu
Set and Rep: 1.　　2.　　3.
Weight (kg):

Lunges
Set and Rep: 1.　　2.
Weight (kg):

¾ Regular press-ups
　　　and
Total:

Half sit-ups:　　×

Single side leg levers:　　×

Pelvic tilts:　　×

Notes: Alison had weak lower abs, so we opted for the beginners exercise, but if you're stronger in your abs try full leg levers.

Alison's notes: Good workout today, I feel my hips strengthening and that was a lot of upper arm work.

Your notes:

TRAINING SESSION **WEEK 1** DAY 3

ALISON'S SESSION

AM Rest

PM Training session CV – Run

Time trained 4.00–4.30 p.m.

Session time 30 minutes

RPE 9/10

WORKOUT
Run: 30 minutes / 3 miles
Actual distance: 2.25 miles
Run time: 30 minutes
Average Pace: 14 m/m

Alison's notes: Ran around Whitecliff for as long as possible, but I couldn't run the full 30 minutes in one go because I was finding it hard to breathe. Gavin broke the run down for me and it did get easier, the trick is to take your mind off your problem, mine was breathing.

Notes: If you are able to run easily for 30 minutes, please try to run for the three miles at the best pace you can. Alison did fartlek training as she was unable to run comfortably for more than five minutes. If you find running hard, please use fartlek training (see page 64).

YOUR SESSION

AM

PM   Training session CV – Run

Time trained

Session time   hour(s)   minutes

RPE   /10

WORKOUT
Run: 30 minutes / 3 miles
Actual distance: miles
Run time: minutes
Average Pace: m/m

Your notes:

TRAINING SESSION **WEEK 1** DAY 5

ALISON'S SESSION

AM Rest

PM Training session Circuits

Time trained 7.00–8.20 p.m.

Session time 1 hour 20 minutes

RPE 7/10

WORKOUT

Each exercise is timed for one minute.

You will notice the first exercise is weights, the second exercise is with a step box, the third exercise is on the mat (floor) and the fourth exercise is running.

When running, run as fast as you can for the three minutes to cover the most amount of distance. If you cannot run, then walk as fast as you can and put in an incline.

Complete the cycles in order:

Cycle 1
Jog: 5 minutes (to warm-up)

Cycle 2
Dumbbell press
Step box
Half sit-ups
3 minute run
Weight: 7.5lb (step-ups)

Cycle 3
Bent-over rows
Step box
Reverse curls
3 minute run
Weight 15lb (down, down, up, up)

YOUR SESSION

AM

PM   Training session Circuits – Whole body

Time trained

Session time   hour(s)   minutes

RPE   /10

WORKOUT

Cycle 1
Jog: minutes

Cycle 2
Dumbbell press
Step box
Half sit-ups
        minute run
Weight: kg (step-ups)

Cycle 3
Bent-over rows
Step box
Reverse curls
3 minute run
Weight: kg (down, down, up, up)

Cycle 4
Press-ups
Step box
Heel taps
3 minute run
Weight: 12.5lb (side lunge)

Cycle 5
Arm curl
Step box
Glute extensions
3 minute run
Weight: 7.5lb (back lunge)

Cycle 6
Dips
Step box
Plank
3 minute run
No weight (knee raise step-up)
Alison's running distance: 1.9 miles

Notes: Complete all four exercises in cycles in a row with no rest if possible, before moving on to the next cycle. You can rest in between cycles if you wish, but remember the less time you rest between cycles the fitter you become. This will be your first hard workout. Do not be put off, just give it your best, and when you come to your next circuit session believe me it will not be as hard. Good luck.

Alison's notes: I found the running really hard as Gavin told me to push my body to the maximum.

Cycle 4
Press-ups
Step box
Heel taps
3 minute run
Weight: kg (side lunge)

Cycle 5
Arm curl
Step box
Glute extensions
3 minute run
Weight: kg (back lunge)

Cycle 6
Dips
Step Box
Plank
3 minute run
No weight (knee raise step-up)
Your running distance: miles

Your notes:

WEEK 1 TESTS

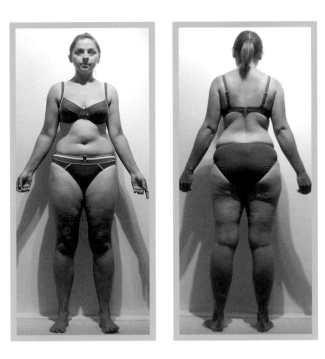

Take a photo of yourself from front and back to help gauge your progress.

ALISON'S WEEKLY TESTS

Weight (kg)	55.5
Height (cm)	157.3
BMI	22.4
RHR	68
BP	112/68
Fat (%)	30.8

Measurements (cm)

Neck	30.48	
Chest	88.90	
Arms	R: 29.21	L: 28.57
Navel	79.37	
Hips	00.90	
Thighs	R: 59.05	L: 58.42
Calves	R: 35.56	L: 35.56

YOUR WEEKLY TESTS

Weight (kg)	
Height (cm)	
BMI	
RHR	
BP	
Fat (%)	

Measurements (cm)

Neck		
Chest		
Arms	R:	L:
Navel		
Hips		
Thighs	R:	L:
Calves	R:	L:

WEEK TWO NUTRITION PLAN WEEK 2

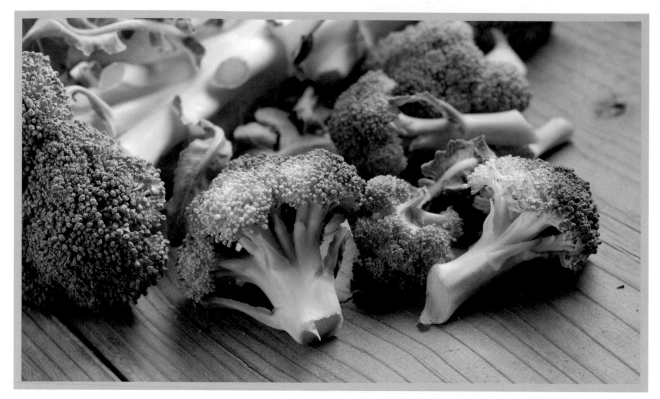

WEEK 2 OVERVIEW

Day	Breakfast	Lunch	Dinner
1	Fruit salad	Beetroot salad	Lamb ratatouille
2	Muesli with fresh fruit	Lamb with feta/goat's cheese	Chilli fish
3	Scrambled eggs with wild mushrooms	Tuna salad with sweet potato	Turkey stir fry with orange
4	Fruit porridge	Vegetable soup	Tuna steak and cannellini bean salad
5	Fresh fruit and seeds	Beef salad pitta	Tandoori turkey salad
6	Fruit smoothie 1	Bean salad	Swordfish with Mediterranean vegetables
7	Omelette	Tuna and olive salad	Hot bean soup with butternut squash

SHOPPING LIST **WEEK 2**

CARBOHYDRATES
75g butter beans
400g cannellini beans
50g tinned chickpeas
250g couscous
475g kidney beans
490g muesli
10 new potatoes
1 bag of pine nuts
400g pinto beans
8 wholemeal or brown
Pitta breads
320g porridge oats
1 bag of sunflower seeds
1 bag of pumpkin seeds
8 sweet potatoes
4 bags of wild rice

DAIRY AND NON-DAIRY ALTERNATIVES
20 eggs
40g feta/goat's cheese
1520ml skimmed/soya/rice/oat milk
2kg soya yoghurt

FISH
8 anchovy fillets
4 plaice fillets
200g (× 4) swordfish
4 small tuna cans
750g tuna steaks

MEAT
400g cooked roast beef
6 lamb chops
400g lean ham
8 turkey breasts

FRUIT
7 apples
2 apricots
6 bananas
1 punnet of blueberries
2 lemons
1 lime
2 mangos
1 orange
2 peaches
1 large pineapple
1 punnet of raspberries

VEGETABLES
2 avocados
4 baby aubergines
2 bags of baby spinach
4 cooked beetroots
25g black olives
175g broccoli
250g cherry tomatoes
1 butternut squash
6 carrots
4 celery sticks
5 courgettes
1 cucumber
175g French beans
3 lettuces
50g mangetout
8 mushrooms
3 onions
135g plum tomatoes
2 red onions
8 red peppers
10 red tomatoes
100g rocket salad
10 spring onions
4 shallots
1 bag of sweet corn
1 yellow pepper

HERBS
Basil
Black pepper
Cayenne pepper
Chilli powder
Chinese five-spice
Chives
Coriander
Coriander seeds
Cumin
Fresh ginger
Garam masala
1 garlic bulb
Ground coriander
Ground pepper
Mint
Parsley
1 red chilli
Rosemary
Turmeric

OTHER
Balsamic vinegar
Chicken stock
Chilli sauce
Cold-pressed extra virgin olive oil
Corn flour
Dijon mustard
Ginger wine
Muscovado sugar
Soy sauce
Sesame oil
Tandoori paste
Tomato purée
Vegetable stock
White wine vinegar
Wholegrain mustard

SNACKS
Fruit
Wholegrain crispbread/crackers
Flat breads
Small bowl of muesli
Yoghurt/soya yoghurt
Nuts (cashew, pine or occasionally mixed nuts)
Soya nuts
Seeds (pumpkin or sunflower)

FRUIT DRINKS
1 carton fruit juice

RECIPES **WEEK 2** DAY 1

BREAKFAST FRUIT SALAD

See page 84

LUNCH BEETROOT SALAD

100g brown rice
100g wild rice
4 shallots, peeled and halved
2 teaspoons olive oil
4 beetroot, finely diced cooked
Juice of 1 lemon
2 tablespoons fresh mint, chopped
2 tablespoons fresh chives, chopped

1 Preheat oven to 200°C (400°F). Place brown/wild rice in medium saucepan of water, bring to boil and simmer for 20–30 minutes.
2 Put the shallots on a baking tray, drizzle with olive oil and roast for 8–10 minutes.
3 Drain the rice and allow to cool. Gently mix together the beetroot, lemon juice and mint.
4 Stir in shallots and chives and serve.

DINNER LAMB RATATOUILLE

8 lamb steaks, lean diced
1 tablespoon olive oil
250g couscous
Spices:
1 tablespoon pepper, freshly ground
2 teaspoons coriander seeds, whole
1 teaspoon garam masala
1 teaspoon chilli powder
For the ratatouille:
2 teaspoons olive oil
4 baby aubergines
1 onion, finely chopped
1 clove garlic, chopped
1 red pepper, deseeded and sliced
1 courgette, sliced
115ml chicken stock
2 tomatoes
1 tablespoon parsley, chopped

1 Mix all the spices in a bowl and brush the steaks with a little olive oil and coat with spice mixture, cover with cling film and refrigerate for 1 hour.
2 To make ratatouille, heat the olive oil in a large frying pan over medium heat.
3 Add aubergines and cook for 4 minutes or until golden. Then add the onion and garlic and cook until lightly coloured.
4 Next add the red pepper and courgette and cook for a further minute. Then pour on the chicken stock and add the tomatoes and bring to boil. Cook for a further 5 minutes, add parsley and season to taste.
5 Bring water to the boil and add the couscous, cover with a lid and allow to settle.
6 Heat oil in a frying pan over high heat and cook lamb for 3 minutes on each side.
7 Serve the lamb with ratatouille and couscous.

Lunch for tomorrow
LAMB RATATOUILLE
Save some lamb ratatouille for tomorrow's lunch.

RECIPES **WEEK 2** DAY 2

BREAKFAST MUESLI WITH FRESH FRUIT

See page 79

LUNCH LAMB WITH FETA/ GOAT'S CHEESE

4 pitta breads, 1 per person (serve hot or cold)

Ratatouille and sauce from last night's dinner

Lettuce

Feta/goat's cheese, small amount

Soya/plain yoghurt

1 Slice open pitta bread and fill with lamb, ratatouille, lettuce and sprinkle with feta/goat's cheese.
2 Drizzle the soya/plain yoghurt over the top.

DINNER CHILLI FISH

4 plaice fillets

1 tablespoon olive oil

1 tablespoon fresh coriander

2 tablespoons lime juice

300ml water

1 tablespoon chilli sauce

2 tablespoons tomato purée

1cm ginger, grated

1 teaspoon muscovado sugar

Lemon wedges, to serve

1 tablespoon white wine vinegar

Brown rice

1 Place fish in a dish, add olive oil, coriander and lime juice and coat well. Cover in cling film and place in the fridge to marinate.
2 Preheat the grill to medium heat. Place water, tomato purée, chilli sauce, white wine vinegar, ginger and sugar in small saucepan. Stir and simmer for 5–8 minutes or until thick.
3 Meanwhile, remove the fish from the marinade and cook under the grill for 5–8 minutes or until the flesh flakes easily.
4 Transfer fish to plates and spoon over the sauce.
5 Serve with brown rice and garnish with lemon wedges.

Lunch for tomorrow
TUNA SALAD WITH SWEET POTATO
See the following page and consider preparing sweet potatoes for your lunch in advance.

RECIPES **WEEK 2** DAY 3

BREAKFAST SCRAMBLED EGGS WITH WILD MUSHROOMS

8 wild mushrooms, large

8 eggs

200ml serving of milk (soya/rice/oat or skimmed milk)

1 tablespoon chives, chopped

2 teaspoons olive oil

Ground black pepper

1 Preheat the grill to high heat. Brush mushrooms with olive oil and season with pepper. Grill for about 10 minutes or until tender.
2 Meanwhile, in a bowl lightly whisk eggs and milk together and lightly season with black pepper.
3 Heat a non-stick frying pan over medium heat and pour in the egg mixture and cook. Keep stirring until the egg is cooked, then stir in chives. Place eggs on the mushrooms and serve.

LUNCH TUNA SALAD WITH SWEET POTATO

See page 81

DINNER TURKEY STIR FRY WITH ORANGE

4 turkey breasts, sliced

1 tablespoon of sesame oil

1 tablespoon olive oil

2 large carrots, thinly sliced

175g small florets of broccoli

2 teaspoons ginger, crushed

2 teaspoons garlic, crushed

4 spring onions, finely sliced

1 tablespoon corn flour

For the marinade:

1 tablespoon wholegrain mustard

2 red peppers, sliced

2 tablespoons soy sauce

1 large orange, finely grated and juiced

Brown rice

1 Marinade: mix together the soy sauce, mustard, orange rind and juice into a small bowl. Stir in the turkey and set aside to marinade. Boil the rice.
2 Heat the olive and sesame oil in a wok or large frying pan over a high heat. Add the carrots and broccoli and cook for 3 minutes.
3 Remove the turkey from mix and add to the wok. Add the garlic, ginger, spring onions and red pepper and stir fry for another 4 minutes.
4 Mix the corn flour and the reserve of the marinade to make a smooth sauce and pour over the turkey.
5 Stir fry for a further 1–2 minutes until the broccoli is tender, serve immediately with brown rice.

Lunch for tomorrow
VEGETABLE SOUP
See the following page and consider preparing your lunch in advance.

RECIPES **WEEK 2** DAY 4

BREAKFAST FRUIT PORRIDGE   *See page 80*

LUNCH VEGETABLE SOUP

1 litre vegetable stock

2 carrots, sliced

2 celery sticks, chopped

1 onion, chopped

1 tablespoon fresh parsley, chopped

400g tinned tomatoes

1 tablespoon basil, chopped

1 tablespoon rosemary, finely chopped

1 Bring stock to boil in a large saucepan.
2 Add the carrots, celery, onion, parsley and tomatoes and simmer gently for 30 minutes.
3 Stir through basil and rosemary, and season with black pepper.

DINNER TUNA STEAK AND CANNELLINI BEAN SALAD

1 tablespoon pine nuts

4 × 100g tuna steaks

½ tablespoon olive oil

1 garlic clove, crushed

400g white cannellini beans, drained and rinsed

1 tablespoon basil, finely sliced

½ tablespoon parsley

2 spring onions, finely sliced

Generous amount of mixed salad leaves

1 Heat a small non-stick frying pan over medium heat, add the pine nuts and stir until toasted and golden, then set aside.
2 Heat a large non-stick frying pan over high heat and add the olive oil.
3 Place tuna steaks in frying pan and cook for 2–3 minutes each side. The tuna should still be a little pink in middle. Allow to cool slightly.
4 Place the remaining ingredients and pine nuts in bowl and mix.
5 Serve the tuna with bean salad on the side.

Dinner for tomorrow
TANDOORI TURKEY SALAD
See the following page and consider preparing your lunch in advance.

RECIPES **WEEK 2** DAY 5

BREAKFAST FRESH FRUIT AND SEEDS

See page 81

LUNCH BEEF SALAD PITTA

4 wholemeal pitta breads (serve hot or cold)

400g cold roast beef, finely sliced

Green salad, generous amounts of

4 large tomatoes, sliced

1 red pepper, sliced

½ red onion, finely sliced

2 tablespoons chopped basil

For the dressing:

2 tablespoons olive oil

1 tablespoon balsamic vinegar

1 teaspoon Dijon mustard

Season with black pepper

1 In a small bowl mix together all the dressing ingredients.
2 Put the remaining ingredients in a large salad bowl and mix well.
3 Slice open the pitta bread and fill with beef and salad.
4 Pour the dressing over the top.

DINNER TANDOORI TURKEY SALAD

4 sweet potatoes, peeled and chopped

½ tablespoon olive oil

400g turkey breasts

100g baby spinach

4 plum tomatoes, thinly sliced

½ cucumber

Coriander, small handful

Lemon wedges

For the marinade:

1 tablespoon tandoori paste

50g of soya/plain yoghurt

1 Mix the tandoori paste and yoghurt in a bowl.
2 Add the turkey and coat thoroughly. Cover and chill for 30 minutes – leave overnight if you have time.
3 Meanwhile, preheat the oven to 190°C (375°F).
4 Place sweet potatoes in an ovenproof dish and drizzle with olive oil. Cook for 20–30 minutes or until soft.
5 Preheat grill and cook turkey over a medium heat for 6 minutes each side or until cooked. Remove from the heat and let turkey rest for 5 minutes then slice the turkey into strips.
6 Place the spinach, tomatoes and cucumber in large salad bowl and put turkey strips over the top.

For the dressing:

150g of soya/plain yoghurt

2 tablespoons fresh mint

½ tablespoon olive oil

2 tablespoons lemon juice

7 Mix the dressing ingredients together in a small bowl and drizzle the dressing over salad.

8 Garnish with coriander and lemon wedges and serve.

Lunch for tomorrow
BEAN SALAD
Consider preparing the eggs in advance.

RECIPES **WEEK 2** DAY 6

BREAKFAST FRUIT SMOOTHIE 1

See page 85

LUNCH BEAN SALAD

4 eggs

2 avocados, stoned and peeled

400g tinned kidney beans

400g tinned pinto beans

1 red onion, finely sliced

Coriander, large handful chopped

250g cherry tomatoes, halved

For the dressing:

1 red chilli, finely sliced

½ teaspoon ground cumin

1 tablespoon of lime juice

3 tablespoons olive oil

1 Boil eggs for 6½ minutes, then place in cold water to cool.

2 Slice avocados and place in bowl with the beans, onions, coriander and tomatoes.

3 Mix the dressing ingredients in a small bowl.

4 Once eggs have cooled but are still warm, peel off shells and cut into quarters.

5 Mix the salad with the dressing and place the eggs on top and serve.

DINNER SWORDFISH WITH MEDITERRANEAN VEGETABLES

2 tablespoons olive oil

1 clove of garlic, chopped

2 teaspoons balsamic vinegar

1 tablespoon parsley, chopped

1 tablespoon basil

Juice of ½ lemon

4 × 200g swordfish steaks

1 red pepper, sliced and deseeded

1 yellow pepper, sliced and deseeded

2 courgettes, sliced

1 red onion, sliced

10 new potatoes, thinly sliced

Lemon wedges

1 Preheat the grill to high.
2 Add new potatoes in a baking tray and drizzle with olive oil. Place under the grill for 10–15 minutes.
3 Add the peppers, courgettes and onion into a bowl with half the olive oil and mix.
4 Transfer vegetables to the grill with the new potatoes and cook for 3–5 minutes, turning occasionally until slightly charred.
5 Place cooked vegetables and potatoes into a bowl.
6 To make the mixture for the fish, add garlic, balsamic vinegar, parsley, basil, lemon juice and rest of olive oil and mix together in another bowl.
7 Place fish in foil, add the mixture and wrap.
8 Grill the fish for 2–3 minutes each side or until cooked.
9 Divide vegetables and new potatoes between four plates and place fish on top.
10 Garnish with lemon wedges and serve immediately.

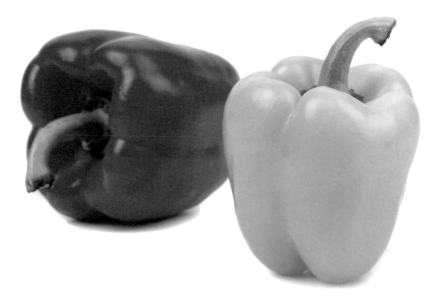

RECIPES **WEEK 2** DAY 7

BREAKFAST OMELETTE

See page 86

LUNCH TUNA AND OLIVE SALAD

See page 80

DINNER HOT BEAN SOUP WITH BUTTERNUT SQUASH

1–2 tablespoons olive oil

1 medium onion, chopped and peeled

2 cloves of garlic, peeled and finely chopped

1 butternut squash, peeled and chopped small

2 large carrots, peeled and chopped

2 celery sticks, trimmed and chopped

1 large courgette, sliced

2 red peppers, deseeded and chopped

1.5 litres (2.5 pints) vegetable stock

50g tinned chickpeas

75g red tinned kidney beans

1 teaspoon cayenne pepper

1 teaspoon turmeric powder

1 Heat the olive oil in large pan over medium heat, add onion and garlic and cook for 2–3 minutes.
2 Add cayenne pepper and turmeric and stir for 2 minutes.
3 Add butternut squash, carrots and celery and cook for a further 4–5 minutes.
4 Next add the courgette and peppers and cook for 2 minutes.
5 Add in the chickpeas, kidney beans, butternut squash and vegetable stock.
6 Cover the pan with lid and simmer gently for 40 minutes to an 1 hour.

Lunch for tomorrow
CHICKEN WRAP
See the page 115 and consider preparing the chicken in advance.

TRAINING DIARY **WEEK 2**

WEEK 2 OVERVIEW
Day 1: Weights – whole body; cellulite massage
Day 2: Rest
Day 3: CV – run
Day 4: Rest
Day 5: Circuits
Day 6: Rest
Day 7: CV – walk; myo stretch

ALISON'S DIARY

Day 1 (Monday)
Feeling good today, I had no aches or pains at all. I was, however, tempted by a large Bakewell tart (my favourite) but I remained strong and resisted temptation – I am very proud of myself. Had a cellulite massage today on my legs and Gavin was right, the second time round was not as painful.
Tiredness 8
Stress 6
Sleep 6 hours 30 minutes

Day 2 (Tuesday)
Day off today but loads to catch up on so still busy. The skin on my face is improving – spots clearing up. I am mentally preparing myself for the run tomorrow.
Tiredness 7
Stress 5
Sleep 6 hours 30 minutes

Day 3 (Wednesday)
Working early today and celebrated my birthday at work with a very posh afternoon tea. Usually I would dive at the cakes but I didn't fancy anything sweet so just had a scone and a few sandwiches (with a small Bakewell slice to finish).
Tiredness 8
Stress 5
Sleep 6 hours

Day 4 (Thursday)
I cooked for the family and had a really lovely meal taken from the nutrition programme.
Tiredness 8
Stress 5
Sleep 7 hours 30 minutes

Day 5 (Friday)
Had a really stressful day at work today mostly due to who I was working with. The exercise helped me release some of the stress though.
Tiredness 8
Stress 7
Sleep 6 hours 30 minutes

Day 6 (Saturday)
I thought I would be stiff today after my circuit workout yesterday but I feel fine – arms and shoulders aching a little but in a good way. I had a bad moment and had a fat scone covered with jam.
Tiredness 6
Stress 5
Sleep 8 hours 30 minutes

Day 7 (Sunday)
Bored to death at work today, really quiet. I didn't want breakfast this morning before work because it was about 6.15 a.m. but I forced it down. Test day again, Gavin was pleased with the results, which I was happy about, and we went for a walk out to the Purbecks.
Tiredness 7
Stress 4
Sleep 6 hours 30 minutes

TRAINING SESSION **WEEK 2** DAY 1

ALISON'S SESSION

AM Rest

PM **Training session** Weights – Whole body

Time trained 4.00–4.45 p.m.

Session time 45 minutes

RPE 6/10

WORKOUT
Superset
Alternate squat thrusts   Set and Rep: 3 × 10
Wide squat thrusts   Set and Rep: 3 × 10

Superset
Glute extension   Set and Rep: 3 × 10
Dirty dogs   Set and Rep: 3 × 10

Deadlift (using dumbbells in each hand)
1 × 20 warm-up – no weight
Set and Rep: 1. 12   2. 12   3. 12
Weight (lb):   7.5   12.5   12.5

Pec fly
Set and Rep: 1. 15   2. 13   3. 13
Weight (lb):   7.5   7.5   7.5

Dumbbell press
Set and Rep: 1. 15   2. 13   3. 15
Weight (lb):   7.5   7.5   7.5

YOUR SESSION

AM

PM   **Training session** Weights – Whole body

Time trained

Session time   hour(s)   minutes

RPE   /10

WORKOUT
Superset
Alternate squat thrusts   Set and Rep: ×
Wide squat thrusts   Set and Rep: ×

Superset
Glute extension   Set and Rep: ×
Dirty dogs   Set and Rep: ×

Deadlift (using dumbbells in each hand)
1 × 20 warm-up – no weight
Set and Rep: 1.   2.   3.

Pec fly
Set and Rep: 1.   2.   3.
Weight (lb):

Dumbbell press
Set and Rep: 1.   2.   3.
Weight (lb):

Straight arm pull-overs (using one dumbbell)
Set and Rep: 1. 15   2. 14   3. 13
Weight (lb):   7.5   7.5   7.5

Reverse shrugs (using one dumbbell behind you)
Set and Rep: 1. 15   2. 15   3. 15
Weight (lb):   22.5   22.5   22.5

Alison's notes: Great weight training session. Gavin gave me some 'compound exercises' such as deadlifts that utilise more than one muscle group at a time. This is a great arm and shoulder workout.

Straight arm pull-overs (using one dumbbell)
Set and Rep: 1.   2.   3.
Weight (lb):

Reverse shrugs (using one dumbbell behind you)
Set and Rep: 1.   2.   3.
Weight (lb):

Your notes:

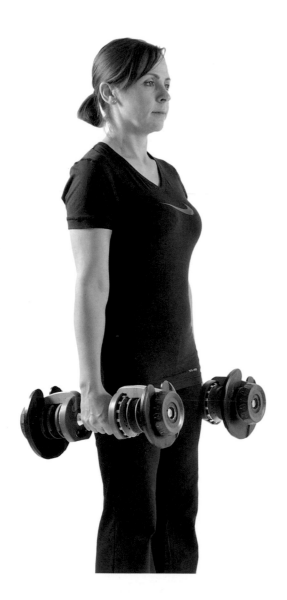

TRAINING SESSION **WEEK 2** DAY 3

ALISON'S SESSION

AM Rest

PM Training session CV – Run

Time trained 7.15–7.45 p.m.

Session time 30 minutes

RPE 8/10

WORKOUT
Run – 30 minutes/3 miles
Actual distance: 2.25 miles
Run time: 30 minutes
Average Pace: 14 m/m

Alison's notes: I ran the same route as last week because I wanted to do better than I did last time. This time I ran for as long as possible, but I still couldn't run the full 30. I did run for the remaining 14 minutes back to the car, then I collapsed. I realise now how important it is to stretch properly – I do this before and after running now.

Notes: Alison showed a great determination to push herself past her previous run; this time she ran for 15 minutes non-stop. The running pace was still 14m/m, the same as before, but she chose to run at a slightly slower pace to see if she could run the full distance without stopping too many times. This is a slightly slower pace than normal, so if you can run at a faster pace please do so, but you should aim not to stop as frequently as you did on your last run. You should not worry about speed, mileage and timings at this early stage, because as you increase the mileage your minute/mile pace will naturally increase so you are running faster.

YOUR SESSION

AM

PM Training session CV – Run

Time trained

Session time   hour(s)   minutes

RPE   /10

WORKOUT
Run – 30 minutes/3 miles
Actual distance: miles
Run time: minutes
Average Pace: m/m

Your notes:

TRAINING SESSION **WEEK 2** DAY 5

ALISON'S SESSION

AM Training session Circuits

Time trained 11.00 a.m.–12.15 p.m.

Session time 1 hour 15 minutes

RPE 9/10

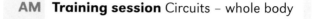

PM Rest

WORKOUT

Start on cycle 1 following the exercises 1 to 3 in set 1, then go to set 2 etc. Complete all three sets and exercises before moving on to the run and the next cycle. Do this until you have completed all six cycles.

1st set   use a slightly lighter weight for the high reps.

2nd set   use a moderate weight.

3rd set   use a heavy weight for the lower reps.

Complete the cycles in order:

Cycle 1
Set 1 30   **Set 2** 20   **Set 3** 10
1. Dumbbell press – weight (lb): 7.5   7.5   10
2. Step box – step-ups
3. Half sit-ups
Run 3 mins

Cycle 2
Set 1 30   **Set 2** 20   **Set 3** 10
1. Bent-over rows – weight (lb): 10   12.5   15
2. Step box – down, down, up, up
3. Heel taps
Run 3 mins

YOUR SESSION

AM   **Training session** Circuits – whole body

Time trained

Session time   hour(s)   minutes

RPE   /10

PM

WORKOUT

Cycle 1
Set 1 30   **Set 2** 20   **Set 3** 10
1. Dumbbell press – weight (kg):
2. Step box – step-ups
3. Half sit-ups
Run 3 mins

Cycle 2
Set 1 30   **Set 2** 20   **Set 3** 10
1. Bent-over rows – weight (kg):
2. Step box – down, down, up, up
3. Heel taps
Run 3 mins

Cycle 3

Set 1 30   **Set 2** 20   **Set 3** 10

1. Supinated curl – weight (lb): 7.5   10   12.5
2. Step box – box jumps
3. Press-ups (as many full, then into ¾)
Run 3 mins

Cycle 4

Set 1 30   **Set 2** 20   **Set 3** 10

1. Triceps kickbacks – weight (lb): 7.5   7.5   10
2. Star jumps
3. Reverse curls
Run 3 mins

Cycle 5

Set 1 30   **Set 2** 20   **Set 3** 10

1. Squats – weight (lb): 15   17.5   20
2. Spotty dogs
3. Wide squat thrusts
Run 3 mins

Cycle 6

Set 1 30   **Set 2** 20   **Set 3** 10

1. Calf raises – weight (lb): 15   17.5   20
2. Jumping oblique twists
3. Leg levers
Run 3 mins
My running distance: 1.7 miles

Alison's notes: I really loved this, it was a tough workout. I was quite tired half way through and by the end my legs felt like jelly.

Cycle 3

Set 1 30   **Set 2** 20   **Set 3** 10

1. Supinated curl – weight (kg):
2. Step box – box jumps
3. Press-ups (as many full, then into ¾)
Run 3 mins

Cycle 4

Set 1 30   **Set 2** 20   **Set 3** 10

1. Triceps kickbacks –
   weight (kg):
2. Star jumps
3. Reverse curls
Run 3 mins

Cycle 5

Set 1 30   **Set 2** 20   **Set 3** 10

1. Squats – weight (kg):
2. Spotty dogs
3. Wide squat thrusts
Run 3 mins

Cycle 6

Set 1 30   **Set 2** 20   **Set 3** 10

1. Calf raises – weight (kg):
2. Jumping oblique twists
3. Leg levers
Run 3 mins
Your running distance: miles

Your notes:

TRAINING SESSION **WEEK 2** DAY 7

ALISON'S SESSION

AM **Training session** CV – Walk

Time trained 8.00–10.20 a.m.

Session time 2 hours 20 minutes

RPE 7/10

PM Off

WORKOUT
Walk: 8 miles
Actual distance: 7 miles
Time: 2 hours 20 minutes
Average Pace: 20 m/m

YOUR SESSION

AM **Training session** Walk

Time trained

Session time   hour(s)   minutes

RPE   /10

PM

WORKOUT
Walk
Actual distance: miles
Time: minutes
Average Pace: m/m

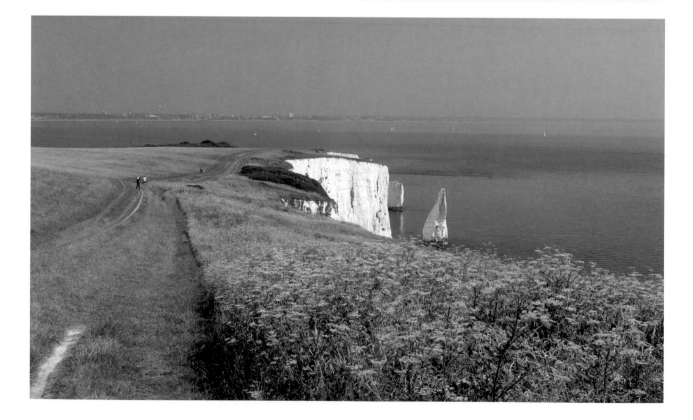

Equipment

Food
2 bananas
3 apples
1 bag soya nuts
4 litres water

Clothing
Cross-country trainers
Shorts
T-shirt
Training top
Walking socks

Spare clothing
Sandals
Warm jacket/top
Gloves
Hat and scarf

Other
First aid kit
First field dressing
Torch
Map and compass
Money
Mobile phone
Whistle

Alison's notes: I went walking with Gavin on this sunny but windy day. We both carried our own bags and mine weighed 15lb. I followed what Gavin said about what to take with me such as spare clothing and food, as the weather can change so quickly in the Purbecks and you wouldn't want to be stranded out there.

Equipment

Food

Clothing

Spare clothing

Other

Your notes

WEEK 2 TESTS

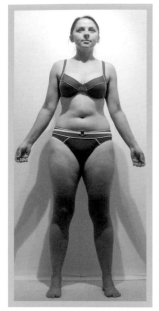

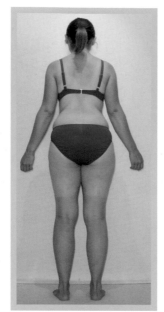

Front view of Alison at the end of week 2.

Back view of Alison at the end of week 2.

ALISON'S WEEKLY TESTS

Weight (kg)	55
Height (cm)	157.3
BMI	22.2
RHR	70
BP	112/65
Fat (%)	30.4

Measurements (cm)

Neck	30.48	
Chest	87.63	
Arms	R: 29.21	L: 29.21
Navel	78.10	
Hips	86.36	
Thighs	R: 59.05	L: 58.42
Calves	R: 35.56	L: 35.56

YOUR WEEKLY TESTS

Weight (kg)	
Height (cm)	
BMI	
RHR	
BP	
Fat (%)	

Measurements (cm)

Neck		
Chest		
Arms	R:	L:
Navel		
Hips		
Thighs	R:	L:
Calves	R:	L:

WEEK **THREE** NUTRITION PLAN **WEEK 3**

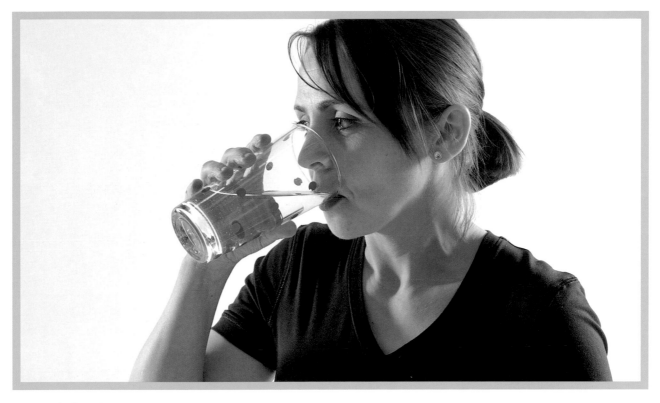

WEEK 3 OVERVIEW

Day	Breakfast	Lunch	Dinner
1	Fruit salad	Chicken wrap	Lemon sole
2	Fruit porridge	Tuna salad with sweet potato	Chicken hot pot
3	Muesli with fresh fruit	Chicken hot pot pitta	Cod and spinach parcels
4	Wheat biscuits or muesli with fruit	Egg salad	Stir fried pork
5	Fresh fruit and seeds	Salmon salad	Chicken yoghurt
6	Omelette	Butternut squash and coriander soup	Lime tuna steaks
7	Fruit smoothie 1	Chicken salad pitta	Beef and sweet potato pie

SHOPPING LIST **WEEK 3**

CARBOHYDRATES
1 bag of brown rice
240g of muesli
10 Charlotte potatoes
10 new potatoes
1 bag of pine nuts
8 wholemeal or brown pitta breads
560g porridge oats
1 bag of rice noodles
1 bag of sunflower and pumpkin seeds
4 organic tortilla wraps
6 sweet potatoes
Wheat biscuits

DAIRY AND NON-DAIRY ALTERNATIVES
12 eggs
680ml skimmed/soya/rice/oat milk
1.7kg soya yoghurt

FISH
200g × 4 cod fillets
4 cooked salmon fillets
4 lemon sole
175g × 4 tuna steaks
4 small tins tuna

MEAT
800g lean minced beef
16 chicken breasts
800g chicken thigh fillets
400g lean ham
450g pork fillets

FRUIT
3 apples
2 apricots
8 bananas
1 lemon
2 limes
3 oranges

2 mangos
1 melon
1 punnet of raspberries

VEGETABLES
2 avocados
115g baby corn
4 baby gem lettuce
600g baby spinach
400g bamboo shoots
175g broccoli
200g button mushrooms
300g cherry tomatoes
2 butternut squash
8 carrots
7 celery sticks
2 courgettes
1 cucumber
3 leeks
3 lettuces
450g mangetout
11 onions
225g frozen peas
1 red onion
4 red peppers
14 red tomatoes
100g rocket salad
13 spring onions
6 yellow peppers

HERBS
Basil
Black pepper
Coriander
Cumin
Dill
Fresh ginger
1 garlic bulb
1 lemon thyme sprig
Nutmeg
Parsley
Rosemary
Turmeric

OTHER
Balsamic vinegar
Beef stock
Chicken stock
Chinese rice wine
Cider vinegar
Cold-pressed extra virgin olive oil
Corn flour
Dijon mustard
Plain flour
Dark soy sauce
115ml red wine
Soy sauce
400g tinned tomatoes
Vegetable stock
115ml white wine
White wine vinegar

SNACKS
Fruits
Wholegrain crispbread/crackers
Crackers/flat breads
Small bowl of muesli
Yoghurt/soya yoghurt
Nuts (cashew, pine or occasionally mixed nuts)
Soya nuts
Seeds (pumpkin or sunflower)

FRUIT DRINKS
1 carton fruit juice

RECIPES **WEEK 3 DAY 1**

BREAKFAST FRUIT SALAD

See page 84

LUNCH CHICKEN WRAP

4 chicken breasts, cooked and cut into strips

4 organic wholewheat tortilla wraps (served hot or cold)

200g mixed salad

4–5 tomatoes, sliced

1 red onion, finely chopped

1 yellow pepper, cut into strips

2 tablespoons of soya/plain yoghurt

1 Heat ½ tablespoon extra virgin olive oil in a frying pan over a medium heat.
2 Cook four chicken breasts for 8–12 minutes or until cooked.
3 Place mixed salad, red onion, yellow pepper, tomatoes and chicken in salad bowl and mix well.
4 Place tortilla wraps on plates, add mixture from salad bowl and roll wrap.
5 Drizzle over soya/plain yoghurt.

DINNER LEMON SOLE

1 small onion, finely chopped

4 lemon sole fillets (175g each)

2 garlic cloves, sliced thinly

4 lemon thyme sprigs

1 lemon, grated rind and juice

2 tablespoons olive oil

Brown rice

Vegetables of your choice (courgettes, spring onions, etc.)

1 Preheat oven to 180°C (350°F). Boil the rice and grill the vegetables you have chosen.
2 Place sole fillets in large ovenproof dish and sprinkle onion on top. Add garlic and two lemon thyme sprigs on top of the fillets and season with pepper.
3 Mix lemon juice and olive oil in a small bowl and pour over fish.
4 Bake in oven for 15 minutes or until fish flakes easily.
5 Sprinkle on the lemon rind and the rest of the lemon thyme sprigs and serve with rice.

Lunch for tomorrow
TUNA SALAD WITH SWEET POTATO
Consider preparing the sweet potatoes in advance.

RECIPES **WEEK 3** DAY 2

BREAKFAST FRUIT PORRIDGE

See page 80

LUNCH TUNA SALAD WITH
SWEET POTATO

See page 81

DINNER CHICKEN HOT POT

Olive oil, 2 tablespoons

800g chicken thigh fillets, diced

225ml chicken stock

400g tinned chopped tomatoes

115ml white wine

2 cloves garlic, crushed

Corn flour

2 celery sticks, chopped

2 tablespoons rosemary, chopped

2 carrots, finely sliced

2 leeks, washed and sliced

Charlotte potatoes

1 Heat olive oil in large pan over high heat.
2 Add the chicken in batches and cook for
5 minutes or until brown, and remove from pan
once cooked.
3 Reduce heat to medium, add the leeks and cook
for 8 minutes or until soft.
4 Add the carrots, celery and garlic and cook for a
further 10–12 minutes until soft.
5 Add the stock, wine and tomatoes and bring
to boil.
6 Reduce heat to low and return chicken with
some corn flour (to thicken the sauce) and
simmer gently for 35 minutes.
7 Add herbs to taste and serve with Charlotte
potatoes.

Lunch for tomorrow
CHICKEN HOT POT PITTA
See opposite and consider preparing your lunch
in advance.

RECIPES **WEEK 3** DAY 3

BREAKFAST MUESLI WITH
FRESH FRUIT

See page 79

LUNCH CHICKEN HOT POT PITTA

4 chicken breasts, cooked and diced

4 wholemeal pitta breads (served hot or cold)

Sauce from last night's dinner

Lettuce, 4 handfuls washed and chopped

1 red pepper, sliced

1 yellow pepper, sliced

½ red onion, finely sliced

1 Use any remaining chicken and sauce from the hot pot.
2 Heat ½ tablespoon extra virgin olive oil in a frying pan over a medium heat.
3 Cook the chicken for 8–12 minutes or until cooked.
4 Slice open the pitta bread and fill with chicken and salad and pour in the sauce.
5 Serve with salad.

DINNER COD AND SPINACH PARCELS

4 × 200g cod (or barramundi), with skin removed

200g baby spinach leaves

1 tablespoon, ginger

3 spring onions, finely sliced

2 tablespoons soy sauce

Coriander, handful

Lime wedges

Broccoli

Brown rice

1 Preheat oven to 220°C (425°F). Boil the rice and broccoli.
2 Get a large sheet of foil and place half of the spinach leaves in the middle. Add a piece of fish on top then sprinkle with a quarter of ginger, spring onion and drizzle with 2 teaspoons of soy sauce.
3 Wrap the fish in the foil, folding the corners in to ensure the foil is well sealed.
4 Repeat this process with the rest of the fish for each person.
5 Place the four parcels in a baking dish and bake for 15 minutes.
6 Carefully open each parcel and slide contents on to plate.
7 Serve with broccoli and brown rice.

Lunch for tomorrow
EGG SALAD
Consider boiling your eggs in advance.

RECIPES **WEEK 3** DAY 4

BREAKFAST WHEAT BISCUITS OR MUESLI WITH FRUIT

See page 82

LUNCH EGG SALAD

4 baby gem lettuces

200g baby spinach

150g cherry tomatoes, halved

4 shelled hard-boiled eggs, cut into quarters

½ cucumber, sliced

1 yellow pepper, deseeded and sliced

For the dressing:

1 tablespoon Dijon mustard

1 tablespoon olive oil

2 teaspoons cider vinegar

1 teaspoon water

1 Arrange the lettuce, spinach, tomatoes, yellow pepper and cucumber on plates.
2 Mix the mustard and water together, combine with the olive oil and vinegar in a small bowl.
3 Put the eggs on top of the salad, drizzle with the dressing and serve.

DINNER STIR FRIED PORK

450g lean pork fillet, cut into strips

1 tablespoon, olive oil,

16 button mushrooms

115g baby corn

1 garlic clove, finely chopped

Fresh ginger, 2.5cm finely chopped

400g mangetout

400g bamboo shoots, drained and sliced

2 teaspoons dark soy sauce

2 teaspoons Chinese rice wine

225ml vegetable or chicken stock

2 teaspoons corn flour

1 tablespoon water

1 carrot, finely sliced

1–2 spring onions, trimmed and cut lengthways

Rice or rice noodles

For the marinade:

1 tablespoon dark soy sauce

1 tablespoon Chinese rice wine

2 teaspoons corn flour

Pepper

1 Mix the marinade ingredients together in a dish and season with pepper.
2 Add the pork to the marinade, cover and chill for 20 minutes.
3 Blanch the baby corn in boiling water for a few minutes.
4 Drain and refresh in cold water.
5 Heat half the olive oil in a preheated wok and add the pork. Stir fry for 5 minutes until browned. Remove and reserve.
6 Wipe the wok and add the remaining oil and heat. Next, place in the garlic and cook until golden, adding the ginger, mangetout, bamboo shoots and mushrooms and fry for 3 minutes.
7 Stir in the soy sauce, Chinese rice wine, stock and the reserved liquid from pork.
8 Cook for 2–3 minutes then mix the corn flour and water and stir until thickened.
9 Return the pork to the heat stirring in the carrot.
10 Garnish with spring onions and serve with rice or rice noodles.

RECIPES **WEEK 3** DAY 5

BREAKFAST FRESH FRUIT AND SEEDS

See page 81

LUNCH SALMON SALAD

200g mixed salad leaves

¼ cucumber, roughly chopped

4 cooked poached salmon fillets,
bite-size pieces

2 yellow peppers, sliced

2 tablespoons coriander, chopped

250g cherry tomatoes, halved

For the dressing:

500g soya/plain yoghurt

2 tablespoons coriander, chopped

1 garlic clove, finely chopped

4 teaspoons lemon juice

1 teaspoon cumin, ground

1 For the dressing, place all ingredients in a bowl and mix together; season with black pepper.
2 Cover and refrigerate for 5–10 minutes before using (if the sauce is too thick, add some water to thin out).
3 Arrange salad leaves, cherry tomatoes, spring onions, salmon, cucumber and yellow pepper in a salad bowl and toss.
4 Add salmon on top of salad.
5 Drizzle the dressing over and serve.

DINNER CHICKEN YOGHURT

1 tablespoon plain flour

4 lean chicken breasts, diced skinless

1 tablespoon olive oil

8 small onions, chopped

2 garlic cloves, crushed

225ml chicken stock

2 carrots, chopped

2 celery sticks, chopped

225g frozen peas

1 yellow pepper, sliced and deseeded

115g button mushrooms, sliced

125ml low fat soya/plain yoghurt

3 tablespoons fresh parsley, chopped

10 new potatoes

1 Spread flour over a dish and season with pepper and add chicken. Coat with flour.
2 Heat olive oil in large saucepan and add the onions and garlic and cook over low heat, stirring occasionally for 5 minutes.
3 Add chicken and cook for 10 minutes continuously stirring.
4 Stir in the chicken stock, carrots, peas and celery.
5 Bring to boil and then reduce the heat. Cover and simmer for 5 minutes.
6 Add the peppers and mushrooms, cover and simmer for a further 10 minutes.
7 Stir in the soya/plain yoghurt and chopped parsley and cook for a further 1–2 minutes.
8 Serve with new potatoes.

RECITES **WEEK 3** DAY 6

BREAKFAST OMELETTE

See page 86

LUNCH BUTTERNUT SQUASH AND CORIANDER SOUP

See page 87

DINNER LIME TUNA STEAKS

4 × 175g tuna steaks, trim the skin

2 teaspoons, olive oil

½ teaspoon grated lime zest

1 garlic glove, crushed

1 teaspoon ground cumin

1 teaspoon ground coriander

1 tablespoon lime juice

Small handful of fresh coriander, chopped

Salad leaves

For the relish:

2 avocados, peeled and chopped

1 tablespoon lime juice

½ red onion, cut finely

2 tomatoes, chopped

1 Mix the avocados, lime juice, red onion and tomatoes together in a small bowl.
2 To make the paste, mix lime zest, olive oil, garlic, ground cumin and ground coriander in bowl.
3 Spread paste thinly on both sides of the tuna while heating a non-stick pan until hot, and press the tuna steaks into pan to seal them.
4 Reduce heat and cook for 5 minutes. Turn tuna steaks over and cook for a further 4–5 minutes, or until cooked through.
5 Remove tuna from pan and drain on kitchen paper.
6 Transfer fish to plates, serve with salad leaves and relish.
7 Sprinkle 1 tablespoon of lime juice over the top, garnish with fresh coriander.

RECIPES **WEEK 3** DAY 7

BREAKFAST FRUIT SMOOTHIE 1

See page 85

LUNCH CHICKEN SALAD PITTA

4 pitta breads, hot or cold

½ tablespoon olive oil

4 lean chicken breasts, sliced into strips

1 Pour the olive oil in a frying pan or wok, on a medium heat.

4 tablespoons fresh basil, chopped

1 red pepper

2 spring onions, finely chopped

150g cherry tomatoes, halved

2 tablespoons pine nuts

200g baby spinach

For the dressing:

¼ of a cucumber, finely grated

4 tablespoons soya/plain yoghurt

1 tablespoons olive oil

1 teaspoon balsamic vinegar

2 teaspoons black pepper

2 teaspoons dried dill

2 Add chicken strips and cook for 8 minutes, or until golden brown. Keep stirring.

3 Add the red pepper, spring onions, tomatoes and pine nuts and cook for a few minutes, while stirring.

4 Place all dressing ingredients in a small bowl and mix well.

5 Slice open the pitta bread and add the chicken, vegetables and spinach. Drizzle over dressing and garnish with basil.

DINNER BEEF AND SWEET POTATO PIE

800g lean minced beef

2 tablespoons olive oil

1 onion, finely chopped

1 leek, finely chopped

1 carrot, finely chopped

1 stick celery, finely chopped

4 tomatoes, diced

2 sweet potatoes, peeled and chopped

1 medium butternut squash, peeled and chopped

2 cloves of garlic, finely chopped

115ml beef stock

1 tablespoon flour

115ml red wine

1 tablespoon rosemary, chopped

Salad leaves

1 Preheat the oven to 180°C (350°F). Heat a large pan of water, boil the sweet potatoes and butternut squash for 10 minutes, or until soft when pierced with knife.

2 Heat a large pan, add olive oil and brown the mince in small batches.

3 Once the mince is cooked, add the onion, leek, carrot, celery and garlic, and cook for 4 minutes.

4 Add stock, flour, wine, tomatoes and rosemary and bring to boil. Simmer for 25 minutes.

5 Mash the sweet potatoes and butternut squash in a bowl.

6 Put mince mixture in large ovenproof dish and place mash on top.

7 Cook for 20 minutes and serve with salad.

Lunch for tomorrow *BEAN SALAD*

Consider preparing your eggs in advance.

TRAINING DIARY **WEEK 3**

WEEK 3 OVERVIEW
Day 1: Weights – upper body
Day 2: CV – cycle
Day 3: Rest
Day 4: CV – run
Day 5: Circuits; cellulite massage
Day 6: CV – walk; myo massage
Day 7: CV – myo stretch

ALISON'S DIARY

Day 1 (Monday)
Feeling a bit lethargic today, due to work shortly.
Tiredness 6
Stress 4
Sleep 7 hours 30 minutes

Day 2 (Tuesday)
We ended up cycling in the rain with a light wind, but it was so nice to be outside. I felt my chest tighten a little bit on the cycle so we slowed down so I could catch my breath.
Tiredness 7
Stress 5
Sleep 8 hours

Day 3 (Wednesday)
Had a day off. I really need today off from exercising as I'm working really hard at the moment and exercising more than I have ever done.
Tiredness 7
Stress 8
Sleep 6 hours 30 minutes

Day 4 (Thursday)
My legs were feeling tired during my run and I ended up getting a stitch halfway through. I wasn't too happy with my run but Gavin said I was better today than I was last week.
Tiredness 7
Stress 6
Sleep 8 hours 30 minutes

Day 5 (Friday)
I'm looking forward to my bed tonight because I did a hard circuit session today with a cellulite massage, and when I was on my late shift at work I found myself to be quite drowsy and dopey. Had a flapjack to eat to give me a bit of an energy kick – only wanted to eat half but by the time I realised, I had already polished it all off.
Tiredness 7
Stress 5
Sleep 7 hours

Day 6 (Saturday)
I had a really good night's sleep last night and could have slept the whole day, but I had things to do and the weather was beautiful. Went for the walk and when I got back Gavin gave me a myo massage to sort my body out. I have suffered in my lower back, and hips for a few years, but Gavin said I had to tighten and exercise my muscles first for a few weeks before he could manipulate and release my back and hips.
Tiredness 6
Stress 5
Sleep 7 hours 30 minutes

Day 7 (Sunday)
I had my tests this morning before I had to go off to work. I was quite impressed with the photos compared to last week's results and it feels nice that the weight is dropping off me. Gavin pointed out that I was snacking on the sweet things again when I feel stressed or tired, so I'm going to be working on that next week.
Tiredness 5
Stress 4
Sleep 6 hours

TRAINING SESSION **WEEK 3** DAY 1

ALISON'S SESSION

AM Training session Weights – Upper body

Time trained 11.30 a.m.–12.25 p.m.

Session time 55 minutes

RPE 8/10

PM Rest

WORKOUT
Dumbbell bench press
1 × 20 warm-up with 7.5 lb
Set and Rep: 1. 15   2. 15   3. 15
Weight (lb):   10   12.5   15

Incline fly
Set and Rep: 1. 15   2. 15   3. 15
Weight (lb):   7.5   10   10

Low pull
Set and Rep: 1. 15   2. 15   3. 15
Weight (kg):   10   15   20

Boxing
Complete the first set for each one and then go
back to the start to complete the second set for
each boxing exercise.

Alternate: 2 × 30
Straight: 2 × 30
Wide: 2 × 30
Reverse: 2 × 30
Upper cuts: 2 × 30
Reverse: 2 × 30

YOUR SESSION

AM Training session Weights – Upper body

Time trained

Session time   hour(s)   minutes

RPE   /10

PM

WORKOUT
Dumbbell bench press
1 × 20 warm-up with 7.5 lb
Set and Rep: 1.   2.   3.
Weight (kg):

Incline fly
Set and Rep: 1.   2.   3.
Weight (kg):

Low pull
Set and Rep: 1.   2.   3.
Weight (kg):

Boxing

Alternate: ×
Straight: ×
Wide: ×
Reverse: ×
Upper cuts: ×
Reverse: ×

Lat pull-downs
Set and Rep: 1. 15   2. 12   3. 15
Weight (total kg):   12.5   12.5   12.5

Superset
Leg levers   Sets and Reps: 3 × 10
Reverse curls   Sets and Reps: 3 × 10
Dorsal raise: 3 × 10
Bench dips: 3 × 20

Lat raise
Set and Rep: 1. 12   2. 12   3. 12
Weight (lb):   7.5   7.5   7.5

Reverse shrug (used one dumbbell)
Set and Rep: 1. 15   2. 15   3. 15
Weight (lb):   25   25   30

Alison's notes: I really enjoyed the boxing, so much fun. It's also a great way to get out a little pent-up aggression too.

Lat pull-downs
Set and Rep: 1.   2.   3.
Weight (total kg):

Superset
Leg levers   Sets and Reps: ×
Reverse curls   Sets and Reps: ×
Dorsal raise: ×
Bench dips: ×

Lat raise
Set and Rep: 1.   2.   3.
Weight (kg):

Reverse shrug
Set and Rep: 1.   2.   3.
Weight (kg):

Your notes:

TRAINING SESSION **WEEK 3** DAY 2

ALISON'S SESSION

AM Rest

PM Training session CV – Cycle

Time trained 2.15–3.15 p.m.

Session time 1 hour

RPE 7/10

WORKOUT
Cycle: 1 hour/10 miles
Actual distance: 9.7 miles

Alison's notes: I really enjoyed the cycle today – great to be outside and there was a very refreshing light wind and rain.

I cycled as hard as I could, especially when I was on the flat. There was one major hill that I tackled successfully, but the smaller one just afterwards nearly forced me to get off the bike and push it.

Some of the cycle was off-road, which is what I really enjoy, especially when I'm riding my mountain bike.

My quads and knee stiffened as soon as I had finished the bike ride, but I stretched them immediately and they were fine.

YOUR SESSION

AM

PM Training session CV – Cycle

Time trained

Session time   hour(s)   minutes

RPE   /10

WORKOUT
Cycle: 1 hour/10 miles
Actual distance: miles

Your notes:

TRAINING SESSION **WEEK 3** DAY 4

ALISON'S SESSION

AM Rest

PM **Training session** CV – Run

Time trained 7.15–8.00 p.m.

Session time 45 minutes

RPE 9/10

YOUR SESSION

AM

PM **Training session** CV – Run

Time trained

Session time   hour(s)   minutes

RPE   /10

WORKOUT

Run: 30 minutes/3 miles
Actual distance: 3 miles
Run time: 41 minutes
Average pace: 13.4 m/m

Alison's notes: I gave my run a 9.5/10 – I tried so hard to make it a good run, which it was. I did feel a bit sick half way through the run and a little later when I was stretching. I think I will enjoy the running a lot more than I do now, as soon as I conquer my breathing pattern.

Notes: If you are able to run the 30 minutes comfortably, please try to run the three mile distance instead at the best pace you can. We ran three miles for the first time to push Alison's comfort limits as she is improving with every run. The unfortunate thing for Alison was the weather, it blew in our faces the whole way round. Alison ran for 15 minutes continuously before walking. We then did the fartlek running again (ran for five minutes fast and then two minutes at walking pace). Alison repeated this four times.

WORKOUT

Run: 30 minutes/3 miles
Actual distance: miles
Run time: minutes
Average pace: m/m

Your notes:

TRAINING SESSION **WEEK 3** DAY 5

ALISON'S SESSION

AM Rest

PM Training session Circuits

Time trained 6.00–7.10 p.m.

Session time 1 hour 10 minutes

RPE 7/10

WORKOUT

This is a mentally tough workout because you have to complete the first set all the way through, and then you have to do it again for the second set all the way through.

Start with the 0.5 mile run first before moving on to cycle 1. Complete each exercise in numerical order before you move on to the next run.

After completing cycle 2 move back to cycle 1 and complete the 2nd set, following it as before.

Finish the circuit with a run at the end.

1st set 30 reps
2nd set 40 reps
Run/sprint 0.5 miles (5 minutes)

Cycle 1
1. Wide squats thrusts
2. Squat jumps
3. Alt squat thrusts
4. Dips
5. Crunches
6. Press-ups
Run/sprint – 0.25 miles (3 minutes)

YOUR SESSION

AM

PM Training session Circuits

Time trained

Session time   hour(s)   minutes

RPE   /10

WORKOUT

1st set   reps
2nd set   reps
Run/sprint   miles (minutes)

Cycle 1
1. Wide squats thrusts
2. Squat jumps
3. Alt squat thrusts
4. Dips
5. Crunches
6. Press-ups
Run/sprint   miles (minutes)

Cycle 2

7. Glute extensions
8. Dirty Dogs
9. Deadlift
10. Jumping oblique twists
11. Star Jumps
12. Spotty Dogs

Pull-ups
Set and Rep: 1. 5   2. 5   3. 4

Run: 0.5 miles

Alison's notes: Another good workout, a mixture of light running and circuit training with some stretches – my legs were very stiff and aching afterwards. Looking forward to the walk tomorrow, need a good night's sleep though.

Cycle 2

7. Glute extensions
8. Dirty Dogs
9. Deadlift
10. Jumping oblique twists
11. Star Jumps
12. Spotty Dogs

Pull-ups
Set and Rep: 1.   2.   3.

Run: miles

Your notes:

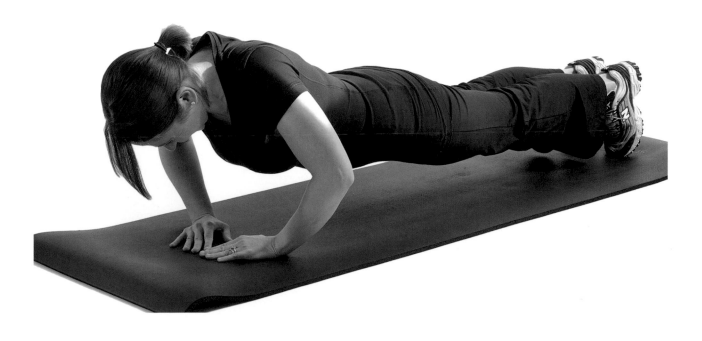

TRAINING SESSION **WEEK 3** DAY 6

ALISON'S SESSION

AM Training session Walk

Time trained 9.00 a.m.–10.08 a.m.

Session time 1 hour 8 minutes

RPE 7/10

PM Off

WORKOUT
Walk: 4 miles
Actual distance: 4.25 miles
Time: 1 hour 8 minutes
Average pace: 16 m/m

Alison's notes: Lovely walk, beautiful weather.
We walked about five miles around the Purbecks
through fields and along the coastline. Legs and
knees a little sore on the last hill but used the steps
which was much easier.

YOUR SESSION

AM   Training session Walk

Time trained

Session time   hour(s)   minutes

RPE   /10

PM

WORKOUT
Walk: 4 miles
Actual distance: miles
Time: hour   minutes
Average pace: m/m

Your notes:

WEEK 3 TESTS

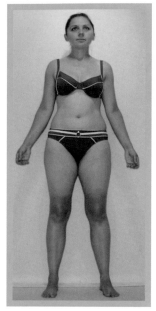

Front view of Alison at the end of week 3.

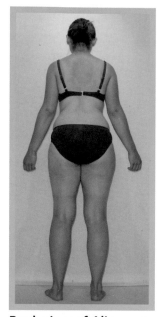

Back view of Alison at the end of week 3.

ALISON'S WEEKLY TESTS

Weight (kg)	55	
Height (cm)	157.3	
BMI	22.2	
RHR	68	
BP	112/64	
Fat (%)	29.1	
Measurements (cm)		
Neck	30.48	
Chest	84.45	
Arms	R: 28.57	L: 28.57
Navel	76.83	
Hips	85.09	
Thighs	R: 58.42	L: 58.42
Calves	R: 35.56	L: 35.56

YOUR WEEKLY TESTS

Weight (kg)		
Height (cm)		
BMI		
RHR		
BP		
Fat (%)		
Measurements (cm)		
Neck		
Chest		
Arms	R:	L:
Navel		
Hips		
Thighs	R:	L:
Calves	R:	L:

WEEK **FOUR** NUTRITION PLAN **WEEK 4**

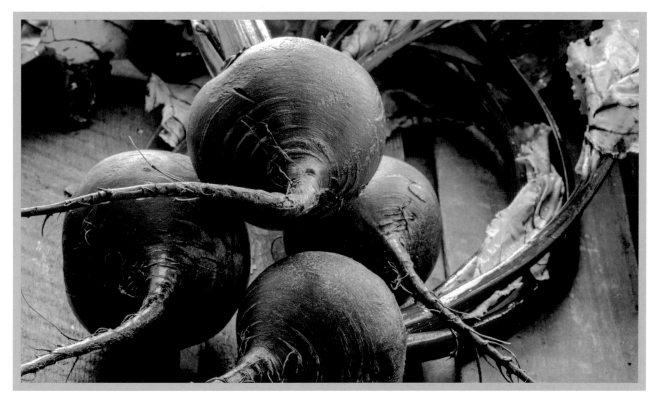

WEEK 4 OVERVIEW

Day	Breakfast	Lunch	Dinner
1	Fresh fruit and seeds	Bean salad	Mediterranean steaks
2	Wheat biscuits or muesli with fruit	Tuna salad	Stir fried turkey ginger
3	Fruit salad	Beetroot soup	Baked trout
4	Fruit porridge	Chicken wrap	Pork and baked apples
5	Muesli with fresh fruit	Mackerel and potato salad	Tuna pak choi
6	Omelette	Tomato and pepper soup	Ratatouille lamb chops
7	Fruit smoothie 1	Tuna and olive salad	Lemon roasted chicken

SHOPPING LIST **WEEK 4**

CARBOHYDRATES
400g baked potatoes
1 bag of brown rice
810g kidney beans
250g couscous
240g of muesli
400g pinto beans
400g new potatoes
520g porridge oats
1 bag of rice noodles
1 bag of sunflower and
pumpkin seeds
4 organic tortilla wraps
1 bag of sesame seeds
8 sweet potatoes
Wheat biscuits

DAIRY AND NON-DAIRY ALTERNATIVES
12 eggs
680ml skimmed/soya/rice/
oat milk
1.7kg soya yoghurt

FISH
8 anchovy fillets
4 × 200g cod fillets
4 cooked mackerel fillets
4 × 200g tuna steaks
4 small tins tuna
4 whole trout

MEAT
4 chicken breasts
1 large whole chicken
400g lean ham
800g lamb chop
800g pork fillet
4 turkey breasts

FRUIT
12 apples
8 bananas
1 punnet of blueberries
5 lemons

2 limes
2 mangos
1 melon
1 punnet of raspberries
1 punnet of strawberries

VEGETABLES
4 aubergines
2 avocados
8 asparagus
500g raw beetroot
16 × 25g black olives
500g cherry tomatoes
2 carrots
2 celery sticks
4 courgettes
½ cucumber
225g French beans
250g green beans
2 lettuces
50g mangetout
7 onions
3 pak choi
4 parsnips
50g frozen peas
115g plum tomatoes
3 red onions
12 spring onions
7 red peppers
750g red tomatoes
100g rocket salad
200g savoy cabbage
1 turnip
1 yellow pepper

HERBS
Basil
1 Bay leaf
Black pepper
Black peppercorns
Chilli powder
Chives
Cinnamon
Coriander
Coriander seeds
Cumin

Dill
Fresh ginger
Garam masala
1 garlic bulb
Ground fennel
Mint
Oregano
Parsley
Red chilli
Rosemary

OTHER
Balsamic vinegar
Chicken stock
Chinese rice wine
Cold-pressed extra virgin
olive oil
Corn flour
Dijon mustard
Fish stock
Peanut oil
Red wine vinegar
Sun-dried tomatoes
Soy sauce
Brown sugar
400g tinned tomato paste
Tomato purée
Vegetable stock
White wine vinegar

SNACKS
Fruit
Wholegrain crispbread crackers
Flat breads
Small bowl of muesli
Yoghurt/soya yoghurt
Nuts (cashew, pine or
occasionally mixed nuts)
Soya nuts
Seeds (pumpkin or sunflower)

FRUIT DRINKS
1 carton Fruit juice

RECIPES **WEEK 4** DAY 1

BREAKFAST FRESH FRUIT AND SEEDS

See page 81

LUNCH BEAN SALAD

See page 101

DINNER MEDITERRANEAN STEAKS

4 cod steaks – 140g per steak
150ml fish stock
1 bay leaf
6 black peppercorns
Lemon rind
Lemon wedges
1 small onion, sliced
Parsley
Couscous
For the sauce:
400g chopped tomatoes canned
1 garlic clove, finely chopped
1 tablespoon sun-dried tomato paste
16 black olives (optional)

1 To make the sauce, place the chopped tomatoes, garlic, tomato paste and olives in a large heavy-based saucepan over a low heat. Heat gently, stirring occasionally.
2 Meanwhile, place the fish in a shallow ovenproof casserole dish and pour over the fish stock and add the peppercorns, bay leaf, lemon rind and onion. Bring to the boil, cover and simmer for 10 minutes.
3 Transfer cod to a serving plate and keep warm while water boils for the couscous.
4 Next, sieve the fish stock into the sauce and stir over a medium heat until reduced.
5 Pour the sauce over the fish, garnish with parsley and lemon wedges.

Lunch for tomorrow *TUNA SALAD*

Consider preparing your sweet potatoes in advance.

RECIPES **WEEK 4** DAY 2

BREAKFAST WHEAT BISCUITS OR MUESLI WITH FRUIT

See page 82

LUNCH TUNA SALAD

4 cooked sweet potatoes

4 small tinned tuna

1 tablespoon balsamic vinegar

1 tablespoon olive oil

Side salad:

100g of rocket leaves

4 tomatoes, roughly chopped

¼ cucumber, roughly chopped

50g mangetout

1 red pepper, sliced

1 Preheat oven to 190°C (375°F).
2 Cut the sweet potatoes into small chunks, drizzle olive oil over the top and place into the oven for 30–40 minutes.
3 Once cooked, allow to cool and place into the fridge for tomorrow's lunch.
4 Place rocket leaves, mangetout, tomatoes, cucumber and red pepper in a salad bowl and gently mix with balsamic vinegar and olive. Serve with the tuna and sweet potatoes.

DINNER STIR FRIED TURKEY GINGER

2 teaspoons sesame seeds

1 tablespoon sesame oil

800g skinless turkey breasts, cut into thin strips

1 onion, quartered

1 red pepper, deseeded and sliced

2 tablespoons soy sauce

Chinese rice wine, splash of

1 pak choi, halved

1 3cm piece of ginger

1 garlic clove, crushed

1 red chilli, finely sliced

Brown rice

1 Heat a wok/large frying pan over medium heat, add the sesame seeds, stir until lightly toasted and then set aside.
2 Steam pak choi in a steamer for 2–3 minutes, then remove and set aside. Boil water for the rice.
3 Add the turkey to the wok/frying pan and stir fry for 6–8 minutes, or until the turkey is cooked. Remove from wok and set aside. Wipe out wok with paper towel.
4 Return wok to heat and add the rest of the sesame oil with the ginger, garlic, chilli, onion and red pepper, and stir fry for 2 minutes.
5 Return turkey to wok, add rice wine, soy sauce and stir. Add pak choi and stir.
6 Serve with rice and a sprinkle the toasted sesame seeds.

Lunch for tomorrow
BEETROOT SOUP
Consider preparing your lunch in advance.

RECIPES **WEEK 4** DAY 3

BREAKFAST FRUIT SALAD

See page 84

LUNCH BEETROOT SOUP

2 onions, peeled and roughly chopped

2 large carrot, peeled and roughly chopped

1 large turnip peeled and roughly chopped

2 celery sticks, roughly chopped

500g raw beetroot, peeled and chopped

400g potatoes, washed and chopped

200g savoy cabbage

3 garlic cloves, finely sliced

2 litres of vegetable stock

410g tin kidney beans

1 tablespoon red wine vinegar

150g soya/plain yoghurt

1 Put onions, carrots, turnips, celery, beetroot, garlic and vegetable stock in large pan.
2 Bring to the boil and simmer for 30 minutes.
3 Add the potatoes, cabbage, beans and simmer for a further 20–30 minutes or until potatoes are tender.
4 Stir in the vinegar and the yoghurt.
5 Serve soup in bowls.

DINNER BAKED TROUT

4 sweet potatoes, roughly chopped

1 courgette, roughly chopped

2 red peppers, roughly chopped

250g cherry tomatoes

1 medium red onion, roughly chopped

4 fresh trout, gutted

Black pepper

2 teaspoons coriander

1 teaspoon cinnamon

2 teaspoons oregano

2 teaspoons basil

1 clove garlic, finely chopped

1 tablespoon olive oil

1 Preheat the oven to 190°C (375°F).
2 Pre-boil the sweet potatoes in saucepan of water, until potatoes are slightly soft. Drain water.
3 Place the sweet potatoes, courgette, tomatoes red pepper, all the herbs, garlic and onion in a baking dish and drizzle over the olive oil.
4 Bake for 10–15 minutes, or until the vegetables are cooked, stirring vegetables occasionally.
5 Meanwhile, preheat grill to medium/high and place the fish on grill tray.
6 Drizzle over a little olive oil and season with black pepper and cook for 5–6 minutes each side, or until fish is cooked.
7 Arrange vegetables on serving plate and place fish on top.

RECIPES **WEEK 4** DAY 4

BREAKFAST FRUIT PORRIDGE

See page 80

LUNCH CHICKEN WRAP

See page 115

DINNER PORK AND BAKED APPLES

1 × 800g lean pork fillet, remove fat

2 tablespoon ground fennel

2 tablespoons olive oil

2 apples, cored and quartered

2 teaspoons brown sugar

2 tablespoons water

4 parsnips, peeled and chopped into chunks

Rosemary, 4 sprigs

200g green beans

1 Preheat oven to 180°C (350°F).
2 Season the pork with pepper and roll in the fennel.
3 Wrap in cling film and refrigerate for 10–15 minutes.
4 Heat a large frying pan over a high heat and cook the pork with half the olive oil on each side for 3 minutes, or until golden. Set aside and cover.
5 Place apples in an ovenproof dish, sprinkle the brown sugar and water. Cover with foil and set aside.
6 Place parsnip, rosemary and remaining oil in a baking dish and toss to coat. Bake for 10 minutes.
7 Place apples into the oven, and at the same time add the pork to the parsnip dish. After a further 10 minutes of cooking the parsnips should be golden, the pork cooked and the apples soft.
8 Meanwhile, bring a small saucepan of water to the boil and add the beans. Cook for 5 minutes.
9 Serve immediately.

Lunch for tomorrow
MACKEREL AND POTATO SALAD
Consider preparing your potatoes in advance.

RECIPES **WEEK 4** DAY 5

BREAKFAST MUESLI WITH FRESH FRUIT

See page 79

LUNCH MACKEREL AND POTATO SALAD

4 mackerel fillets (250g each)
4 teaspoons Dijon mustard
Serve with green beans
For the potato salad:
400g new potatoes
4 spring onions, roughly chopped
1 tablespoon fresh dill, chopped
1 tablespoon chives, chopped
1 tablespoon parsley, chopped

1 Steam the potatoes for 20 minutes or until tender.
2 Mix the spring onions, dill, chives, parsley, lemon juice, potatoes and fromage frais in a salad bowl.
3 Preheat the grill to high and wash the mackerel. Pat dry with kitchen towel, making sure the black skin from the gut has been removed.
4 Lay the fillets skin-side down and spread the mustard on the flesh.
5 Grill the mackerel for 5 minutes until the flesh is no longer translucent.
6 Serve with potato salad and green beans.

DINNER TUNA PAK CHOI

4 × 200g tuna steaks
2 teaspoons peanut oil
2 pak choi, leaves separated and washed
4 spring onions, finely sliced
1 tablespoon fresh coriander
1 tablespoon mint leaves
Lime wedges
For the dressing:
2 tablespoon light soy sauce
2 teaspoons lime juice
1 teaspoon ginger, grated

1 In a small bowl mix all the dressing ingredients.
2 Heat frying pan over medium heat and brush tuna steaks with peanut oil.
3 Add tuna to pan and cook for 4 minutes on each side.
4 Use a steamer to cook pak choi for 2–3 minutes.
5 Arrange the pak choi on a serving plate and place tuna on top.
6 Sprinkle with spring onion, coriander and mint, and drizzle the dressing on top.
7 Use lime wedges to garnish and serve.

RECIPES **WEEK 4** DAY 6

BREAKFAST OMELETTE   *See page 86*

LUNCH TOMATO AND PEPPER SOUP

2 red peppers, deseeded and halved

2 tablespoons olive oil

1 large onion, finely sliced

2 cloves of garlic, crushed

1 tablespoon tomato paste

750g tomatoes, roughly chopped

450ml vegetable stock

Basil, handful

1 Preheat oven to 180°C (350°F).
2 Place red peppers in baking tray, skin-side up and drizzle with half the olive oil.
3 Roast for 25 minutes, or until soft and remove from oven. Allow to cool slightly, then roughly chop.
4 Heat the rest of the oil in a large saucepan, over a medium heat.
5 Add the onion and cook until soft.
6 Add garlic and tomato paste and cook for 2 minutes, stirring continuously.
7 Add red pepper, tomato and stock, cover and simmer for 15 minutes.
8 Allow the soup to cool slightly, and gently stir. Season with basil and serve.

DINNER RATATOUILLE LAMB CHOPS

8 lean lamb chops, diced

1 tablespoon olive oil

250g couscous

Spices:

1 tablespoon ground pepper

2 teaspoons coriander seeds

1 teaspoon garam masala

1 teaspoon chilli powder

For the ratatouille:

2 teaspoons olive oil

4 baby aubergines

1 onion, finely chopped

1 red pepper, deseeded and sliced

1 courgette, sliced

1 Mix all the spices in a bowl and brush the chops with a little olive oil. Coat chops with spice mixture, cover with cling film and refrigerate for 1 hour.
2 To make ratatouille, heat the olive oil in a large frying pan over medium heat. Add aubergines and cook for 4 minutes or until golden.
3 Add onion and garlic and cook until lightly coloured. Next add the red pepper and courgette and cook for further minute.
4 Add chicken stock and tomatoes and bring to boil, cook for a further 5 minutes and add parsley and season to taste.
5 Bring water to a boil and add the couscous, cover with a lid and allow to settle.
6 Heat oil in a frying pan over high heat and cook lamb for 3 minutes each side.

115ml chicken stock

2 tomatoes, sliced

1 tablespoon parsley, chopped

1 clove garlic, finely chopped

7 Serve the lamb chops with ratatouille and couscous.

RECIPES **WEEK 4** DAY 7

BREAKFAST FRUIT SMOOTHIE 1

See page 85

LUNCH TUNA AND OLIVE SALAD

See page 80

DINNER LEMON ROASTED CHICKEN

4 lemons, 2 × grated zest, 2 × cut into quarters

1 large chicken

1 onion, roughly chopped

50g peas (fresh or frozen)

50g French beans, trimmed

1 courgette, sliced

6–8 asparagus heads, trimmed

600ml chicken stock

Fresh basil, 1 handful chopped

Brown rice

1 Preheat oven to 180°C (350°F). Rub the lemon rind on the chicken and place in a casserole dish.

2 Squeeze lemon juice all over the chicken. Add the vegetables and basil around the chicken.

3 Pour over the stock and put the chicken in oven and cook for 1½ hours.

4 Serve with brown rice.

Lunch for tomorrow
YELLOW SPLIT PEA SOUP
Soak the yellow split peas overnight.

TRAINING DIARY **WEEK 4**

WEEK 4 OVERVIEW
Day 1: Weights – whole body
Day 2: Rest
Day 3: CV – run
Day 4: CV – cycle PT
Day 5: Myo massage
Day 6: CV – walk
Day 7: Test day
Any day: myo stretch

ALISON'S DIARY

Day 1 (Monday)
Had a great night's sleep. This then helped me for the rest of the day. I did a heavy workout during which I realised it's physically impossible to lift the heavy weights when laughing.
Tiredness 6
Stress 5
Sleep 8 hours

Day 2 (Tuesday)
Busy day off. Had my bike serviced and then took the car to get its MOT. While I was waiting, I went for a little walk around Poole.
Tiredness 6
Stress 5
Sleep 8 hours

Day 3 (Wednesday)
A bad night's sleep because it was broken all night. I did however have a really good run which I was so proud of.
Tiredness 7
Stress 8
Sleep 6 hours

Day 4 (Thursday)
My first cycle PT. I felt really strong and I love all the different types of exercise. I felt that good I didn't even need my inhaler.
Tiredness 6
Stress 7
Sleep 7

Day 5 (Friday)
Had a lovely lunch, which set me up all day. I had another myo massage to keep my muscles released. Since last week's myo massage and this exercise, I have not suffered with my backache at all.
Tiredness 6
Stress 5
Sleep 7 hours

Day 6 (Saturday)
I'm really worried that I am jeopardising my results by snacking on too many bad things. Gavin is going to go through my eating plan with a fine-toothed comb today, so I have nothing to hide.
Tiredness 6
Stress 5
Sleep 8 hours

Day 7 (Sunday)
I had all the tests today. I couldn't believe that the results were so good compared with all the other weeks. It was like a weight had been lifted from my shoulders and I know I'm heading in the right direction. I also had the day off and relaxed with Gavin at Beaulieu.
Tiredness 5
Stress 3
Sleep 7 hours

TRAINING SESSION **WEEK 4** DAY 1

ALISON'S SESSION

AM Training session Weights – Whole body

Time trained 11.30 a.m.–12.30 p.m.

Session time 1 hour

RPE 7/10

PM Off

YOUR SESSION

AM Training session Weights – Whole body

Time trained

Session time hour(s) minutes

RPE /10

PM

WORKOUT

This is a heavy weight training session, so please try to push yourself and lift as much weight as you comfortably can without losing form and technique.

Dumbbell bench press
1 × 15 warm-up with 5 lb
Set and Rep: 1. 10   2. 10   3. 10   4. 10
Weight (lb):   10   15   15   15

Dumbbell press
Set and Rep: 1. 10   2. 10   3. 10   4. 10
Weight (lb):   7.5   10   10   10

Deadlift (total weight includes bar)
Set and Rep: 1. 15   2. 10   3. 10   4. 10   5. 9
Weight (kg):   25   30   35   35

Superset
Static lunges (bosu) Sets and Reps: 3 × 15
Squats   Sets and Reps: 3 × 15

Calf raises
Set and Rep: 1. 15   2. 15   3. 15
Weight (lb):   25   25   25

WORKOUT

Dumbbell bench press
1 × 15 warm-up with 5 lb
Set and Rep: 1.   2.   3.   4.
Weight (kg):

Dumbbell press
Set and Rep: 1.   2.   3.   4.
Weight (kg):

Deadlift (total weight includes bar)
Set and Rep: 1.   2.   3.   4.   5.
Weight (kg):

Superset
Static lunges (bosu) Sets and Reps: 3 × 15
Squats   Sets and Reps: 3 × 15

Calf raises
Set and Rep: 1.   2.   3.
Weight (kg):

¾ *Regular press-ups*
1–6 and 6–1
Total: 42

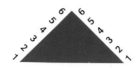

For the next two exercises pick a moderate weight to do maximum reps for three sets.

Cable arm curl
Set and Rep:	1. 16	2. 15	3. 12
Weight (kg):	5	5	5

Rope triceps press-down
Set and Rep:	1. 21	2. 23	3. 19
Weight (kg):	5	5	5

¾ *Regular press-ups*
_____ and _____
Total: 42

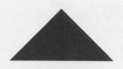

Cable arm curl
Set and Rep:	1.	2.	3.
Weight (kg):			

Rope triceps press-down
Set and Rep:	1.	2.	3.
Weight (kg):			

Your notes:

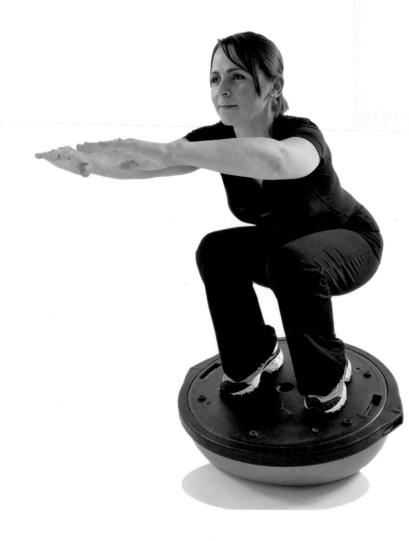

TRAINING SESSION **WEEK 4** DAY 3

ALISON'S SESSION

AM Rest

PM Training session CV – Run

Time trained 5.00–5.32 p.m.

Session time 32 minutes

RPE 8/10

WORKOUT
Run: 30 minutes/3 miles
Actual distance: 3 miles
Run time: 32 minutes 15 seconds
Average Pace: 11.45 m/m

Alison's notes: Did a really good continuous run around Baiter park, Whitecliff and Poole park – I was very proud of myself.

Notes: If you are able to run the 30 minutes comfortably, please try to run for the three miles instead at the best pace you can. Alison ran the whole way without stopping and had a bit of rain and wind to make it even harder. If you are getting the same response from your running as Alison, you are on your way to being able to run a 10km run, possibly under a 10 m/m pace.

YOUR SESSION

AM

PM Training session Run

Time trained

Session time   hour(s)   minutes

RPE   /10

WORKOUT
Run: 30 minutes/3 miles
Actual distance: miles
Run time: minutes   seconds
Average Pace: m/m

Your notes:

TRAINING SESSION **WEEK** 4 DAY 4

ALISON'S SESSION

AM Rest

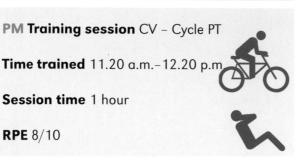

PM Training session CV – Cycle PT

Time trained 11.20 a.m.–12.20 p.m.

Session time 1 hour

RPE 8/10

WORKOUT

Cycle for 2 miles before going into the cycle sprints

Cycle sprints: find either a 125m straight bit of road/track or time yourself for 20 seconds on a stationary bike. Sprint as hard and fast as you can for the distance/time required. Rest for 30 seconds and then sprint again. Repeat until you have sprinted the amount required.

Alison opted for the distance of 125m as she wanted to beat her time each time she sprinted.

5 × cycle sprints
Times: 1. 18.25   2. 18.17   3. 18.49
       4. 19.10   5. 18.12

Boxing × 3
1. Alternate: × 30
2. Upper cuts: × 30
3. Wide: × 30
4. Reverse: × 30

Deadlift superset squats
Sets and Reps: 1.15   2.15   3.15/1.15
               4.15   5.15
Weight (lb):   12.5   12.5   12.5/15
               15   15

YOUR SESSION

AM

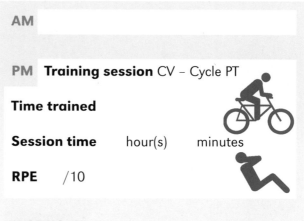

PM Training session CV – Cycle PT

Time trained

Session time   hour(s)   minutes

RPE   /10

WORKOUT

5 × cycle sprints
Times: 1.   2.   3.
       4.   5.

Boxing × 3
1. Alternate: ×
2. Upper cuts: ×
3. Wide: ×
4. Reverse: ×

Deadlift superset squats
Sets and Reps: 1.   2.   3.
               4.   5.
Weight (kg):

Leg workout × 3
1. Squats: × 20
2. Static lunges: × 20
3. Frog hops: × 20
4. Jumps overs: × 20
5. Calf raise: × 20

5 × cycle sprints
Times: 1. 18.25   2. 18.17   3. 18.49
       4. 19.10   5. 18.12

Boxing × 2
1. Alternate: × 30
2. Upper cuts: × 30
3. Wide: × 30
4. Reverse: × 30

Cycle 2 miles at the end to finish.

Alison's notes: There was quite a strong wind and I found the cycling quite easy – in one direction – the other direction was when the wind was blowing in my face and I was barely moving, it felt really odd.

Leg workout × 3
1. Squats: ×
2. Static lunges: ×
3. Frog hops: ×
4. Jumps overs: ×
5. Calf raise: ×

5 × cycle sprints
Times: 1.   2.   3.
       4.   5.

Boxing × 2
1. Alternate: ×
2. Upper cuts: ×
3. Wide: ×
4. Reverse: ×

Cycle   miles at the end to finish.

Your notes:

TRAINING SESSION **WEEK 4** DAY 6

ALISON'S SESSION

AM Training session CV – Walk

Time trained 9.00–10.36 a.m.

Session time 1 hours 36 minutes

RPE 7/10

PM Off

WORKOUT

Walk: 6 miles
Actual distance: 6 miles
Time: 1 hours 36 minutes
Average pace: 16 m/m

Alison's notes: Had a lovely walk with the dogs along the beach, up a fairly steep path and then back through Highcliffe castle via Chewton Glen to home. I was a little achy after yesterday's workout but I feel great for it.

YOUR SESSION

AM **Training session** CV – Walk

Time trained

Session time   hour(s)   minutes

RPE   /10

PM

WORKOUT

Walk: 6 miles
Actual distance: miles
Time: minutes
Average pace: m/m

Your notes:

WEEK 4 TESTS

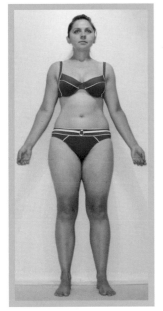 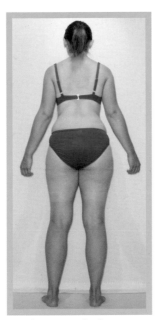

Front view of Alison at the end of week 4.

Back view of Alison at the end of week 4.

ALISON'S WEEKLY TESTS

Weight (kg)	55
Height (cm)	157.3
BMI	22.2
RHR	70
BP	112/65
Fat (%)	30.4

Measurements (cm)

Neck	30.48	
Chest	87.63	
Arms	R: 29.21	L: 29.21
Navel	78.10	
Hips	86.36	
Thighs	R: 59.05	L: 58.42
Calves	R: 35.56	L: 35.56

YOUR WEEKLY TESTS

Weight (kg)	
Height (cm)	
BMI	
RHR	
BP	
Fat (%)	

Measurements (cm)

Neck		
Chest		
Arms	R:	L:
Navel		
Hips		
Thighs	R:	L:
Calves	R:	L:

WEEK 4 HEALTH CHECK

ALISON'S RESULTS

Statistics

Weight (kg)	55
Height (cm)	157.3

Health tests

BMI	22.2
RHR	59
BP	123/67
Fat (%)	28.7
Glucose	6.2
Cholesterol	4.6
Lung function	390

Measurements (cm)

Neck	30.48	
Chest	89.53	
Arms	R: 27.94	L: 27.94
Navel	76.83	
Hips	83.82	
Thighs	R: 57.78	L: 57.78
Calves	R: 35.56	L: 35.56

Calliper test (mm)

Biceps	8
Triceps	16
Waist	11
Subscapularis	15
Total	50
Calliper fat (%)	29.6

Fitness tests

Bleep test (20m) level	5

Maximum reps in one minute

¾ push-ups	24
½ sit-ups	42
Squats	43
Dips	30
Max pull-ups	1

YOUR RESULTS

Statistics

Weight (kg)	
Height (cm)	

Health tests

BMI	
RHR	
BP	
Fat (%)	
Glucose	
Cholesterol	
Lung function	

Measurements (cm)

Neck		
Chest		
Arms	R:	L:
Navel		
Hips		
Thighs	R:	L:
Calves	R:	L:

Calliper test (mm)

Biceps	
Triceps	
Waist	
Subscapularis	
Total	
Calliper fat (%)	

Fitness tests

Bleep test (20m) level	

Maximum reps in one minute

¾ push-ups	
½ sit-ups	
Squats	
Dips	
Max pull-ups	

WEEK **FIVE** NUTRITION PLAN **WEEK 5**

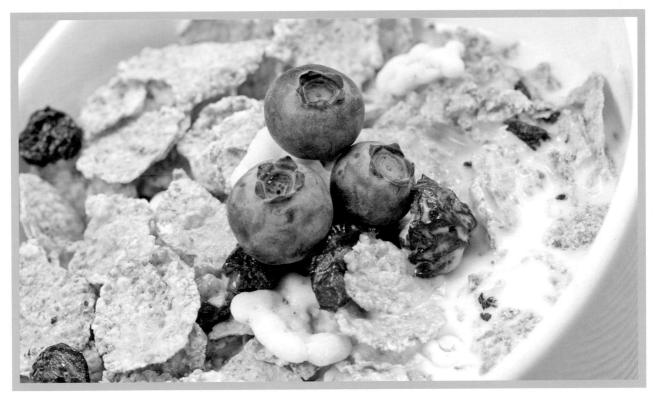

WEEK 5 OVERVIEW

Day	Breakfast	Lunch	Dinner
1	Fresh fruit and seeds	Yellow split pea soup	Prawn stir fry
2	Wheat biscuits or muesli with fruit	Tuna salad	Lamb stew
3	Muesli with fresh fruit	Lamb pitta	Chicken with lemongrass
4	Fruit porridge	Salmon salad	Fillet of beef
5	Fresh fruit and seeds	Chicken wrap	Barramundi curry
6	Omelette	Beef and beetroot salad	Paella
7	Fruit smoothie 2	Vegetable soup	Roasted chicken

SHOPPING LIST **WEEK 5**

CARBOHYDRATES
6 baking potatoes
1 bag of brown rice
260g of muesli
12 new potatoes
480g porridge oats
225g yellow split peas
200g short grain rice
1 bag of rice noodles
1 bag of sunflower and
pumpkin seeds
4 organic tortilla wraps
5 sweet potatoes
Wheat biscuits

DAIRY AND NON-DAIRY ALTERNATIVES
8 eggs
150g Greek yoghurt
50g parmesan cheese/goat's
cheese
1760ml skimmed/soya/rice/
oat milk
2.5kg soya yoghurt

FISH
800g barramundi fillets
150g calamari
200g mussels
600g raw prawns
4 poached salmon fillets
4 small tins tuna
400g white fish of your choice

MEAT
800g beef fillet
400g cooked roast beef
800g chicken on the bone
4 chicken breasts
1 large whole chicken
400g lean ham
600g boneless lamb

FRUIT
7 apples
2 apricots
9 bananas
1 punnet of blueberries
1 bag of green grapes
3 lemons
1 lime
2 peaches
1 punnet of raspberries

VEGETABLES
16 asparagus
4 cooked beetroot
125g frozen broad beans
250g broccoli
250g cherry tomatoes
7 carrots
4 celery sticks
1 courgette
½ cucumber
3 lettuce
250g mangetout
175g mushrooms
8 onions
225g frozen peas
200g runner beans
1 red onion
1 green pepper
2 red peppers
12 red tomatoes
150g rocket salad
150g baby spinach
21 spring onions
150g sugar snap peas
1 yellow pepper

HERBS
Basil
3 bay leaves
Black pepper
Coriander
Cumin
6 dill sprigs
1 fennel bulb
1 garlic bulb

Fresh ginger
11 lemongrass stalks
Mint
Oregano
Paprika
Parsley
6 peppercorns
Red chilli
Rosemary
Saffron
Thyme

OTHER
Balsamic vinegar
Chicken stock
Chinese rice wine
Cold-pressed extra virgin
olive oil
Corn flour
Dijon mustard
Fish sauce
Prawn paste
Soy sauce
Brown sugar
800g tinned tomatoes
Tomato purée
Vegetable stock
115ml white wine
Worcestershire sauce

SNACKS
Fruits
Wholegrain crispbread crackers
Flat breads
Small bowl of muesli
Yoghurt/soya yoghurt
Nuts (cashew, pine or
occasionally mixed nuts)
Soya nuts

FRUIT DRINKS
1 carton fruit juice

RECIPES **WEEK 5** DAY 1

BREAKFAST FRESH FRUIT AND SEEDS

See page 81

LUNCH YELLOW SPLIT PEA SOUP

225g yellow split peas (pre-soak for 12 hours overnight in cold water)

1.5 litres of vegetable stock

1 onion, peeled and sliced

1 sweet potato, peeled and chopped

3 carrots, trimmed, peeled and sliced

Fresh mint, handful

Baby spinach leaves, 4 handfuls

1 Drain the water from the split peas.
2 Boil the vegetable stock in a large saucepan, add split peas, then simmer for 25 minutes, removing any scum that appears.
3 Add all the other vegetables and simmer for a further 15–20 minutes, or until vegetables are tender.
4 Remove from heat and allow to cool.
5 Blend soup with food processor or blender.
6 Serve with fresh mint.

DINNER PRAWN STIR FRY

8 spring onions, finely chopped

1 green pepper, finely chopped

1 red pepper, finely chopped

2 tablespoons olive oil

2 garlic cloves, finely chopped

1 tablespoon ginger, finely cut

200g mangetout

450g raw prawns, thawed and peeled

4 tablespoons Chinese rice wine

Rice noodles

1 Heat the olive oil in a big frying pan or wok over a medium to high heat.
2 Add the spring onions, garlic, ginger and peppers to pan and stir fry for 4 minutes, stirring continuously.
3 Add the mangetout and prawns and stir fry for 4 minutes or until prawns have change colour.
4 Stir in rice wine.
5 Serve with rice noodles.

Lunch for tomorrow
TUNA SALAD
Consider preparing your sweet potatoes in advance

RECIPES **WEEK 5** DAY 2

BREAKFAST WHEAT BISCUITS OR
MUESLI WITH FRUIT   *See page 82*

LUNCH TUNA SALAD   *See page 134*

DINNER LAMB STEW

600g lean boneless lamb, diced
into 2.5cm cubes
1 onion, chopped
6 peppercorns
1 fennel bulb
115g mushrooms
1 teaspoon corn flour
1 tablespoon soya milk
150ml soya/plain yoghurt
6 baking potatoes
6 fresh dill sprigs
1 bay leaf
Half a lemon, grated rind and juice

1 Place lamb in large saucepan and cover with cold water.
2 Bring to boil over medium heat, remove any scum that rises to the surface.
3 Add the onion, two dill sprigs, bay leaf and peppercorns. Reduce heat, cover and simmer for 45 minutes.
4 Add the fennel, potatoes and mushrooms and simmer for a further 30 minutes, or until lamb is tender.
5 Using a slotted spoon, transfer the lamb, onion, fennel and mushrooms to a dish and keep warm.
6 Sieve the cooking liquid and reserve 300ml. Pour the reserved cooking liquid into a pan and bring to boil. Mix the corn flour and milk until smooth, then add to the cooking liquid.
7 Reduce the heat and simmer for 5 minutes, keep stirring until thickened.
8 Add the lemon rind and juice to the sauce.
9 Return the lamb, onion, fennel and mushrooms to the sauce pan and simmer for 5 minutes.
10 Meanwhile, mix the yoghurt, and four fresh dill sprigs in a small bowl, then add to the stew.
11 Serve with the potatoes.

Lunch for tomorrow
LAMB PITTA
Leave some of the lamb and sauce for lunch tomorrow.

RECIPES **WEEK 5** DAY 3

BREAKFAST MUESLI WITH FRESH FRUIT

See page 79

LUNCH LAMB PITTA

4 pitta breads (1 per person)

Use some of last night's dinner including sauce

Rocket leaves, handful per person

4 tomatoes, sliced

1 Slice open the pitta bread
2 Place last night's dinner into the pitta bread with the rocket leaves and sliced tomatoes.

DINNER CHICKEN WITH LEMONGRASS

800g lean chicken pieces on the bone

150g sugar snap peas

16 asparagus

4 spring onions, finely sliced

Lime wedges

Brown rice

For the marinade:

1 lemongrass stalk, finely chopped

2 cloves garlic, crushed

2 teaspoons ginger, grated

2 tablespoons soy sauce

115ml chicken stock

2 teaspoons olive oil

2 tablespoons Chinese rice wine

1 Mix all the marinade ingredients in a bowl.
2 Coat the chicken thoroughly with the marinade.
3 Cover with cling film and refrigerate for up to 2 hours or overnight and, if possible, turn occasionally.
4 Preheat oven 180°C (350°F).
5 Place chicken and marinade into dish and cook for 30 minutes, turning occasionally.
6 Bring a small saucepan of water to the boil and cook asparagus and sugar snap peas for 2–3 minutes.
7 Drain and serve meat, juices and vegetables.

RECIPES **WEEK 5** DAY 4

BREAKFAST FRUIT PORRIDGE

See page 80

LUNCH SALMON SALAD

See page 119

DINNER FILLET OF BEEF

800g beef fillet
3 onions, finely sliced
2 teaspoons olive oil
2 teaspoons balsamic vinegar
8 mushrooms, peeled and stems removed
115ml white wine
100g fresh mixed salad leaves

1. Preheat oven to 180°C (350°F).
2. Cook the onions in olive oil over a medium heat for 20–25 minutes, or until soft. Add the balsamic vinegar and cook for a further 5 minutes.
3. Heat a non-stick frying pan over high heat. Sear fillet on both sides and transfer beef to a baking dish.
4. Place mushrooms on second baking tray, pour over the wine and cover with foil.
5. Place both dishes in the oven and cook for 15 minutes.
6. Remove the beef from oven, cover with foil and leave to rest for 10 minutes.
7. At the same time, remove the foil from the mushrooms and bake for a further 10 minutes.
8. Divide the meat into four portions, serve with mixed salad leaves, caramelised onions and mushrooms.

Lunch for tomorrow
CHICKEN WRAP
Consider preparing the chicken in advance.

RECIPES **WEEK 5** DAY 5

BREAKFAST FRESH FRUIT AND SEEDS

See page 81

LUNCH CHICKEN WRAP   *See page 115*

DINNER BARRAMUNDI CURRY

1 tablespoon olive oil

800g barramundi fillet, diced

1 teaspoon brown sugar

115ml chicken stock

1 tablespoon fish sauce

200g runner beans

Handful of coriander

Rice or vegetables

For the curry paste:

1 red chilli, roughly chopped

1 lemongrass stalk, finely chopped

2 spring onions, finely chopped

1 clove garlic, roughly chopped

2 teaspoons finely grated ginger

2 teaspoons coriander

1 teaspoon of prawn paste

1 Place all curry paste ingredients in food processor and blend to a fine paste.
2 Boil the rice, and grill the vegetables under a medium heat.
3 Heat olive oil in large non-stick frying pan over a medium heat.
4 Add the curry paste and fish and stir fry for 3 minutes, turning fish carefully to coat with paste.
5 Add the sugar, chicken stock, fish sauce and beans.
6 Cook for a further 5 minutes.

RECIPES **WEEK 5** DAY 6

BREAKFAST OMELETTE   *See page 86*

LUNCH BEEF AND BEETROOT SALAD

4 cooked beetroots

50g Parmesan, shaved

400g lean finely sliced cold roast beef

Generous amount of salad and baby spinach

Basil, small handful, chopped

For the dressing:

1 tablespoon balsamic vinegar

2 tablespoons olive oil, cold pressed

1 clove of garlic, chopped

1 teaspoon Dijon mustard

1　Add all dressing ingredients into bowl and whisk well.

2　Add the remaining ingredients into large salad bowl and mix together

3　Pour dressing over the top.

DINNER PAELLA

2 tablespoons olive oil

1 onion, finely chopped

3 tomatoes, roughly chopped

200g short grain rice

1 litre chicken stock

400g fish of your choice

150g uncooked prawns, peeled

200g mussels, bearded and washed

150g calamari

150g peas

Spices and herbs:

1 teaspoon saffron

1 teaspoon paprika

2 cloves of garlic, crushed

Small handful of parsley, roughly chopped

Ground black pepper

Lemon wedges

1　In a small non-stick frying pan, lightly toss saffron and transfer to a cup.

2　Crush and add paprika and 60ml boiling water. Stir to dissolve and set aside.

3　Heat olive oil in large pan over medium heat.

4　Add garlic and onion, and cook for 5 minutes, or until soft.

5　Add the tomatoes and cook for a further 3minutes.

6　Add rice and cook for 5 minutes, stirring continuously. Meanwhile bring the stock to a boil in a large saucepan.

7　Add the stock and saffron liquid to the rice mixture, stir well and simmer for 15 minutes.

8　Add fish, prawns, mussels and calamari on top of rice, cover with foil and cook for10 minutes.

9　Add peas, re-cover pan and cook for a further 5 minutes.

10 Sprinkle with parsley, season with pepper and serve with lemon wedges.

RECIPES **WEEK 5** DAY 7

BREAKFAST FRUIT SMOOTHIE 2

4 tablespoons of nut and seed muesli

1200ml milk (soya/rice/oat or skimmed milk)

2 bananas

2 apricots

2 peaches

1 Mix the muesli and milk in a blender until nearly smooth.
2 Add the bananas, peaches and apricots and blend until completely smooth.
3 If the smoothie is too thick, add more water.

LUNCH VEGETABLE SOUP

See page 99

DINNER ROASTED CHICKEN

1 tablespoon olive oil

1.5kg lean chicken

1 onion, peeled and roughly chopped

2 cloves of garlic, finely chopped

2 celery stalks, cut into chunks

2 large carrots, cut into chunks

12 new potatoes

1 tablespoon fresh thyme

2 bay leaves

400g tinned chopped tomatoes

1 tablespoon Worcestershire sauce

300ml chicken stock

125g frozen broad beans

125g frozen peas

250g broccoli florets

Freshly ground black pepper

1 Preheat oven to 190°C (375°F).
2 Heat the olive oil in an oven-proof dish, remove any excess fat and set the chicken breast side up in the dish.
3 Add the onion, garlic, celery, carrots, potatoes, thyme and bay leaves.
4 Pour in chopped tomatoes, Worcestershire sauce and stock. Mix together and bring to a simmer.
5 Cover and cook for 1 hour or until chicken is cooked.
6 Carefully remove chicken from casserole dish.
7 Add the frozen peas, broad beans and broccoli, season with pepper and cook for 10 minutes.
8 Carve and serve vegetables with tomato sauce.

Lunch for tomorrow
CHICKEN SALAD
Keep enough chicken left over from dinner for tomorrow's lunch.

TRAINING DIARY **WEEK 5**

WEEK 5 OVERVIEW
Day 1: Weights – whole body
Day 2: CV – run PT
Day 3: Rest; myo lymphatic massage
Day 4: Circuits
Day 5: CV – run
Day 6: Rest
Day 7: Rest
Any day: Myo stretch

ALISON'S DIARY

Day 1 (Monday)
I had a tough weights session and was introduced to the Olympic bar. Found it all hard but felt the benefits pretty much straight away.
Tiredness 6
Stress 3
Sleep 8 hours

Day 2 (Tuesday)
I printed off some of my photos from weeks 1 and 4 to have a closer look at my change, there was already quite a difference – I love the way it's going. Again my body feels tired so I've booked in a massage tomorrow and I'm having the day off.
Tiredness 8
Stress 5
Sleep 8 hours

Day 3 (Wednesday)
I had my first proper lymphatic massage to help boost my immune system and get rid of some of my water retention. I drank lots of water and also visited the ladies room a lot, which flushed out some of my toxins – I was told this was going to happen and is good for me.
Tiredness 6
Stress 7
Sleep 6 hours 45 minutes

Day 4 (Thursday)
Well, I'm impressed, my work clothes seem to feel looser especially around my thighs and I have a bit more energy – not sure if this was just the massage but if it is, it must be magic.
Tiredness 4
Stress 6
Sleep 8 hours

Day 5 (Friday)
Feeling as though I have a bit more energy, but when I went for the run I found it incredibly hard. I had a cellulite massage.
Tiredness 4
Stress 5
Sleep 6 hours

Day 6 (Saturday)
Up early as I have lots to do this morning before going to work. I'm still not feeling myself and it feels like I have a foggy mind. I'm going out tonight with my friends but I don't finish work until 9.00 p.m.
Tiredness 5
Stress 5
Sleep 6 hours 40 minutes

Day 7 (Sunday)
I didn't drink last night, but I was still up until the early hours of this morning. I still had to get up for the test. I have a spa day booked soon – a great reward for doing so well.
Tiredness 5
Stress 4
Sleep 3 hours

TRAINING SESSION **WEEK 5** DAY 1

ALISON'S SESSION

AM Training session Weights – Whole body

Time trained 11.00 a.m.–12.00 p.m.

Session time 1 hour

RPE 9/10

PM

YOUR SESSION

AM Training session Weights – Whole body

Time trained

Session time   hour(s)   minutes

RPE   /10

PM

WORKOUT
Squats
Alison used an Olympic 7ft bar (weighs 20kg).
Weight seen below is the total weight including
the bar.

Set and Rep: 1. 16   2. 16   3. 16   4. 16   5. 16
Weight (kg): No Bar   Bar   Bar   30   30

Lunges (bosu)
Set and Rep: 1. 15   2. 15   3. 15
Weight: No   No   No

Bench press
Set and Rep: 1. 10   2. 10   3. 10
Weight (kg): Bar   Bar   Bar

Dumbbell press
Set and Rep: 1. 10   2. 10   3. 10
Weight (lb): 5   5   5

WORKOUT
Squats

Set and Rep: 1.   2.   3.   4.   5.
Weight (kg):

Lunges (bosu)
Set and Rep: 1.   2.   3.
Weight (kg):

Bench press
Set and Rep: 1.   2.   3.
Weight (kg):

Dumbbell press
Set and Rep: 1.   2.   3.
Weight (kg):

Regular pull-ups
1–5 and 5–1
Total: 15

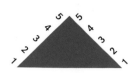

Regular pull-ups

_____ and _____

Total: _____

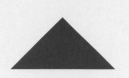

Alison's notes: I was properly introduced to the bar in today's tough weight session. I worked hard today in the gym but wow, I felt great afterwards. It's amazing how quickly you can feel the benefit from some of these workouts and exercises. It's a positive morale booster and encourages you to want to go to the gym more.

Your notes:

TRAINING SESSION **WEEK 5** DAY 2

ALISON'S SESSION

AM Rest

PM Training session CV – Run PT

Time trained 8.40–9.25 p.m.

Session time 45 minutes

RPE 8/10

Actual distance 2.52 miles

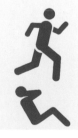

YOUR SESSION

AM

PM   Training session CV – Run PT

Time trained

Session time   hour(s)   minutes

RPE   /10

Actual distance   miles

WORKOUT

Run for half a mile before you get on to station 1. Complete all exercises in station 1 then run as fast as you can to the next station to complete those exercises in the same way.

Run: 0.5 miles first to station 1
Press-ups × 10
Wide press-ups × 10
Dips × 10

Run: 0.25 miles to station 2
Half sit-ups × 10
Leg levers × 10
Reverse curls × 10

Run: 0.25 miles to station 3
Jumping oblique twists × 10
Oblique side crunches × 10
Heel taps × 10

Run: 0.25 miles to station 4
Spotty dogs × 10
Star jumps × 10
Squat thrusts × 10

Run: 0.75 miles to finish

Alison's notes: Good luck with this one – the main thing is to keep going. Try not to look at what you have left to do, think about what you have already done.

WORKOUT

Run:　　　miles first to station 1
Press-ups ×
Wide press-ups ×
Dips ×

Run:　　　miles first to station 2
Half sit-ups ×
Leg levers ×
Reverse curls ×

Run:　　　miles first to station 3
Jumping oblique twists ×
Oblique side crunches ×
Heel taps ×

Run:　　　miles first to station 4
Spotty dogs ×
Star jumps ×
Squat thrusts ×

Run:　　　miles to finish

Your notes:

TRAINING SESSION **WEEK 5** DAY 4

ALISON'S SESSION

AM Rest

PM Training session Circuits

Time trained 8.00–8.55 p.m.

Session time 55 minutes

RPE 7/10

YOUR SESSION

AM

PM Training session

Time trained

Session time ____ hour(s) ____ minutes

RPE ____ /10

WORKOUT

Complete 100 reps as best as you can for each exercise below.

For example, you may not do 100 reps in one hit, but you can break that down into four lots of 25 or five lots of 20, or do as many as you can (e.g. do 60 reps and then do the last 40 reps after a short rest).

This circuit has been left in this manner so you push yourself as far as you can. The more you push, the better your end results. (Below you will see how Alison managed to break down the 100 reps.)

Step-ups
100 in one go

Lat pull-downs (weight 10kg total)
50, 50

Press-ups regular ¾
25, 25, 25, 25

Squats
100 in one go

Calf raises
80, 20

WORKOUT

Step-ups

Lat pull-downs (weight 10kg total)

Press-ups regular ¾

Squats

Calf raises

Half sit-ups
60, 20, 20

Reverse curls
100 in one go

Arm haulers
35, 35, 30

Dips
60, 20, 10,10

Alison's notes: This is quite a misleading workout – there are not many exercises, but quite a lot of reps for each one. I found the step-ups, squats and calf raises quite easy to do all in one go, but I had to break down the press-ups and dips.

Half sit-ups

Reverse curls

Arm haulers

Dips

Your notes:

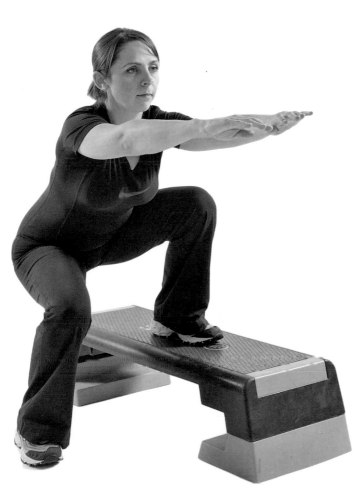

TRAINING SESSION **WEEK 5** DAY 5

ALISON'S SESSION

AM Rest

PM Training session CV – Run

Time trained 4.20–5.00 p.m.

Session time 40 minutes

RPE 9/10

YOUR SESSION

AM

PM **Training session** CV – Run

Time trained

Session time   hour(s)   minutes

RPE   /10

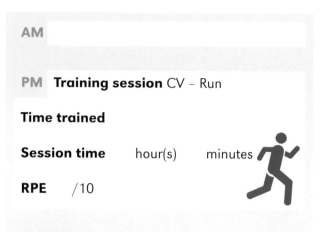

WORKOUT

Run: 4 miles
Actual distance: 3.5 miles
Run time: 42 minutes
Average Pace: 12 m/m

Alison's notes: This was a hard run for me as the weather was so hot and I think Gavin thought I was being a little on the lazy side and started pushing me even harder. I do remember saying afterwards that I never wanted to run again after this one, but it didn't last long.

Notes: Alison chose to run for 40 minutes and managed to do the full 42-minute run in one go without stopping because she choose to run at a slightly slower pace. She is going to aim for this distance from now on as her fitness is much improved, and this will gain greater results for the end 10km run.

If you are able to run for 40 minutes quite comfortably, then run the four miles stated at the best pace that you can.

WORKOUT

Run: 4 miles
Actual distance: miles
Run time: minutes
Average Pace: m/m

Your notes:

WEEK 5 TESTS

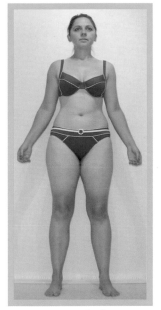 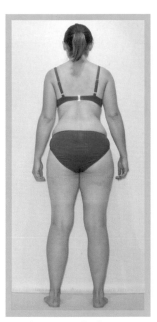

Front view of Alison at the end of week 5.

Back view of Alison at the end of week 5.

ALISON'S WEEKLY TESTS

Weight (kg)	54.8
Height (cm)	157.3
BMI	22.1
RHR	59
BP	103/64
Fat (%)	28.4

Measurements (cm)

Neck	29.84	
Chest	84.45	
Arms	R: 27.94	L: 27.94
Navel	76.20	
Hips	82.55	
Thighs	R: 57.78	L: 57.78H
Calves	R: 35.56	L: 35.56

YOUR WEEKLY TESTS

Weight (kg)	
Height (cm)	
BMI	
RHR	
BP	
Fat (%)	

Measurements (cm)

Neck		
Chest		
Arms	R:	L:
Navel		
Hips		
Thighs	R:	L:
Calves	R:	L:

WEEK SIX NUTRITION PLAN WEEK 6

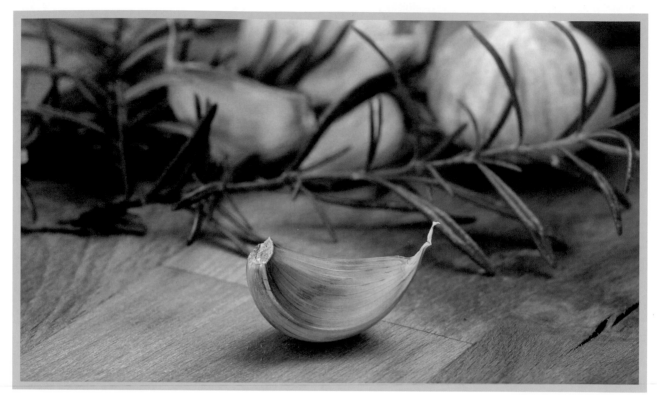

WEEK 6 OVERVIEW

Day	Breakfast	Lunch	Dinner
1	Fruit porridge	Chicken salad	Spicy prawns
2	Wheat biscuits or muesli with fruit	Vegetable soup	Greek chicken salad
3	Muesli with fresh fruit	Chicken wrap	Lamb with rosemary and garlic
4	Fruit smoothie 2	Tuna salad	Butternut squash and spinach frittata
5	Fresh fruit and seeds	Turkey and pine nut salad	Green fish curry
6	Omelette	Rice and salad with beetroot	Beef in black bean sauce
7	Fruit salad	Butternut squash and coriander soup	Kedgeree

SHOPPING LIST **WEEK 6**

CARBOHYDRATES
1 bag of black beans
1 bag of brown basmati rice
1 bag of brown rice
1 bag of wild rice
1 tin of chickpeas
1 bag of long grain rice
250g of muesli
320g porridge oats
1 bag of rice noodles
1 bag of sunflower seeds
1 bag of pumpkin seeds
4 organic tortilla wraps
1 bag of pine nuts
8 Maris Piper potatoes
4 sweet potatoes
225g water chestnuts
8 wholemeal/brown pitta breads
Wheat biscuits

DAIRY AND NON-DAIRY ALTERNATIVES
200g feta/goat's cheese
50g goat's cheese
17 eggs
1.88 litres skimmed/soya/rice/oat milk
2kg soya yoghurt

FISH
225g haddock fillets
225g smoked haddock fillets
700g cooked prawns
4 tinned tuna cans
225g × 4 white fish

MEAT
400g rump beef
8 chicken breasts
400g lean ham
1.5kg leg of lamb
4 turkey breasts

FRUIT
7 apples
2 apricots
6 bananas
1 punnet of blackberries
1 punnet of blueberries
4 lemons
4 peaches
1 large pineapple
1 punnet of raspberries

VEGETABLES
1 avocado
115g baby corn
300g baby spinach
4 cooked beetroot
12 black olives
225g broccoli
1.4kg butternut squash
6 cherry tomatoes
4 carrots
4 celery sticks
1 cos lettuce
1 courgette
2 cucumbers
1 green pepper
2 leeks
2 lettuces
50g mangetout
3 onions
8 plum tomatoes
2 red onions
3 red peppers
8 red tomatoes
175g rocket salad
4 shallots
20 spring onions
1 turnip
3 yellow peppers

HERBS
Basil
Black pepper
Chilli powder
Coriander
Ground coriander
Coriander seeds
Ground cumin seeds
Fresh ginger
2 green chillies
1 garlic bulb
Mint
Nutmeg
Paprika
Parsley
4 red chillies
Rosemary
Turmeric

OTHER
Balsamic vinegar
150ml coconut milk
Chicken stock
Chinese rice wine
Cold-pressed extra virgin olive oil
Peanut oil
Soy sauce
Brown sugar
Tahini
800g tinned tomatoes
Vegetable stock
115ml white wine

SNACKS
Fruit
Wholegrain crispbread crackers
Flat breads
Small bowl of muesli
Yoghurt/soya yoghurt
Nuts (cashew, pine or occasionally mixed nuts)
Soya nuts
Seeds (pumpkin or sunflower)

FRUIT DRINKS
1 carton fruit juice

RECIPES **WEEK 6** DAY 1

BREAKFAST FRUIT PORRIDGE

See page 80

LUNCH CHICKEN SALAD

Cooked chicken from previous night, cut into pieces

Generous amount of salad leaves

1 red pepper, sliced

1 yellow pepper, sliced

2 spring onions, finely chopped

1 Prepare the salad and place chicken over the top.
2 Serve immediately.

DINNER SPICY PRAWNS

2 garlic cloves, finely chopped

2cm piece of fresh ginger, thinly sliced

4 fresh red chillies, deseeded and finely chopped

Olive oil, 1 tablespoon

4 spring onions, chopped

2 green peppers, deseeded and sliced

400g tin tomatoes

½ tablespoon brown sugar

700g cooked prawns, peeled

4 spring onions, finely sliced to garnish

Rice and vegetables of your choice

1 Heat the olive oil in a large wok or frying pan over medium heat.
2 Add ginger, chilli and garlic, stir constantly for 1 minute – do not brown.
3 Add the spring onions and green peppers, stir for 5 minutes.
4 Add the tinned tomatoes and sugar, bring to boil and stir constantly. If sauce is too thick, add a little water.
5 Reduce heat and simmer for 5 minutes.
6 Stir in the prawns and cook for 4 minutes.
7 Transfer food to plates, garnish with spring onions and serve with rice/vegetables.

Lunch for tomorrow
VEGETABLE SOUP
Consider preparing your lunch in advance.

RECIPES **WEEK 6** DAY 2

BREAKFAST WHEAT BISCUITS OR
MUESLI WITH FRUIT   *See page 82*

LUNCH VEGETABLE SOUP   *See page 99*

DINNER GREEK CHICKEN SALAD

1 cos lettuce, cut into large pieces

1 cucumber, roughly chopped

1 green pepper, deseeded and finely chopped

12 olives (optional)

½ red onion, finely sliced

8 plum tomatoes

1 tablespoon lemon juice

1 tablespoon olive oil

200g low fat feta/goat's cheese

4 chicken breasts

8 wholemeal pitta breads (2 per person)

For the tzatziki:

1 clove of garlic, crushed

200g soya/plain yoghurt

¼ cucumber, finely grated

½ small red onion, finely chopped

1 tablespoon parsley, chopped

1 tablespoon mint, chopped

For the humous:

1 large tin chickpeas, drained

2 cloves garlic, peeled

2–3 tablespoons olive oil

1 dessertspoon tahini

1. Put the lettuce, cucumber, pepper, olives, tomatoes and onion into a large salad bowl.
2. Add the olive oil and lemon juice and mix well.
3. Crumble the feta/goat's cheese or mature goat's cheese over the top.
4. Prepare the tzatziki by mixing all the ingredients together in a small bowl.
5. Prepare humous by placing all the ingredients in a blender and blend until a smooth paste.
6. Meanwhile, grill the chicken on a medium heat for 8–12 minutes, or until thoroughly cooked.
7. Allow to cool for a couple of minutes and cut into pieces.
8. Toast the pitta bread before serving then fill with chicken, salad, tzatziki and humous.

Lunch for tomorrow
CHICKEN WRAP
Consider preparing the chicken in advance.

RECIPES **WEEK 6** DAY 3

BREAKFAST MUESLI WITH FRESH FRUIT

See page 79

LUNCH CHICKEN WRAP

See page 115

DINNER LAMB WITH ROSEMARY AND GARLIC

1.5kg lean leg of lamb (200g per person)

1 tablespoon olive oil

2 sprigs rosemary

2 cloves garlic, peeled and halved

2 lemons, quartered

115ml white wine

Serve with your favourite vegetables or beans and 8 roast potatoes (2 per person)

1 Preheat oven to 180°C (350°F).
2 Rub meat with olive oil.
3 Place rosemary, garlic and lemon in a baking dish and pour in the white wine.
4 Add lamb on top and bake for 1 to 1½ hours depending on taste.
5 Cook your vegetables and roast the potatoes.
6 Remove from oven, cover with foil and set aside for 10 minutes before carving.

Lunch for tomorrow
TUNA SALAD
Consider preparing the sweet potatoes in advance.

RECIPES **WEEK 6** DAY 4

BREAKFAST FRUIT SMOOTHIE 2

See page 157

LUNCH TUNA SALAD   *See page 134*

DINNER BUTTERNUT SQUASH AND
SPINACH FRITTATA

400g butternut squash, peeled and cut
into 3cm cubes

1 tablespoon olive oil

1 teaspoon soy sauce

2 leeks, finely chopped and washed

2 cloves garlic, crushed

300g baby spinach

8 eggs

400g soya/plain yoghurt

50g matured/goat's cheese, grated

Salad leaves

1 Preheat oven to 170°C (330°F). Grease a small
baking dish with a little olive oil.
2 Place butternut squash in baking tray, add 1
teaspoon of olive oil and soy sauce and roast for
25 minutes.
3 Heat the rest of the olive oil over a medium
heat.
4 Add the leek and cook for 5 minutes, or until
soft. Then add the garlic and spinach leaves and
cook until spinach has wilted.
5 Whisk eggs, soya/plain yoghurt and cheese
together in large bowl.
6 Then add the butternut squash and spinach
mixture and gently stir.
7 Pour the mixture into a baking dish and cook for
20 minutes, or until set. Serve with a salad.

Lunch for tomorrow
TURKEY AND PINE NUT SALAD
Consider preparing the turkey breasts in
advance (refrigerate overnight).

RECIPES **WEEK 6** DAY 5

BREAKFAST FRESH FRUIT
AND SEEDS   *See page 81*

LUNCH TURKEY AND PINE NUT SALAD

½ tablespoon olive oil

3–4 tablespoons of pine nuts

4 cooked turkey breasts, cut into pieces

Generous amount of salad leaves

1 avocado, sliced

1 red pepper, sliced

1 yellow pepper, sliced

2 spring onions, finely chopped

1 Heat the olive oil in a frying pan over a medium heat.
2 Cook the turkey breasts for 8–12 minutes, or until cooked.
3 Allow turkey to cool.
4 Prepare the salad and arrange the cooked turkey on top of the leaves.
5 Sprinkle with the pine nuts.
6 Drizzle with balsamic vinegar and serve immediately.

DINNER GREEN FISH CURRY

1 tablespoon olive oil

2 spring onions, sliced

1 teaspoon ground cumin seeds

2 green chillies, finely chopped

1 teaspoon coriander seeds

4 tablespoons fresh coriander

4 tablespoons fresh mint

150ml coconut milk

4 white fish fillets (225g each)

Basmati rice or vegetables of your choice

1 Heat the olive oil in a large frying pan over a medium heat. Add the spring onions and cook for 2 minutes or until soft.
2 Stir in ground cumin, chillies and coriander seeds and cook until the spices are fragrant.
3 Add the fresh coriander, mint, and coconut milk.
4 Carefully cook fish in frying pan 10–15 minutes or until the flesh flakes easily when tested with a fork.
5 Transfer the fish on to plates and serve with rice and vegetables of your choice.
6 Garnish with fresh mint.

Dinner for tomorrow
BEEF IN BLACK BEAN SAUCE
See the following page and consider marinating the beef overnight.

RECIPES WEEK 6 DAY 6

BREAKFAST OMELETTE

See page 86

LUNCH RICE AND SALAD WITH BEETROOT

100g brown rice

100g wild rice

4 shallots, peeled and halved

2 teaspoons olive oil

4 cooked beetroots, finely diced

1 lemon, juice of

2 tablespoons fresh mint, chopped

2 tablespoons fresh parsley, chopped

1 Preheat oven to 200°C (400°F). Place brown and wild rice in saucepan of water, bring to boil and simmer for 20 minutes.
2 Place the shallots on a baking tray, drizzle with olive oil and roast for 8–10 minutes.
3 Drain the rice and allow to cool. Mix the beetroot, lemon juice and mint. Stir in shallots and parsley, then serve.

DINNER BEEF IN BLACK BEAN SAUCE

400g lean rump steak, remove fat, cut into chunks

1 tablespoon olive oil

225g broccoli, cut into florets

115g baby corns, cut in half

4 spring onions, sliced diagonally

225g tinned water chestnuts

Rice or egg noodles

For the marinade:

1 tablespoon black beans, soaked in cold water for 5–10 minutes

2 tablespoons dark soy sauce

2 tablespoons Chinese rice wine

1 tablespoon peanut oil

1 teaspoon brown sugar

1 garlic clove, thinly sliced

1 tablespoon ginger, finely chopped

1 To make marinade: mash black beans in a bowl with a fork, stir in the remaining marinade ingredients and blend with a food processor.
2 Pour the marinade over steak and coat thoroughly in a baking dish. Cover with cling film and leave in fridge for 6 hours or more.
3 Heat the olive oil in large wok or frying pan. Drain the steak and reserve the marinade.
4 Stir fry the steak over a medium/high heat for 3 minutes, then transfer to a plate.
5 Add the broccoli and baby corn to the wok and stir in 3 tablespoons of water, cover and steam for 5 minutes, or until the vegetables are tender.
6 Add spring onions and water chestnuts to the wok and stir fry for a further 2 minutes.
7 Return the steak to the wok and pour in the reserved marinade.
8 Cook and keep stirring, until heated through. Serve with noodles of your choice.

RECIPES **WEEK 6 DAY** 7

BREAKFAST FRUIT SALAD   *See page 84*

LUNCH BUTTERNUT SQUASH AND CORIANDER SOUP   *See page 87*

DINNER KEDGEREE

225g haddock fillet
225g smoked haddock fillet
1 tablespoon olive oil
1 onion, chopped
225g long grain rice
1 hard-boiled egg, cut into quarters
2 tablespoons fresh parsley
Spices:
½ teaspoon ground turmeric
½ teaspoon cumin
½ teaspoon chilli powder
¼ teaspoon ground ginger

1 Place the haddock and smoked haddock in large frying pan.
2 Pour enough water to cover, and poach gently over a low heat for 10–15 minutes.
3 Remove from heat and allow to cool.
4 Sieve the cooking liquid into a measuring jug and make it up to 600ml if necessary.
5 Heat the olive oil in a large frying pan.
6 Add the onions and cook on low heat for 3 minutes, or until soft.
7 Mix in the spices, add the rice and cook. Stir until well coated.
8 Gently stir in the reserved liquid and bring to boil.
9 Cover and cook over low heat for 20 minutes, or until the liquid has been absorbed into the rice.
10 Meanwhile, skin the fish and remove any remaining bones.
11 Flake the flesh and fold the fish into the rice.
12 Transfer to a serving dish and garnish with a boiled egg.
13 Sprinkle over the chopped parsley and serve immediately.

TRAINING DIARY **WEEK 6**

WEEK 6 OVERVIEW
Day 1: CV – run
Day 2: CV – walk; myo lymphatic massage
Day 3: CV – cycle PT
Day 4: Weights – upper body
Day 5: Rest
Day 6: CV – walk
Day 7: Myo massage
Any day: Myo stretch

ALISON'S DIARY
Day 1 (Monday)
I did the run today and felt really strong considering I only had three hours sleep on Saturday night. I didn't take any of my inhalers for my asthma, and didn't need them for the rest of the day either.
Tiredness 7
Stress 5
Sleep 6 hours

Day 2 (Tuesday)
Day off from work today. I went for a dog walk in the morning and had another amazing lymphatic massage. I then had a power walk in the evening.
Tiredness 7
Stress 4
Sleep 7 hours

Day 3 (Wednesday)
Early shift today, and I reckon I'm becoming allergic to my job. I'm now going to start to look for a new one – I'm not sure what I want to do, but I can't keep going with the frame of mind I have, it's not healthy.
Tiredness 4
Stress 5
Sleep 6 hours 30 minutes

Day 4 (Thursday)
I sat in the sun for a bit today. I felt really good and it set me up to work for the rest of the day. Went for a lovely dog walk before going to the gym.
Tiredness 5
Stress 5
Sleep 8 hours

Day 5 (Friday)
Still aching and feeling slightly tender in some of my muscles from yesterday's workout, but in a good way. We went for another dog walk, but I couldn't tell you for how long.
Tiredness 5
Stress 5
Sleep 7 hours 30 minutes

Day 6 (Saturday)
We went for a long walk on the Isle of Purbeck today with a couple of the family dogs. Again it is so nice to get outside no matter what the weather, it's so refreshing. We went to a wedding this evening which was really nice too, and an excuse to buy a new dress to show off my better figure.
Tiredness 4
Stress 4
Sleep 7 hours 30 minutes

Day 7 (Sunday)
Day off. Had a myo massage. I always feel so much taller and relaxed when I have one. I have had no pain in my lower back and hip for two weeks now.
Tiredness 3
Stress 4
Sleep 8 hours 30 minutes

TRAINING SESSION **WEEK 6** DAY 1

ALISON'S SESSION

AM Rest

PM Training session CV – Run

Time trained 7.00–7.51 p.m.

Session time 51 minutes

RPE 8/10

WORKOUT

Run: 40 minutes/4 miles
Actual distance: 4.25 miles
Run time: 51 minutes
Average Pace: 12 m/m

Alison's notes: Felt very strong on the run today, I didn't stop until the end and my breathing was fairly controlled throughout.

Notes: Instead of the 40-minute time allocated, the workout was changed to run the four miles due to how well she ran last time. Alison managed to do the full four miles in one go without stopping.

YOUR SESSION

AM

PM Training session CV – Run

Time trained

Session time   hour(s)   minutes

RPE   /10

WORKOUT

Run: 40 minutes/4 miles
Actual distance: miles
Run time: minutes
Average Pace: m/m

Your notes:

TRAINING SESSION **WEEK 6** DAY 2

ALISON'S SESSION

AM Training session CV – Walk

Time trained 8.10–9.00 a.m.

Session time 50 minutes

RPE 4/10

PM Rest

WORKOUT
Walk: 3 miles
Actual distance: 3 miles
Time: 50 minutes
Average pace: 16.40 m/m

Alison's notes: Had a lovely evening walk along the coastal path, it was such a fresh evening – I swear I slept like a log that night because of it.

YOUR SESSION

AM Training session CV – Walk

Time trained

Session time   hour(s)   minutes

RPE   /10

PM

WORKOUT
Walk: 3 miles
Actual distance: miles
Time: minutes
Average pace: m/m

Your notes:

TRAINING SESSION **WEEK 6** DAY 3

ALISON'S SESSION

AM Rest

PM Training session CV – Cycle PT

Time trained 7.30–8.40 p.m.

Session time 1 hour 10 minutes

RPE 8/10

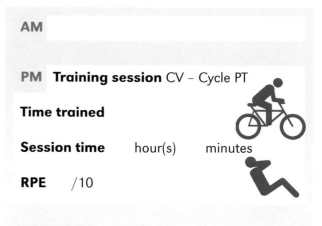

WORKOUT

You have a time limit of 1 minute and 30 seconds for each exercise.

Complete all the number 1 exercises before moving on to the number 2 exercises, then number 3 exercises, and so on until you have finished all eight exercises.

Always use your stronger leg to lead when you are performing your step box exercises to stop bad technique.

Give yourself minimal rest before moving on to the 25-minute cycle.

Leg exercises
1. Squat
2. Squat (bosu)
3. Squat
4. Squat (bosu)
5. Squat
6. Standing glute extension
7. Standing glute extension
8. Squat (deep)

YOUR SESSION

AM

PM Training session CV – Cycle PT

Time trained

Session time   hour(s)   minutes

RPE   /10

WORKOUT

Leg exercises
1. Squat
2. Squat (bosu)
3. Squat
4. Squat (bosu)
5. Squat
6. Standing glute extension
7. Standing glute extension
8. Squat (deep)

Mat work

1. Reverse crunch
2. Reverse curl
3. Half sit-ups
4. Crunches
5. Heel taps
6. Dirty dogs
7. Spotty dogs
8. V sit-ups

Step box exercises

1. Step-up left leg first
2. Step-up right leg first
3. Toe taps
4. Side lunge left leg
5. Side lunge right leg
6. Down down up up left leg
7. Down down up up right leg
8. Back lunge

Cycle for 25 minutes, trying to keep your RPM between 80 and 90. You can either cycle on a turbo trainer (or a spinning bike) inside or cycle outside.

Alison's notes: Gavin's advice to me was to give everything I had for each exercise, and that's what I did. I had such a rush at the end, but what a lot of work to get it.

Notes: Cycled outside battling against all the elements, like the horrible wind we had today. We still managed to keep the RPM around 80–90 most of the way, and cycled about four miles.

Mat work

1. Reverse crunch
2. Reverse curl
3. Half sit-ups
4. Crunches
5. Heel taps
6. Dirty dogs
7. Spotty dogs
8. V sit-ups

Step box exercises

1. Step-up left leg first
2. Step-up right leg first
3. Toe taps
4. Side lunge left leg
5. Side lunge right leg
6. Down down up up left leg
7. Down down up up right leg
8. Back lunge

Your notes:

TRAINING SESSION **WEEK 6** DAY 4

ALISON'S SESSION

AM Rest

PM Training session Weights – Upper body

Time trained 6.35–7.15 p.m.

Session time 40 minutes

RPE 6/10

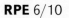

YOUR SESSION

AM

PM Training session Weights – Upper body

Time trained

Session time   hour(s)   minutes

RPE   /10

WORKOUT
Superset

	Close grip pull-downs				Dumbbell press			
Sets	1.	2.	3.	4.	1.	2.	3.	4.
Reps	20	10	10	20	20	10	9	20
Weight (kg)	5	10	10	5	10	15	15	10

Superset

	¾ press-ups				Supinated curl			
Sets	1.	2.	3.	4.	1.	2.	3.	4.
Reps	30	30	30	30	20	10	10	18
Weight (lb)					5	7.5	7.5	5

WORKOUT
Superset

	Close grip pull-downs				Dumbbell press			
Sets	1.	2.	3.	4.	1.	2.	3.	4.
Reps								
Weight (kg)								

Superset

	¾ press-ups				Supinated curl			
Sets	1.	2.	3.	4.	1.	2.	3.	4.
Reps								
Weight (kg)								

Superset

	Lat raises				Dips			
Sets	1.	2.	3.	4.	1.	2.	3.	4.
Reps	20	15	13	20	30	30	30	30
Weight (lb)	3	5	5	3				

Notes: This is a fast workout that incorporates your whole upper body. With the exercises you will notice Alison starts and finishes with high reps and a moderate weight. The middle two sets are lower reps with a heavier weight. This will make sure you hit all areas of your muscles to help you tone up.

Superset

	Lat raises				Dips			
Sets	1.	2.	3.	4.	1.	2.	3.	4.
Reps								
Weight (kg)								

Your notes:

TRAINING SESSION **WEEK 6** DAY 6

ALISON'S SESSION

AM Rest

PM Training session CV – Walk

Time trained 10.00 a.m.–1.00 p.m.

Session time 3 hours

RPE 7/10

YOUR SESSION

AM

PM Training session CV – Walk

Time trained

Session time   hours   minutes

RPE   /10

WORKOUT
Walk
Actual distance: 11.02 miles
Time: 2 hours 56 minutes
Average pace: 16 m/m

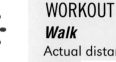

Equipment
Food
2 bananas
2 apples
1 bag soya nuts
1 bag goji berries
2 litres water

Clothing
Walking boots
Walking trousers
Vest
Training T-shirt
Walking socks

Spare clothing
Sandals
Warm jacket/top
Gloves
Hat
Waterproof jacket

Other
First aid kit
First field dressing
Torch
Map and compass
Money
Mobile phone
Whistle

Alison's notes: We went for a three-hour walk to get back outside and into the fresh air. We planned the walk to finish with a pub lunch at the end.

WORKOUT
Walk
Actual distance: _____ miles
Time: _____ minutes
Average pace: _____ m/m

Equipment
Food

Clothing

Spare clothing

Other

Your notes

WEEK 6 TESTS

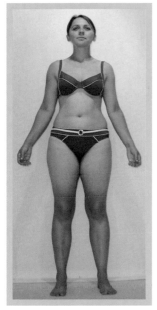 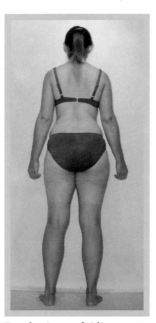

Front view of Alison at the end of week 6.   **Back view of Alison at the end of week 6.**

ALISON'S WEEKLY TESTS

Weight (kg)	54
Height (cm)	157.3
BMI	21.8
RHR	59
BP	103/65
Fat (%)	27.4

Measurements (cm)

Neck	29.84	
Chest	84.45	
Arms	R: 27.30	L: 27.30
Navel	74.93	
Hips	80.64	
Thighs	R: 57.15	L: 57.15
Calves	R: 35.56	L: 35.56

YOUR WEEKLY TESTS

Weight (kg)	
Height (cm)	
BMI	
RHR	
BP	
Fat (%)	

Measurements (cm)

Neck		
Chest		
Arms	R:	L:
Navel		
Hips		
Thighs	R:	L:
Calves	R:	L:

WEEK **SEVEN** NUTRITION PLAN **WEEK 7**

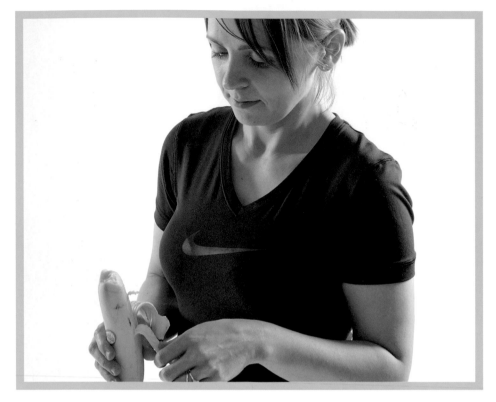

WEEK 7 OVERVIEW

Day	Breakfast	Lunch	Dinner
1	Wheat biscuits or muesli with fruit	Beef salad pitta	Snapper with basil
2	Fruit salad	Yellow split pea soup	Chicken with roasted tomatoes
3	Muesli with fresh fruit	Chicken wrap	Lamb with baked fennel
4	Fruit porridge	Egg salad	Citrus baked cod
5	Fresh fruit and seeds	Tuna salad	Soya/plain yoghurt baked chicken
6	Omelette	Tomato and pepper soup	Vegetarian stir fry
7	Fruit smoothie 1	Salmon salad	Spiced barramundi fillets

SHOPPING LIST **WEEK 7**

CARBOHYDRATES
1 bag of brown rice
12 charlotte potatoes
240g of muesli
560g porridge oats
1 bag of rice noodles
1 bag of sunflower seeds
1 bag of pumpkin seeds
4 organic tortilla wraps
1 bag of sesame seeds
5 sweet potatoes
4 wholemeal/brown pitta breads
225g yellow split peas
Wheat biscuits

DAIRY AND NON-DAIRY ALTERNATIVES
12 eggs
60g feta/goat's cheese
680ml skimmed/soya/rice/oat milk
2kg soya yoghurt

FISH
200g × 4 barramundi
175g × 4 cod/hake
200g × 4 snapper fillets
4 poached salmon fillets
4 small tins tuna

MEAT
400g cooked roast beef
12 chicken breasts
400g lean ham
1.4kg lamb cutlets

FRUIT
3 apples
4 bananas
2 lemons
2 limes
2 mangos
1 melon
1 orange
1 large pineapple
1 punnet of raspberries

VEGETABLES
100g baby corn
3 bags of baby spinach
55g button mushrooms
1 broccoli floret
350g cabbage
400g cherry tomatoes
3 carrots
1 courgette
2 cucumbers
2 fennel bulbs
1 green pepper
4 lettuce
200g mangetout
150g mushrooms
6 onions
2 red onions
4 red peppers
100g rocket salad
20g snow pea pods
11 spring onions
750g tomatoes
21 red tomatoes
5 yellow peppers

HERBS
Basil
Black pepper
Cardamom seeds
Chilli powder
Chinese five-spice
Cinnamon
Coriander
Cumin
Fresh ginger
1 garlic bulb
Mint
Oregano
Parsley
1 red chilli
Rosemary
Tarragon

OTHER
Balsamic vinegar
Cider vinegar
Cold-pressed extra virgin olive oil
Dijon mustard
Oyster sauce
Peanut oil
Sesame oil
Soy sauce
Tomato purée
Vegetable stock
60ml white wine

SNACKS
Wholegrain crispbread crackers
Crackers/flat breads
Small bowl of muesli
Yoghurt/soya yoghurt
Nuts (cashew, pine or occasionally mixed nuts)
Soya nuts
Seeds (pumpkin or sunflower)

FRUIT DRINKS
1 carton fruit juice

RECIPES **WEEK 7** DAY 1

BREAKFAST WHEAT BISCUITS OR
MUESLI WITH FRUIT

See page 82

LUNCH BEEF SALAD PITTA

See page 100

DINNER SNAPPER WITH BASIL

4 × 200g snapper fillets

2 tablespoons olive oil

1 clove garlic, crushed

½ red chilli, finely chopped

4 spring onions, finely chopped

2 tablespoons basil, roughly chopped

1 tablespoon dried oregano

60ml white wine

4 tomatoes, roughly chopped

Green salad

1. Preheat oven to 180°C (350°F).
2. Heat half the olive oil in a small saucepan over a medium heat.
3. Add the chilli, garlic and spring onions and stir fry for 2 minutes, or until garlic is golden.
4. Reduce the heat to medium low and add the herbs and white wine, stirring occasionally for 5 minutes.
5. Remove from heat and stir in the chopped tomatoes.
6. Heat a large non-stick frying pan over a high heat and brush the fish with the remaining oil.
7. Sear each side for 2 minutes and transfer to an ovenproof baking dish and spoon sauce over fish.
8. Bake for 6–8 minutes or until fish is cooked. The flesh will flake away easily when pressed with a fork when the fish is ready. Serve with salad.

Lunch for tomorrow
YELLOW SPLIT PEA SOUP
Soak the yellow split peas for tomorrow's lunch.

RECIPES **WEEK 7** DAY 2

BREAKFAST FRUIT SALAD

See page 84

LUNCH YELLOW SPLIT PEA SOUP

See page 151

DINNER CHICKEN WITH ROASTED TOMATOES

4 large tomatoes, cut into quarters

1 tablespoon olive oil

1 small onion, sliced

1 tablespoon fresh basil, roughly chopped

4 × 200g skinless chicken breasts

60g goat's or mature cheese, cut into chunks

Salad or vegetables of your choice

1. Preheat oven to 180°C (350°F). Line a baking tray with baking paper and place tomatoes on tray.
2. Place in a hot oven for 15 minutes. Meanwhile, heat the olive oil in a frying pan over medium heat.
3. Add the onion and basil and cook for 5 minutes or until onion is soft.
4. Drain and reserve the oil and place onion and basil on a plate.
5. Return pan to heat and add the reserved oil.
6. Add chicken and cook for 6 minutes each side, or until lightly browned on both sides.
7. Heat grill to medium.
8. Divide the chicken into four portions and cover the chicken with a layer of the tomato and onion mixture.
9. Top with feta/goat's cheese and place under grill until the cheese has melted.
10. Serve with either salad or vegetables.

Lunch for tomorrow
CHICKEN WRAP
Consider preparing extra chicken in advance.

RECIPES **WEEK 7** DAY 3

BREAKFAST MUESLI WITH FRESH FRUIT

See page 79

LUNCH CHICKEN WRAP

See page 115

DINNER LAMB WITH BAKED FENNEL

1.4kg lamb cutlets (200g meat per person) with fat trimmed off

2 fennel bulbs, sliced

2 red onions, cut into wedges

1 tablespoon olive oil

100g baby spinach leaves

8–12 Charlotte potatoes

For the marinade:

2 tablespoons rosemary, chopped

2 teaspoons tarragon, chopped

2 teaspoons parsley

1 tablespoon olive oil

1 Mix the marinade ingredients together and pour into a shallow dish.
2 Add the meat to the marinade and coat thoroughly.
3 Cover and allow to marinate for 30 minutes.
4 Preheat oven to 180°C (350°F).
5 Place fennel and onion in a baking dish and drizzle with olive oil and bake for 20 minutes.
6 Roast the potatoes.
7 Preheat grill to high and cook the lamb cutlets to your liking.
8 Once cooked, set aside to rest. Toss the spinach leaves through the hot vegetables.
9 Arrange the vegetables on serving plates and place the lamb on top.
10 Serve with potatoes.

Lunch for tomorrow
EGG SALAD
See the following page and consider preparing the eggs in advance.

RECIPES WEEK 7 DAY 4

BREAKFAST FRUIT PORRIDGE

See page 80

LUNCH EGG SALAD

See page 118

DINNER CITRUS BAKED COD

4 × cod or hake cutlets (175g/6oz each)

2 tablespoons lime juice

1 green pepper, deseeded and cut into strips

1 tablespoon olive oil

1 onion, finely chopped

1 Place fish in a shallow ovenproof dish and pour over lime juice.
2 Cover and leave to marinade in the refrigerator for 15–25 minutes.
3 Preheat oven to 180°C (350°F).
4 Heat olive oil in a frying pan and cook onion, garlic, green pepper and pumpkin seeds. Cook until onion is soft.

1 clove garlic, crushed

40g pumpkin seeds

1 lime, grated zest

1 tablespoon coriander, chopped

55g button mushrooms, finely sliced

2 tablespoons fresh orange juice
or white wine

Broccoli

5 Gently stir in the lime zest, chopped coriander and mushrooms.
6 Spoon this mixture over fish and pour over the orange juice.
7 Cover and bake in oven for 30 minutes, or until fish is tender.
8 Serve with steamed broccoli.

Lunch for tomorrow
TUNA SALAD
Consider preparing the sweet potatoes in advance.

RECIPES **WEEK 7** DAY 5

BREAKFAST FRESH FRUIT AND SEEDS   *See page 81*

LUNCH TUNA SALAD   *See page 134*

DINNER SOYA/PLAIN YOGHURT BAKED CHICKEN

1 tablespoon olive oil

4 × 200g skinless chicken breasts

For the salad:

½ cucumber, sliced

4 large tomatoes, sliced

½ small red onion, finely sliced

½ tablespoon mint leaves

1 teaspoon lemon juice

For the marinade:

½ teaspoon Chinese five-spice powder

1 teaspoon chilli powder

2 teaspoons soy sauce

1 glove garlic, crushed

1 tablespoon olive oil

200g soya/plain yoghurt

1 In a bowl fold the five-spice powder, chilli powder, soy sauce, garlic and olive oil through the soya/plain yoghurt.
2 Coat the chicken with the mixture and leave to marinate for up to 4 hours.
3 Preheat the oven to 180°C (350°F).
4 Line a baking dish with baking paper.
5 Heat the olive oil in a non-stick frying pan over medium heat.
6 Add the chicken and cook for 2 minutes each side.
7 Transfer the chicken to the prepared baking dish and bake for 6–8 minutes or until cooked.
8 Remove from oven and allow to rest for 5 minutes.
9 Cut into thick slices.
10 Prepare the salad adding all the ingredients in salad bowl and mix.
11 Serve salad with the chicken.

RECIPES **WEEK 7 DAY 6**

BREAKFAST OMELETTE

See page 86

LUNCH TOMATO AND PEPPER SOUP

See page 138

DINNER VEGETARIAN STIR FRY

1 tablespoon peanut oil

1 clove garlic

1 teaspoon ginger, grated

1 onion, sliced

150g mangetout

150g mushrooms

350g cabbage, shredded

1 Heat a large wok or frying pan over high heat.
2 Add peanut oil, and once pan is smoking add the garlic, ginger and onion.
3 Stir fry for 2–3 minutes or until the onion begins to soften.
4 Next, add the mangetout, mushrooms, cabbage and baby corn and stir fry for a further 5 minutes, or until almost cooked.

100g baby corn

2 tablespoons oyster sauce

1 tablespoon soy sauce

2 tablespoons coriander leaves

Brown rice

5 Add the oyster sauce, soy sauce and coriander and cook for 1 minute.

6 Serve immediately with brown rice.

RECIPES **WEEK 7** DAY 7

BREAKFAST FRUIT SMOOTHIE 1

See page 85

LUNCH SALMON SALAD

See page 119

DINNER SPICED BARRAMUNDI STEAKS

1 tablespoon olive oil

4 × 200g barramundi fillets

1 tablespoon sesame oil

20g snow pea pods (string removed)

1 tablespoon sesame seeds

1 large yellow pepper, cut into thin strips

Brown rice

For the paste:

Freshly ground pepper

1 teaspoon ground cumin

½ teaspoon ground cardamom

½ teaspoon ground cinnamon

1 clove garlic, chopped

1 tablespoon fresh coriander

1 tablespoon parsley

1 lemon, juice and finely grated zest

1 Preheat oven to 180°C (350°F). Pat fish with paper towel, brush with half the olive oil and season.

2 Place fish in a single layer in an ovenproof baking dish.

3 Next, mix the remaining olive oil with the cumin, coriander, cardamon, cinnamon, garlic, parsley, and lemon juice and zest until you have a loose paste and spread evenly over the top of the fish.

4 Cover dish with foil and bake for 10–15 minutes, or until fish is cooked. Boil the rice.

5 Heat the sesame oil over medium to high heat and add the snow pea pods and sesame seeds.

6 Cook for 2 minutes or until snow pea pods are crisp tender. Gently stir in the yellow pepper and cook for a further 2 minutes. Serve immediately with barramundi and rice.

Lunch for tomorrow:
SWEET POTATO AND BEAN SALAD
Consider preparing the eggs and sweet potatoes in advance.

TRAINING DIARY **WEEK 7**

WEEK 7 OVERVIEW
Day 1: Cellulite massage; CV – run
Day 2: Rest
Day 3: CV – run
Day 4: Rest
Day 5: Circuits
Day 6: Weights – upper body
Day 7: CV – cycle; myo lymphatic massage
Any day: Myo stretch

ALISON'S DIARY
Day 1 (Monday)
I had a cellulite massage today before going for my run. Again, this massage is quite painful in places but you can see a noticeable difference.
Tiredness 5
Stress 5
Sleep 8 hours

Day 2 (Tuesday)
I'm feeling really good today, I have more energy and had a really good night's sleep. I went out for a meal tonight and also went to the cinema.
Tiredness 4
Stress 5
Sleep 7 hours

Day 3 (Wednesday)
What beautiful weather. I really enjoyed the run as I can see myself running faster and further without struggling too much.
Tiredness 4
Stress 3
Sleep 10 hours

Day 4 (Thursday)
I had such a lovely day today. I went on a spa with a friend. I relaxed, swam a few lengths and ate really healthily but way too much, felt stuffed coming home.
Tiredness 3
Stress 3
Sleep 7 hours 30 minutes

Day 5 (Friday)
Due to yesterday's spa day I had hardly any stress and lots of energy. This helped me enjoy a really hard workout.
Tiredness 3
Stress 2
Sleep 6 hours

Day 6 (Saturday)
Had such a tough and emotional workout today, I have so much going on at the moment that I can't seem to do anything to fix it and I think the workout just brought it out of me. Unfortunately Gavin got the blame for pushing me too hard. Sorry Gavin, great therapy session though.
Tiredness 3
Stress 4
Sleep 8 hours

Day 7 (Sunday)
Tests today and I've had a terrible food week. I knew I had put weight on due to my bad week, so I ended up slipping back into old habits. As Gavin pointed out, this is easily rectified and by this time next week I could have better results than last week. I can't believe it but Gavin is almost certain. I had a good workout today and also a lymphatic massage to help get rid of some of those unwanted toxins.
Tiredness 6
Stress 4
Sleep 6 hours 30 minutes

TRAINING SESSION **WEEK 7** DAY 1

ALISON'S SESSION

AM Rest

PM Training session CV – Run

Time trained 7.00–7.36 p.m.

Session time 36 minutes

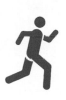

RPE 7/10

WORKOUT

Run: 3 miles
Actual distance: 3.0 miles
Time: 36 minutes
Average pace: 12 m/m

Alison's notes: I had such a good run today, no stops and my breathing was quite relaxed and controlled throughout. I had a cellulite massage just before my run so I don't know if this stimulated the blood flow and made my legs work better, but I take all the credit.

YOUR SESSION

AM

PM   Training session CV – Run

Time trained

Session time   hour(s)   minutes

RPE   /10

WORKOUT

Run: 3 miles
Actual distance: miles
Time: minutes
Average pace: m/m

Your notes:

TRAINING SESSION **WEEK 7** DAY 3

ALISON'S SESSION

AM Rest

PM Training session CV – Run

Time trained 7.00–7.40 p.m.

Session time 40 minutes

RPE 8/10

WORKOUT

Run: 4 miles
Actual distance: 3.5 miles
Time: 40 minutes
Average pace: 11.30 m/m

Alison's notes: On this run I was trying to keep my pace the same as my shorter-distance runs just to push myself. I even decided to do a sprint to the finish on the last section.

YOUR SESSION

AM

PM Training session CV – Run

Time trained

Session time   hour(s)   minutes

RPE   /10

WORKOUT

Run: 4 miles
Actual distance: miles
Time: minutes
Average pace: m/m

Your notes:

TRAINING SESSION **WEEK 7** DAY 5

ALISON'S SESSION

AM Rest

PM Training session Circuits

Time trained 7.00–7.55 p.m.

Session time 55 minutes

RPE 9/10

YOUR SESSION

AM

PM Training session Circuits

Time trained

Session time   hour(s)   minutes

RPE   /10

WORKOUT

You have one minute to perform as many reps as you can for each exercise.

Once you complete all the exercises for the 1st cycle, go back through the exercises again for the 2nd cycle, but this time try to beat your original score from the 1st cycle. I didn't tell Alison this so she pushed herself really hard for the 1st set, which is what I want you to do.

Any exercise where you do not beat or match your score, you should give yourself a forfeit of an extra two reps per rep you went over.

WORKOUT

Your notes:

Exercise	Weight (lb)	1st cycle scores	2nd cycle scores
Squats	10	58	63
Dumbbell press	10	22	16
Upright rows	15	30	32
Bent-over rows	15	30	40
Pull-ups (regular)	–	7 negatives	8 negatives
¾ press-ups	–	30	35
Half sit-ups	–	60	64
Reverse curls	–	51	55
Dumbbell bench press	15	25	25
Arm curl	10	18	19
Dips	–	35	43

Exercise	Weight (lb)	1st cycle scores	2nd cycle scores
Squats			
Dumbbell press			
Upright rows			
Bent-over rows			
Pull-ups (regular)			
¾ press-ups			
Half sit-ups			
Reverse curls			
Dumbbell bench press			
Arm curl			
Dips			

Alison's notes: The circuit session was hard today, especially as I didn't have dinner until afterwards. I did every exercise as quickly as I could without losing technique and thought I had finished after doing the dips, when Gavin informed that I had to do all of the exercises again and I had to beat my original scores.

Notes: When you put your all into it, this workout is extremely tough. Alison worked hard, and as a result only had one exercise that she didn't manage to beat. We had the little forfeit of 12 reps on the dumbbell press, which we completed at the end of the workout.

Your notes:

TRAINING SESSION **WEEK 7** DAY 6

ALISON'S SESSION

AM Rest

PM Training session Weights – Upper body

Time trained 4.00–4.45 p.m.

Session time 45 minutes

RPE 6/10

WORKOUT
Lat pull-downs
Set and Rep: 1. 10   2. 10   3. 10   4. 9
Weight (kg):   10   15   15   17.5

Single arm cable row
Set and Rep: 1. 15   2. 10   3. 10   4. 10
Weight (kg):   2.5   2.5   2.5   2.5

Bench press
Bar = Olympic bar weighing 20kg
Set and Rep: 1. 7   2. 9   3. 8   4. 10
Weight (kg):   Bar   Bar   Bar   Bar

Incline dumbbell press
Set and Rep: 1. 10   2. 10   3. 10   4. 10
Weight (lb):   10   15   15   15

Superset

	Glute extensions				Dirty dogs			
Sets	1.	2.	3.	4.	1.	2.	3.	4.
Reps	15	15	15	15	15	15	15	15

Alison's notes: Had a tough weights session – I needed to take a little longer between each exercise and set so my muscles could recover. I lifted the Olympic bar and at one point I lost communication with my arms completely.

YOUR SESSION

AM

PM Training session Weights – Upper body

Time trained

Session time   hour(s)   minutes

RPE   /10

WORKOUT
Lat pull-downs
Set and Rep: 1.   2.   3.   4.
Weight (kg):

Single arm cable row
Set and Rep: 1.   2.   3.   4.
Weight (kg):

Bench press
Bar = Olympic bar weighing 20kg
Set and Rep: 1.   2.   3.   4.
Weight (kg):   Bar   Bar   Bar   Bar

Incline dumbbell press
Set and Rep: 1.   2.   3.   4.
Weight (kg):

Superset

	Glute extensions				Dirty dogs			
Sets	1.	2.	3.	4.	1.	2.	3.	4.
Reps								

Your notes:

TRAINING SESSION **WEEK 7** DAY 7

ALISON'S SESSION

AM Rest

PM Training session CV – Cycle

Time trained 3.00–3.50 p.m.

Session time 50 minutes

RPE 5/10

WORKOUT
Cycle: 10 miles
Actual distance: 8 miles

Alison's notes: Test day again. We went through my food diary with a fine-toothed comb and realised how naughty I had been this week – I was not proud of this at all. This was definitely my worst week for results, and after speaking with Gavin I know I will try hard next week to make up for this blip.

YOUR SESSION

AM

PM   Training session CV – Cycle

Time trained

Session time   hour(s)   minutes

RPE   /10

WORKOUT
Cycle: 10 miles
Actual distance: miles

Your notes:

WEEK 7 TESTS

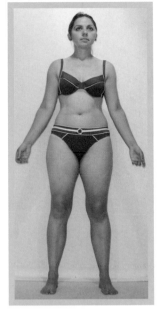 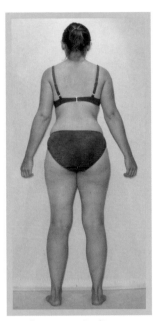

Front view of Alison at the end of week 7.

Back view of Alison at the end of week 7.

ALISON'S WEEKLY TESTS

Weight (kg)	54.5
Height (cm)	157.3
BMI	21.8
RHR	60
BP	105/62
Fat (%)	28.4

Measurements (cm)

Neck	29.84	
Chest	84.45	
Arms	R: 27.30	L: 27.30
Navel	74.93	
Hips	81.28	
Thighs	R: 57.15	L: 57.15
Calves	R: 35.56	L: 35.56

YOUR WEEKLY TESTS

Weight (kg)	
Height (cm)	
BMI	
RHR	
BP	
Fat (%)	

Measurements (cm)

Neck		
Chest		
Arms	R:	L:
Navel		
Hips		
Thighs	R:	L:
Calves	R:	L:

WEEK **EIGHT** NUTRITION PLAN **WEEK 8**

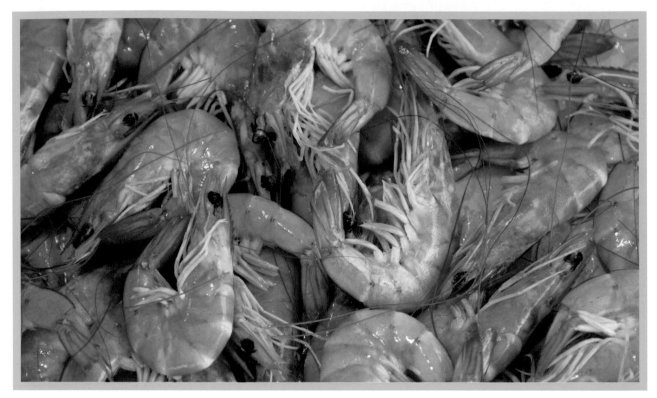

WEEK 8 OVERVIEW

Day	Breakfast	Lunch	Dinner
1	Fresh fruit with seeds	Sweet potato and bean salad	Mackerel and pine nut salad
2	Fruit porridge	Tuna and olive salad	Broccoli and chicken stir fry
3	Muesli with fresh fruit	Vegetable soup	Teriyaki burgers
4	Fruit smoothie 1	Beef salad pitta	Chilli prawns with almonds
5	Fresh fruit and seeds	Mackerel and potato salad	Mustard chicken
6	Omelette	Smoked salmon pitta	Garlic salmon with baked vegetables
7	Wheat biscuits or muesli with fruit	Tuna salad	Lamb casserole

SHOPPING LIST **WEEK 8**

CARBOHYDRATES
80g almonds
1 bag of brown rice
1 bag of couscous
400g kidney beans
240g of muesli
1 bag of pine nuts
125g new potatoes
400g pinto beans
560g porridge oats
12 potatoes
1 bag of sunflower seeds
1 bag of pumpkin seeds
8 sweet potatoes
8 wholemeal/brown pitta breads
Wheat biscuits

DAIRY AND NON-DAIRY ALTERNATIVES
12 eggs
20g feta/goat's cheese
50g soft goat's/low fat cream cheese
880ml skimmed/ soya/rice/oat milk
1.7kg soya yoghurt

FISH
8 anchovy fillets
4 whole mackerel scaled/gutted
225g fresh mackerel
800g cooked prawns
4 salmon fillets
1 pack smoked salmon (for four people)
1.15kg tuna steaks
4 tinned tuna cans

MEAT
500g lean minced beef
400g cooked roast beef
8 chicken breasts
400g lean ham
800g leg of lamb

FRUIT
4 apples
1 apricot
8 bananas
1 punnet of blackberries
1 punnet of blueberries
3 lemons
2 limes
2 mangos
1 melon
2 oranges
1 peach
1 large pineapple
1 punnet of raspberries

VEGETABLES
2 avocados
600g baby spinach
25g black olives
75g broccoli
250g cherry tomatoes
3 carrots
1 celery stick
1 courgette
½ cucumber
175g French beans
2 leeks
3 lettuces
50g mangetout
5 onions
2 parsnips
115g plum tomatoes
3 red onions
4 red peppers
23 tomatoes
100g rocket salad
1 shallot
10 spring onions

HERBS
Basil
2 bay leaves
Black pepper
Chives
Coriander
Cumin
Fresh ginger
1 garlic bulb
Parsley
2 red chillies
Rosemary

OTHER
Balsamic vinegar
Chicken stock
Chinese rice wine
Cold-pressed extra virgin olive oil
Corn flour
Dijon mustard
Light soy sauce
Peanut oil
60ml red wine
Sesame oil
Soy sauce
Brown sugar
400g tinned tomatoes
Tomato purée
Vegetable stock
White wine vinegar
Wholegrain mustard

SNACKS
Fruit
Wholegrain crispbread crackers
Flat breads
Small bowl of muesli
Yoghurt/soya yoghurt
Nuts (cashew, pine or occasionally mixed nuts)
Soya nuts
Seeds (pumpkin or sunflower)

FRUIT DRINKS
1 carton fruit juice

RECIPES **WEEK 8** DAY 1

BREAKFAST FRESH FRUIT AND SEEDS

See page 81

LUNCH SWEET POTATO AND BEAN SALAD

4 cooked sweet potatoes

4 eggs

2 avocados, stoned and peeled

400g tinned kidney beans

400g tinned pinto beans

Coriander, large handful chopped

250g cherry tomatoes, halved

1 small red onion, finely sliced

1 Preheat oven to 190°C (375°F).
2 Boil eggs for 6½ minutes, then place in cold water to cool slightly.
3 Cut the sweet potatoes into small chunks and drizzle with a tablespoon of olive oil and place into oven for 30–40 minutes.
4 Slice avocados and place in bowl with beans, sweet potatoes, onions, coriander and tomatoes.
5 Mix the olive oil, lime juice, chilli and cumin in a small bowl.
6 Once eggs have cooled but are still warm, peel off the shells and cut into quarters.
7 Toss the salad with the dressing, place the eggs on top and serve.

DINNER MACKEREL AND PINE NUT SALAD

4 whole mackerel, scaled and gutted

1 clove of garlic, peeled and sliced

4 tablespoon parsley, chopped

4 spring onions, trimmed and chopped

3 tablespoons pine nuts

1 lemon, zest of

Salad of your choice

1 Preheat the grill to high and cover the grill tray with tin foil.
2 Make two incisions in the side of each mackerel and fill with garlic and parsley and place on a tray.
3 Mix the spring onions, pine nuts and lemon zest in a small bowl and use to stuff the cavity of the mackerel.
4 Place fish under the hot grill and cook for 3–4 minutes on each side or until cooked.
5 Remove the mackerel from the grill and allow to cool for a few minutes. Serve with salad.

RECITES **WEEK 8** DAY 2

BREAKFAST FRUIT PORRIDGE *See page 80*

LUNCH TUNA AND OLIVE SALAD *See page 80*

DINNER BROCCOLI AND CHICKEN STIR FRY

800g skinless chicken breasts, diced

1 head broccoli, broken into florets

1 tablespoon ginger, freshly grated

1 clove garlic, crushed

1 onion, quartered

1 red pepper, deseeded and sliced

2 tablespoons water

2 teaspoons Chinese rice wine

1 tablespoon soy sauce

2 teaspoons corn flour

1 teaspoon sesame oil

1 tablespoon peanut oil

Brown rice

1 Bring a small saucepan of water to the boil and blanch the broccoli for 2 minutes. Drain, and allow to cool.
2 In a cup, mix together the water, Chinese rice wine, soy sauce and corn flour and set aside.
3 Heat a wok or large frying pan over a medium heat.
4 Add sesame and peanut oil, and once smoking add the ginger and garlic and cook for a few seconds, stirring continuously.
5 Add the chicken and stir fry for 6–8 minutes, or until cooked. Remove from wok and set aside.
6 Boil the rice. Add the onion and red pepper to frying pan and stir fry for 5 minutes, or until vegetables begin to soften.
7 Next add the broccoli and corn flour, and stir until sauce has thickened.
8 Return chicken to the frying pan and heat through. Serve with brown rice.

Lunch for tomorrow:
VEGETABLE SOUP
See the following page and consider preparing your lunch in advance.

RECITES **WEEK 8** DAY 3

BREAKFAST MUESLI WITH FRESH FRUIT *See page 79*

LUNCH VEGETABLE SOUP

See page 99

DINNER TERIYAKI BURGERS

500g lean minced beef

2 tablespoons light soy sauce

1 tablespoon fresh ginger, peeled and grated

1 garlic clove, minced

¼ cup onions, chopped

Pinch of pepper

4 baking potatoes, sliced into wedges

Lettuce leaves

3 tomatoes, sliced

1 small red onion, sliced

20g goat's or mature cheese, 5g per person

1. Preheat oven to 190°C (373 F).
2. Boil the potato wedges until partially tender.
3. Place wedges on a baking tray and drizzle over extra virgin olive oil.
4. Cook in the oven until crisp and golden.
5. Combine all the ingredients for the burgers in a bowl.
6. Form into 4–8 patties and grill for 5 minutes one side then turn over.
7. Place the cheese on the uncooked side and cook for a further 5 minutes or until cheese has melted.

RECIPES **WEEK 8** DAY 4

BREAKFAST FRUIT SMOOTHIE 1

See page 85

LUNCH BEEF SALAD PITTA

See page 100

DINNER CHILLI PRAWNS WITH ALMONDS

1 red chilli, finely chopped

1 tablespoon olive oil

1 onion, chopped

2 garlic cloves, roughly chopped

8 tomatoes, roughly chopped

1 teaspoon ground cumin

100ml chicken stock

80g ground almonds

150ml soya/plain yoghurt

1. Heat the olive oil in a frying pan over a medium heat.
2. Add the garlic, chilli and onion and cook until soft.
3. Next add the tomatoes and ground cumin and cook for 10 minutes, stirring occasionally.
4. Add the stock to the mixture and blend in a food processor until smooth.
5. Pour the mixture into a large saucepan, adding the ground almonds, and stir over a low heat for 2 minutes.

800g cooked peeled prawns

1 lime

Brown rice and vegetables of your choice

6 Gently stir in the yoghurt.
7 Squeeze the juice from the lime and stir into sauce.
8 Increase the heat and simmer.
9 Add the prawns and heat for 2–3 minutes until warmed through.
10 Serve with brown rice and vegetables.

Lunch for tomorrow:
MACKEREL AND POTATO SALAD
Consider preparing the potatoes in advance.

RECIPES **WEEK 8** DAY 5

BREAKFAST FRESH FRUIT AND SEEDS

See page 81

LUNCH MACKEREL AND POTATO SALAD

See page 137

DINNER MUSTARD CHICKEN

1 tablespoon olive oil

4 chicken breasts, fat removed

2 large oranges, peeled and cut into segments (reserve the juice)

2 teaspoons cornflour

150ml soya/plain yoghurt

1 teaspoon wholegrain mustard

Parsley to garnish

Couscous, salad or vegetables of your choice

1 Heat the olive oil in a large frying pan and add the chicken breasts.
2 Cook over a medium to high heat for 5 minutes on each side, or until tender and the juices run clear.
3 Season with black pepper, then remove chicken from frying pan and cover with foil and keep warm.
4 Pour the orange juice into a bowl and stir in the corn flour to make a smooth paste.
5 Stir in yoghurt and mustard then pour into the frying pan. Bring to the boil over a low heat while stirring.
6 Add the orange segments to the frying pan and season to taste with pepper.
7 Stir in the juices from the chicken. Spoon the sauce on to four large plates and top with chicken.
8 Serve with salad or vegetables and couscous, and garnish with parsley.

RECIPES **WEEK 8** DAY 6

BREAKFAST OMELETTE   *See page 86*

LUNCH SMOKED SALMON PITTA   *See page 79*

DINNER GARLIC SALMON WITH BAKED VEGETABLES

2 leeks, washed, trimmed and sliced

500g baby spinach leaves

4 × 100g salmon fillets

1 tablespoon olive oil

2 garlic cloves, peeled and finely chopped

1 tablespoon fresh ginger, grated

1 lemon, juice of

Coriander to garnish

Couscous

1   Preheat the oven to 200°C (400°F).
2   Gently boil or steam the leeks for 5 minutes.
3   Arrange the spinach leaves in a baking tray, then add the leeks and place salmon on top.
4   Mix together the olive oil, garlic and ginger in a small bowl and brush mixture over the salmon using pastry brush.
5   Pour over the lemon juice, place in the oven and cook for 10 minutes.
6   Boil and cook couscous.
7   Remove from oven and leave to cool for a few minutes.
8   Serve with couscous and garnish with fresh coriander.

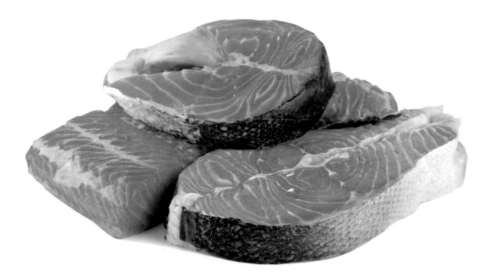

RECIPES **WEEK 8** DAY 7

BREAKFAST WHEAT BISCUITS OR
MUESLI WITH FRUIT

See page 82

LUNCH TUNA SALAD

See page 134

DINNER LAMB CASSEROLE

800g lean lamb leg, diced

2 tablespoons olive oil

1 onion, finely chopped

1 carrot, finely chopped

1 celery stick, finely chopped

2 cloves garlic, crushed

60ml red wine

2 tablespoons tomato purée

450ml chicken stock

1 bay leaf

2 sprigs rosemary

2 parsnips, peeled and chopped

2 tablespoons parsley

New potatoes

1 Preheat oven to 180°C (350°F).
2 Heat a large saucepan over a high heat.
3 Coat lamb with olive oil and cook in small batches for 5 minutes or until browned.
4 Remove from pan and set aside.
5 Add the onion, carrot, celery to the pan and cook for 5 minutes, or until soft.
6 Next, return lamb to pan adding the garlic, red wine and tomato purée and cook for a further 5 minutes.
7 Add the chicken stock, bay leaf, rosemary and enough water to ensure lamb is covered.
8 Cover with lid and bake in the oven for 1 hour.
9 Add the parsnips and cook for a further 40 minutes.
10 Serve with potatoes and sprinkle with parsley.

TRAINING DIARY **WEEK 8**

WEEK 8 OVERVIEW
Day 1: CV – run
Day 2: Rest
Day 3: Weights – upper body
Day 4: Rest
Day 5: CV – cycle
Day 6: Myo lymphatic massage; CV – cycle PT
Day 7: Tests
Any day: Myo stretch

ALISON'S DIARY

Day 1 (Monday)
After Gavin told me some home truths yesterday and put me back on the right track, I was feeling really positive.
Tiredness 5
Stress 3
Sleep 6 hours 45 minutes

Day 2 (Tuesday)
Day off today. I'm feeling really good in myself and ready for the final four weeks, as I really want to show Gavin and myself that I can completed the 12 weeks and look amazing..
Tiredness 3
Stress 2
Sleep 8 hours

Day 3 (Wednesday)
I had a workout before heading up to London with Gavin. Had a really nice meal out and a look around the local sights.
Tiredness 3
Stress 4
Sleep 7 hours

Day 4 (Thursday)
In London all day today and did lots of walking around, but I am having a bit of a low day as I am not fitting my clothes comfortably and I can still see and feel my rolls of fat.
Tiredness 3
Stress 3
Sleep 6 hours

Day 5 (Friday)
Came back from London this morning. I had my cycle and PT session in the evening before going to see my family.
Tiredness 3
Stress 2
Sleep 7 hours

Day 6 (Saturday)
I had the day off work and managed to fit in a lymphatic massage before I had my workout.
Tiredness 3
Stress 1
Sleep 7 hours

Day 7 (Sunday)
Test day today, and I'm feeling really nervous. After all the tests I am really pleased with my results and I can't believe that Gavin was right. My results were even better than they would have been if I hadn't had a bad week 7. This has really boosted my confidence and I'm ready for the final weeks to come.
Tiredness 2
Stress 3
Sleep 7 hours 30 minutes

TRAINING SESSION **WEEK 8** DAY 1

ALISON'S SESSION

AM Rest

PM **Training session** CV – Run

Time trained 7.00–8.00 p.m.

Session time 58 minutes

RPE 8/10

WORKOUT
Run: 5 miles
Actual distance: 4.95 miles
Time: 58 minutes 42seconds
Average pace: 11.40 m/m

Alison's notes: Had a lovely run in the beautiful sunshine along the beach and coast. The first two miles were quite comfortable but I started to struggle after this, had to stop for a drink and get my breath back. Weather a bit too hot to train in, but it was such a beautiful day.

YOUR SESSION

AM

PM **Training session** CV – Run

Time trained

Session time   hour(s)   minutes

RPE   /10

WORKOUT
Run: 5 miles
Actual distance: miles
Time: minutes
Average pace: m/m

Your notes:

TRAINING SESSION **WEEK 8** DAY 3

ALISON'S SESSION

AM Rest

PM Training session Weights – Upper body

Time trained 1.00–2.00 p.m.

Session time 1 hour

RPE 8/10

YOUR SESSION

AM

PM Training session Weights – Upper body

Time trained

Session time   hour(s)   minutes

RPE   /10

WORKOUT

Lat pull-down
Set and Rep: 1. 20   2. 15   3. 15   4. 15   5. 15
Weight (kg):   –   10   15   20   20

Close grip pull-down
Set and Rep: 1. 15   2. 15   3. 12
Weight (kg): 10   10   10

Front arm raise
Set and Rep: 1. 15   2. 15   3. 12
Weight (kg): 10   10   10

Lat raise
Set and Rep: 1. 15   2. 15   3. 12
Weight (kg): 10   10   10

¾ Regular press-ups
1–8 and 8–1
Total: 72

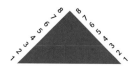

Single arm cable cross overs
Set and Rep: 1. 15   2. 15   3. 12
Set and Rep: 1. 15   2. 15   3. 12

WORKOUT

Lat pull-down
Set and Rep: 1.   2.   3.   4.   5.
Weight (kg):

Close grip pull-down
Set and Rep: 1.   2.   3.
Weight (kg):

Front arm raise
Set and Rep: 1.   2.   3.
Weight (kg):

Lat raise
Set and Rep: 1.   2.   3.
Weight (kg):

¾ Regular press-ups
        and
Total:

Single arm cable cross overs
Set and Rep: 1.   2.   3.
Weight (kg):

Superset

	Dumbbell arm curl			Triceps press-downs		
Sets	1.	2.	3.	1.	2.	3.
Reps	10	10	10	10	10	10
Weight (kg)	52.5	52.5	52.5	10	10	10

Half sit-ups
4 × 25

Reverse curls
4 × 25

Heel taps
4 × 25

Notes: This is a great upper body workout, brilliant for toning. Keep the weights moderate so that you are failing at about 15 reps to get the best out of this workout.

Superset

	Dumbbell arm curl			Triceps press-downs		
Sets	1.	2.	3.	1.	2.	3.
Reps						
Weight (kg)						

Half sit-ups
×

Reverse curls
×

Heel taps
×

Your notes:

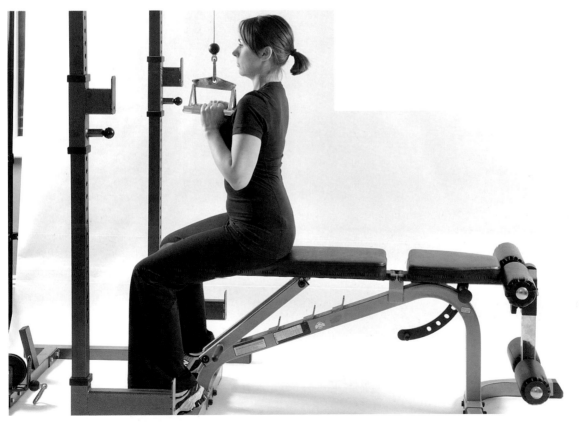

TRAINING SESSION **WEEK 8** DAY 5

ALISON'S SESSION

AM Training session CV – Cycle

Time trained 10.00–11.15 a.m.

Session time 1 hour 15 minutes

RPE 9/10

PM Rest

WORKOUT
Cycle: 10 miles
Actual distance: 10.2 miles

Glute and core workout
Half sit-ups
4 × 15
Leg levers
4 × 15
Dorsal raise
4 × 15
Glute extensions
4 × 15
Dirty dogs
4 × 15

Notes: Alison was still feeling full of energy after the cycle ride outside, so the abdominal exercises were added in to get the most out of the workout.

YOUR SESSION

AM **Training session** CV – Cycle

Time trained

Session time   hour(s)   minutes

RPE   /10

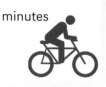

PM

WORKOUT
Cycle: 10 miles
Actual distance: miles

Glute and core workout
Half sit-ups
        ×
Leg levers
        ×
Dorsal raise
        ×
Glute extensions
        ×
Dirty dogs
        ×

Your notes:

TRAINING SESSION **WEEK 8** DAY 6

ALISON'S SESSION

AM **Training session** CV – Cycle PT

Time trained 10.00–11.15 a.m.

Session time 1 hour 15 minutes

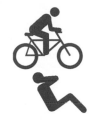

RPE 9/10

Average RPM 80–100

PM Rest

WORKOUT

Cycle for 10 minutes first to warm up.

Each cycle will last for 2 minutes 30 seconds at a specified resistance level, Level 1 being easy and Level 5 being hard (like a hill).

Once you have finished the cycle, move on to the exercise just below it with as little rest as possible. Complete all three sets on that exercise before moving on to the next cycle and level.

Cycle: 10 minutes

Cycle at Level 1: (easy)
RPM: 100 for 2 mins 30 secs
Half sit-ups
(reps and sets): 1. 25   2. 25   3. 25

Cycle – Level 2
Reverse curls
(reps and sets): 1. 25   2. 25   3. 25

Cycle – Level 3
Jumping oblique twists
(reps and sets): 1. 25   2. 25   3. 25

YOUR SESSION

AM **Training session** CV – Cycle PT

Time trained

Session time   hour(s)   minutes

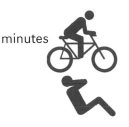

RPE   /10

Average RPM 80–100

PM

WORKOUT

Cycle: 10 minutes

Cycle at Level 1: (easy)
RPM: 100 for 2 mins 30 secs
Half sit-ups
(reps and sets): 1.   2.   3.

Cycle – Level 2
Reverse curls
(reps and sets): 1.   2.   3.

Cycle – Level 3
Jumping oblique twists
(reps and sets): 1.   2.   3.

Cycle – Level 4
Oblique side crunches
(reps and sets): 1. 15   2. 15   3. 15

Cycle – Level 5: (hard) RPM: 80–90
Reverse crunch
(reps and sets): 1. 25   2. 25   3. 25

Cycle – Level 5: (hard) RPM: 80–90
Reverse crunch
(reps and sets): 1. 25   2. 25   3. 25

Cycle – Level 4
Oblique side crunches
(reps and sets): 1. 15   2. 15   3. 15

Cycle – Level 3
Jumping oblique twists
(reps and sets): 1. 25   2. 25   3. 25

Cycle – Level 2
Reverse curls
(reps and sets): 1. 25   2. 25   3. 25

Cycle – Level 1 (easy) RPM: 100
Half sit-ups
(reps and sets): 1. 25   2. 25   3. 25

Notes: Alison rested for no longer than one minute between each cycle and exercise, but as an average she rested for around 40 seconds. This is a brilliant leg, bum and tum workout.

Cycle – Level 4
Oblique side crunches
(reps and sets): 1.   2.   3.

Cycle – Level 5: (hard) RPM: 80–90
Reverse crunch
(reps and sets): 1.   2.   3.

Cycle – Level 5: (hard) RPM: 80–90
Reverse crunch
(reps and sets): 1.   2.   3.

Cycle – Level 4
Oblique side crunches
(reps and sets): 1.   2.   3.

Cycle – Level 3
Jumping oblique twists
(reps and sets): 1.   2.   3.

Cycle – Level 2
Reverse curls
(reps and sets): 1.   2.   3.

Cycle – Level 1 (easy) RPM: 100
Half sit-ups
(reps and sets): 1.   2.   3.

Your notes:

WEEK 8 TESTS

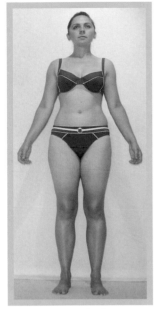 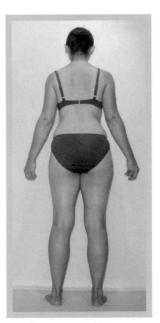

Front view of Alison at the end of week 8.

Back view of Alison at the end of week 8.

ALISON'S WEEKLY TESTS

Weight (kg)	53.5
Height (cm)	157.3
BMI	21.6
RHR	58
BP	110/66
Fat (%)	26.3

Measurements (cm)

Neck	29.84	
Chest	83.18	
Arms	R: 27.30	L: 27.30
Navel	74.29	
Hips	80.01	
Thighs	R: 55.88	L: 55.88
Calves	R: 35.56	L: 35.56

YOUR WEEKLY TESTS

Weight (kg)	
Height (cm)	
BMI	
RHR	
BP	
Fat (%)	

Measurements (cm)

Neck		
Chest		
Arms	R:	L:
Navel		
Hips		
Thighs	R:	L:
Calves	R:	L:

WEEK 8 HEALTH CHECK

ALISON'S RESULTS

Statistics

Weight (kg)	53.5
Height (cm)	157.3

Health tests

BMI	21.6
RHR	58
BP	110/66
Fat (%)	26.3
Glucose	3.8
Cholesterol	3.9
Lung function	420

Measurements (cm)

Neck	29.84	
Chest	83.18	
Arms	R: 27.30	L: 27.30
Navel	74.29	
Hips	80.01	
Thighs	R: 55.88	L: 55.88
Calves	R: 35.56	L: 35.56

Calliper test (mm)

Biceps	6
Triceps	12
Waist	8
Subscapularis	12
Total	38
Calliper fat (%)	26.1

Fitness tests

Bleep test (20m) level	6.7

Maximum reps in one minute

¾ push-ups	35
½ sit-ups	60
Squats	59
Dips	51
Max pull-ups	2.5

YOUR RESULTS

Statistics

Weight (kg)	
Height (cm)	

Health tests

BMI	
RHR	
BP	
Fat (%)	
Glucose	
Cholesterol	
Lung function	

Measurements (cm)

Neck		
Chest		
Arms	R:	L:
Navel		
Hips		
Thighs	R:	L:
Calves	R:	L:

Calliper test (mm)

Biceps	
Triceps	
Waist	
Subscapularis	
Total	
Calliper fat (%)	

Fitness tests

Bleep test (20m) level	

Maximum reps in one minute

¾ push-ups	
½ sit-ups	
Squats	
Dips	
Max pull-ups	

WEEK NINE NUTRITION PLAN **WEEK 9**

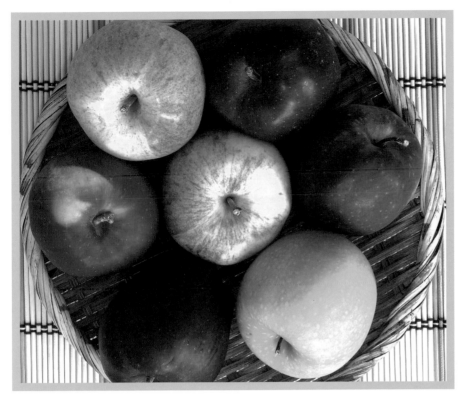

WEEK 9 OVERVIEW

Day	Breakfast	Lunch	Dinner
1	Fresh fruit and seeds	Beetroot salad	Coconut monkfish
2	Fruit smoothie 2	Yellow split pea soup	Chicken with coriander
3	Muesli with fresh fruit	Egg salad	Cajun fish
4	Wheat biscuits or muesli with fruit	Salmon salad	Thai beef salad
5	Fruit porridge	Tuna salad	Spicy tomato chicken
6	Omelette	Butternut squash and coriander soup	Salmon with asparagus
7	Fruit salad	Chicken salad pitta	Ginger turkey curry

SHOPPING LIST **WEEK 9**

CARBOHYDRATES

1 bag of brown rice
1 bag of couscous
260g of muesli
560g porridge oats
1 bag of sunflower seeds
1 bag of pumpkin seeds
5 sweet potatoes
4 wholemeal/brown pitta breads
225g yellow split peas
1 bag of wild rice
Wheat biscuits

DAIRY AND NON-DAIRY ALTERNATIVES

12 eggs
2105ml skimmed/soya/rice/oat milk
2kg soya yoghurt

FISH

6 anchovy fillets
450g monkfish tails
225g raw peeled prawns
4 poached salmon fillets
200g × 4 salmon steaks
4 tins of tuna
800g white fish of your choice

MEAT

800g rump beef steak
500g boneless chicken breasts
8 chicken breasts
400g lean ham
400g turkey breast

FRUIT

8 apples
2 apricots
6 bananas
1 punnet of blackberries
1 punnet of blueberries
4 lemons
2 limes
1 melon
2 oranges
2 peaches
1 large pineapple
1 punnet of raspberries

VEGETABLES

16 asparagus spears
1 avocado
1 baby gem lettuce
350g baby spinach
150g bean sprouts
4 cooked beetroots
1.4kg butternut squash
650g cherry tomatoes
5 carrots
2 celery sticks
1 courgette
1½ cucumbers
3 lettuce
50g mangetout
4 onions
3 red onions
4 red peppers
5 red tomatoes
100g rocket salad
5 shallots
13 spring onions
5 yellow peppers

HERBS

Chilli powder
Chives
Coriander
Ground coriander
Cumin
Curry powder
Fresh ginger
1 garlic bulb
1 green chilli
Mint
Nutmeg
Paprika
Parsley
1 red chilli
Rosemary
Turmeric

OTHER

Balsamic vinegar
Chicken stock
Cider vinegar
150ml coconut milk
Cold-pressed extra virgin olive oil
Corn flour
Dijon mustard
Fish sauce
Honey
115ml lemon juice
8 wooden skewers
Soy sauce
Tomato purée
Vegetable stock
Worcestershire sauce

SNACKS

Fruit
Wholegrain crispbread crackers
Flat breads
Small bowl of muesli
Yoghurt/soya yoghurt
Nuts (cashew, pine or occasionally mixed nuts)
Soya nuts
Seeds (pumpkin or sunflower)

FRUIT DRINKS

1 carton fruit juice

RECIPES **WEEK 9** DAY 1

BREAKFAST FRESH FRUIT AND SEEDS   *See page 81*

LUNCH BEETROOT SALAD   *See page 96*

DINNER COCONUT MONKFISH

450g monkfish tails, cut into chunks

225g raw peeled prawns

1 red pepper, chunks to go on to skewers

1 yellow pepper, chunks to go on to skewers

1 red onion, chunks to go on to skewers

For the marinade:

1 teaspoon olive oil

½ small onion, finely grated

1 teaspoon fresh ginger, grated

150ml canned coconut milk

2 tablespoons fresh coriander, chopped

Serve with salad and couscous

1 To make the marinade, heat the olive oil in a large saucepan and fry the onion and ginger for 5 minutes, or until just soft (not browned).
2 Add the coconut milk to the saucepan and bring to the boil.
3 Boil rapidly for 5 minutes then remove from heat and allow to cool completely.
4 Once cold, stir the coriander into the coconut milk and pour into a shallow dish.
5 Gently stir in monkfish and prawns into the coconut mixture and cover.
6 Leave to marinate in the fridge for 1–4 hours.
7 Preheat grill to medium.
8 Thread the fish and prawns on to skewers with the red onion and peppers.
9 Cook the skewers under the preheated grill for 10–15 minutes, turning frequently.
10 Garnish with toasted desiccated coconut and serve on a bed of salad and couscous.

Lunch for tomorrow:
YELLOW SPLIT PEA SOUP
Pre-soak the yellow split peas overnight in cold water.

RECIPES **WEEK 9** DAY 2

BREAKFAST FRUIT SMOOTHIE 2   *See page 157*

LUNCH YELLOW SPLIT PEA SOUP   *See page 151*

DINNER CHICKEN WITH CORIANDER

1 tablespoon olive oil

4 skinless, boneless chicken breasts 115g each, fat removed

1 teaspoon corn flour

1 tablespoon water

100ml soya/plain yoghurt

175ml chicken stock

2 tablespoons lime juice

2 garlic cloves, finely chopped

1 tomato, peeled, deseeded and chopped

1 shallot, finely chopped

Fresh coriander, 1 bunch chopped

Salad of your choice

1. Heat the olive oil in a large frying pan, then add the chicken and cook over medium heat for 5 minutes each side or until cooked.
2. Remove chicken from frying pan and keep warm.
3. Mix the corn flour and water until smooth. Stir in the yoghurt.
4. Pour the chicken stock and lime juice into frying pan and add the garlic and shallot.
5. Reduce the heat and simmer for 1 minute, then add the tomato and stir into mixture.
6. Cook and stir constantly for 1–2 minutes. Do not let the mixture boil.
7. Stir in the fresh coriander.
8. Serve the chicken with the salad, pour sauce over and garnish with fresh coriander.

Lunch for tomorrow:
EGG SALAD
Consider boiling the eggs in advance.

RECIPES **WEEK 9** DAY 3

BREAKFAST MUESLI WITH FRESH FRUIT

See page 79

LUNCH EGG SALAD

See page 118

DINNER CAJUN FISH

225ml soya/skimmed milk

800g white fish fillets (snapper, whiting, flathead etc.)

2 tablespoons olive oil

400g soya/plain yoghurt

½ cucumber, finely diced

1. Preheat oven to 200°C (400°F).
2. Line a baking tray with baking paper.
3. Pour the milk into a small bowl. In a separate bowl mix the ground spices.
4. Dip the fish fillets into the milk then roll in the mixed spices.
5. Heat the olive oil in a large frying pan over a high heat and fry the fish quickly in batches,

Salad of your choice

Spices:

1 tablespoon paprika

2 teaspoons ground cumin

1 teaspoon chilli powder

for 2 minutes each side, or until golden. Be careful not overcrowd the pan, as the fish will stew.

6 Place the fish fillets on the baking tray and bake for 5 minutes.

7 Mix soya/plain yoghurt and cucumber to make the dressing.

8 Serve the fish with salad and pour over the yoghurt dressing.

RECIPES **WEEK 9** DAY 4

BREAKFAST WHEAT BISCUITS OR MUESLI WITH FRUIT

See page 82

LUNCH SALMON SALAD

See page 119

DINNER THAI BEEF SALAD

800g lean rump steak

1 tablespoon olive oil

For the salad:

100g spinach leaves

1 red pepper, deseeded and finely sliced

150g bean sprouts

4 spring onions, finely sliced

125g fresh coriander

2 tablespoons mint, chopped

For the dressing:

2 tablespoons lime juice

1 tablespoon fish sauce

1 tablespoon soy sauce

1 clove garlic, crushed

1 red chilli, deseeded and chopped

1 Preheat the grill to high.

2 Brush the steak with olive oil and cook for 3–4 minutes each side, or cook to your liking.

3 Remove from the heat and cover steak with tin foil and leave to rest for 5 minutes.

4 Meanwhile, mix all the dressing ingredients in a small bowl.

5 Slice the steak across the grain into thin strips. Place the beef and remaining ingredients in a large bowl.

6 Pour dressing over the salad, gently toss and serve.

Lunch for tomorrow:
TUNA SALAD
Consider preparing the sweet potatoes in advance.

RECIPES **WEEK 9** DAY 5

BREAKFAST FRUIT PORRIDGE

See page 80

LUNCH TUNA SALAD

See page 134

DINNER SPICY TOMATO CHICKEN

500g boneless chicken breasts, diced

3 tablespoons tomato purée

2 tablespoons clear honey

2 tablespoons Worcestershire sauce

1 tablespoon rosemary, chopped

250g cherry tomatoes

8 wooden skewers

Salad of your choice

1 Mix the tomato purée, honey, Worcestershire sauce and rosemary together in a bowl.
2 Add the diced chicken and coat evenly.
3 Preheat the grill to medium.
4 Thread the chicken and the cherry tomatoes on to the wooden skewers and place them on grill rack.
5 Spoon the honey mixture over the chicken skewers and grill for 8–10 minutes, turning occasionally until chicken is cooked through.
6 Serve with a salad.

RECIPES **WEEK 9** DAY 6

BREAKFAST OMELETTE

See page 86

LUNCH BUTTERNUT SQUASH AND CORIANDER SOUP

See page 87

DINNER SALMON WITH ASPARAGUS

400g butternut squash, peeled and cut into thick slices

1 tablespoon olive oil

4 × 200g salmon fillets

16 asparagus spears

1 To make relish, place all the relish ingredients except olive oil in a food processor and lightly process.
2 Add olive oil to form a thick paste.
3 Preheat oven to 180°C (350°F).
4 Place the butternut squash in a bowl and coat with half the amount of olive oil.

For the relish:

Fresh parsley, 1 bunch

6 anchovy fillets

2 lemons, grated zest

115ml lemon juice

60ml olive oil

5 Transfer to baking dish and cook for 20 minutes or until soft.
6 Meanwhile, turn grill to high and lightly brush the salmon with the remaining olive oil.
7 Place salmon in grill and cook for 4 minutes on each side.
8 Remove from heat, cover and set aside.
9 Bring a saucepan of water to the boil, add the asparagus and blanch for 2 minutes, then drain.
10 Arrange the salmon, asparagus and butternut squash slices on a serving plate and serve.

RECIPES **WEEK 9** DAY 7

BREAKFAST FRUIT SALAD

See page 84

LUNCH CHICKEN SALAD PITTA

See page 120

DINNER GINGER TURKEY CURRY

400g turkey fillet

½ tablespoon olive oil

1 onion, sliced

1 green chilli, finely sliced

12cm ginger, peeled and sliced

1 clove garlic, peeled and chopped

3 teaspoons curry powder

300ml chicken or vegetable stock

300g brown or wild rice

Coriander, big bunch

5 tablespoons soya/plain yoghurt

1 Heat the olive oil and add the onion, ginger, chilli and garlic. Cook on medium heat for 10 minutes.
2 Slice the turkey into small pieces, add to the pan with curry powder and cook for 5 minutes.
3 Add the stock, bring to the boil and simmer for 15 minutes.
4 Cook the rice on a medium heat for 15–20 minutes or until cooked.
5 Stir the yoghurt and chopped coriander through the turkey curry and serve with the rice.

Lunch for tomorrow:
BUTTERNUT SQUASH AND CORIANDER SOUP
Consider preparing your lunch in advance.

TRAINING DIARY **WEEK 9**

WEEK 9 OVERVIEW
Day 1: Weights – lower body; myo cellulite
       massage
Day 2: CV – run
Day 3: Rest – myo massage
Day 4: Weights – upper body
Day 5: CV – walk; CV – cycle PT
Day 6: Circuits
Day 7: Rest
Any day: Myo stretch

ALISON'S DIARY

Day 1 (Monday)
I was on such a high from yesterday's test results, especially the bleep test. I felt strong in my session today. and it's good to hit the area that plays on my mind, – my thighs and hips.
Tiredness 2
Stress 3
Sleep 8 hours

Day 2 (Tuesday)
I had a very hard run today in stormy conditions. It was really windy, which made it hard for me to breathe so I did need to stop for a little breather.
Tiredness 3
Stress 5
Sleep 7 hours

Day 3 (Wednesday)
Had a really good massage today to keep my body on track. I'm not feeling as stressed as I was yesterday, and this is really helping me keep focus on the end goal.
Tiredness 3
Stress 3
Sleep 8 hours

Day 4 (Thursday)
I had such a miserable day at work, nothing was going right and the people I was working with were hard work. I finished work late and then just wanted to go to sleep.
Tiredness 4
Stress 5
Sleep 8 hours 45 minutes

Day 5 (Friday)
I'm really enjoying the workouts now and I can feel it all working. We had a long workout today but I wanted to go for a walk first.
Tiredness 3
Stress 4
Sleep 6 hours

Day 6 (Saturday)
A very boring day at work. When I finished work Gavin took me out for the evening to cheer me up and have some fun.
Tiredness 3
Stress 3
Sleep 8 hours

Day 7 (Sunday)
Got up early to do all the tests and pictures before heading off to a theme park for the day. My results are now really starting to look good.
Tiredness 3
Stress 2
Sleep 6 hours

TRAINING SESSION **WEEK 9** DAY 1

ALISON'S SESSION

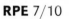 **AM** Rest

PM **Training session** Weights – Lower body

Time trained 12.45–1.30p.m.

Session time 45 minutes

RPE 7/10

YOUR SESSION

 AM

PM **Training session** Weights – Lower body

Time trained

Session time   hour(s)   minutes

RPE   /10

WORKOUT

Complete 90 reps for all the following exercises.

With regard to the rests between sets and exercises, try to limit them. If you can, complete all 90 reps in one go.

Below is how Alison broke down the 90 reps for each exercise. We tried to limit the rest to 5–10 seconds.

Glute extensions
10, 15, 20, 20, 15, 10

Dirty dogs
10, 15, 20, 20, 15, 10

Squats: weight 15lb
90

Lunges: (static, each leg) weight 15lb
30, 20, 20, 20

Wide squat thrust
30, 30, 30

Squat thrust
30, 30, 30

WORKOUT

Glute extensions

Dirty dogs

Squats:

Lunges:

Wide squat thrust

Squat thrust

Standing oblique twists
30, 30, 30

Leg levers
10, 20, 30, 20, 10

Half sit-ups
30, 30, 30

Heel taps
30, 30, 30

Reverse curls
30, 30, 30

Alison's notes: This was a great workout for my legs and bum. I tried to break them up by mixing the exercises together for a bit for variety.

Standing oblique twists

Leg levers

Half sit-ups

Heel taps

Reverse curls

Your notes:

TRAINING SESSION **WEEK 9** DAY 2

ALISON'S SESSION

AM Rest

PM Training session CV – Run

Time trained 8.00–8.48 p.m.

Session time 48 minutes

RPE 8/10

WORKOUT
Run: 4 miles
Actual distance: 4.25 miles
Time: 47.30 minutes
Average pace: 11.12 m/m

Alison's notes: Tonight was such a moody evening, very stormy. The wind came in handy on the first half of the run blowing behind me, it gave me a very false confidence in my running ability because when I turned back and the wind was in my face I soon realised that I hardly had any running ability at all.

Notes: On this run, we were trying to get the pace (minute/miles) down as much as possible by concentrating on putting maximum effort into how fast we could run the four miles.

YOUR SESSION

AM

PM   Training session CV – Run

Time trained

Session time   hour(s)   minutes

RPE   /10

WORKOUT
Run: 4 miles
Actual distance: miles
Time: minutes
Average pace: m/m

Your notes:

TRAINING SESSION **WEEK 9** DAY 4

ALISON'S SESSION

AM Training session Weights – Upper body

Time trained 9.30–10.50 a.m.

Session time 1 hour 20 minutes

RPE 8/10

PM Rest

YOUR SESSION

AM **Training session** Weights – Upper body

Time trained

Session time   hour(s)   minutes

RPE   /10

PM

WORKOUT

Dumbbell press
Set and Rep: 1. 15   2. 15   3. 15   4. 15   5. 13
Weight (lb):   5.5   10   12.5   15

Bench press
Set and Rep: 1. 12   2. 12   3. 8   4. 6
Weight (kg):   bar   bar   2.5   2.5

Deadlift
Set and Rep: 1. 12   2. 12   3. 12   4. 12
Weight (kg):   bar   5   10   15

Superset

	Pec fly			Incline dumbbell press		
Sets	1.	2.	3.	1.	2.	3.
Reps	15	15	15	15	15	15
Weight (kg)	7.5	7.5	7.5	7.5	7.5	7.5

Superset

	Lat pull-down			Low pull		
Sets	1.	2.	3.	1.	2.	3.
Reps	12	12	15	12	15	15
Weight (kg)	10	10	10	10	10	10

WORKOUT

Dumbbell press
Set and Rep: 1.   2.   3.   4.   5.
Weight (kg):

Bench press
Set and Rep: 1.   2.   3.   4.
Weight (kg):

Deadlift
Set and Rep: 1.   2.   3.   4.
Weight (kg):

Superset

	Pec fly			Incline dumbbell press		
Sets	1.	2.	3.	1.	2.	3.
Reps						
Weight (kg)						

Superset

	Lat pull-down			Low pull		
Sets	1.	2.	3.	1.	2.	3.
Reps						
Weight (kg)						

Superset

	Bent-over lat raise			Arm haulers		
	1.	2.	3.	1.	2.	3.
Sets						
Reps	15	15	15	25	25	25
Weight (kg)	5	5	5			

Alison's notes: Wow!

Notes: This is one of the longest weights sessions Alison has done so far (and will ever have to do). It's tough but also satisfying.

Superset

	Bent-over lat raise			Arm haulers		
	1.	2.	3.	1.	2.	3.
Sets						
Reps						
Weight (kg)						

Your notes:

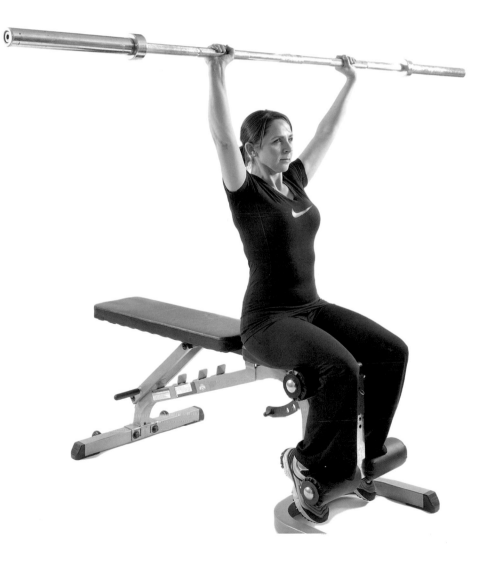

TRAINING SESSION **WEEK 9** DAY 5

ALISON'S SESSION

AM Rest

PM Training session CV – Walk

Time trained 5.00–5.45 p.m.

Session time 45 minutes

RPE 6/10

PM Training session CV – Cycle PT

Time trained 5.45–6.45 p.m.

Session time 1 hour

RPE 6/10

WORKOUT

Once you have finished your walk go straight into the cycle PT. If, however, you do not have time to do both workouts in one go, break them down so you walk in the morning and cycle in the afternoon.

Walk: 3 miles
Actual distance: 3 miles
Time: 45 minutes
Average pace: 15 m/m

Cycle PT

Start off by cycling for 10 minutes then move into the superset exercises. Perform all the sets stated for each of the exercises before moving on to the next 10 minute cycle.

Cycle 10 minutes
Average RPM: 80–100

YOUR SESSION

AM

PM Training session CV – Walk

Time trained

Session time   hour(s)   minutes

RPE   /10

PM Training session CV – Cycle PT

Time trained

Session time   hour(s)   minutes

RPE /10

WORKOUT

Walk: 3 miles
Actual distance: miles
Time: minutes
Average pace: m/m

Cycle PT

Cycle 10 minutes
Average RPM: 80–100

Superset

	Stiff leg deadlifts			Squats		
Sets	1.	2.	3.	1.	2.	3.
Reps	15	15	15	15	15	15
Weight (kg)	20	20	20	20	20	20

Cycle 10 minutes

Superset

	Glute extension			Dirty dogs		
Sets	1.	2.	3.	1.	2.	3.
Reps	15	15	15	15	15	15

Cycle 10 minutes

Superset

	Calf raise			Lunges, static		
Sets	1.	2.	3.	1.	2.	3.
Reps	20	20	20	15	15	15
Weight (kg)	15	15	15	15	15	15

Superset

	Stiff leg deadlifts			Squats		
Sets	1.	2.	3.	1.	2.	3.
Reps						
Weight (kg)						

Cycle 10 minutes

Superset

	Glute extension			Dirty dogs		
Sets	1.	2.	3.	1.	2.	3.
Reps						

Cycle 10 minutes

Superset

	Calf raise			Lunges, static		
Sets	1.	2.	3.	1.	2.	3.
Reps						
Weight (kg)						

Your notes:

TRAINING SESSION **WEEK 9** DAY 6

ALISON'S SESSION

AM Rest

PM Training session Circuits

Time trained 7.00–7.50 p.m.

Session time 50 minutes

RPE 9/10

WORKOUT

Complete cycle 1 first, then cycle 2, and finally cycle 3. You have 1 minute and 30 seconds for each exercise.

Cycle 1
1. Squat
2. Half sit-up
3. Dumbbell press
4. Lunge static
5. Full sit-up
6. Lat raise
7. Stiff leg deadlifts
8. Crunch
9. Arm hauler

Cycle 2
1. Press-ups
2. Reverse curls
3. Alt squat thrusts
4. Dumbbell bench press
5. Leg levers
6. Squat thrusts
7. Incline fly
8. Reverse crunch
9. Wide squat thrust

YOUR SESSION

AM

PM Training session Circuits

Time trained

Session time   hour(s)   minutes

RPE   /10

WORKOUT

Cycle 1
1. Squat
2. Half sit-up
3. Dumbbell press
4. Lunge static
5. Full sit-up
6. Lat raise
7. Stiff leg deadlifts
8. Crunch
9. Arm hauler

Cycle 2
1. Press-ups
2. Reverse curls
3. Alt squat thrusts
4. Dumbbell bench press
5. Leg levers
6. Squat thrusts
7. Incline fly
8. Reverse crunch
9. Wide squat thrust

Cycle 3
1. Oblique side crunch
2. Frog hops
3. Dips
4. Jumping oblique twist
5. Jump overs
6. Supinated curl
7. Heel taps
8. Star jumps
9. Burpees

Notes: Try not to count the number of reps you are performing, just keep going for the time specified. The weight Alison used was 10lb throughout.

Cycle 3
1. Oblique side crunch
2. Frog hops
3. Dips
4. Jumping oblique twist
5. Jump overs
6. Supinated curl
7. Heel taps
8. Star jumps
9. Burpees

Your notes:

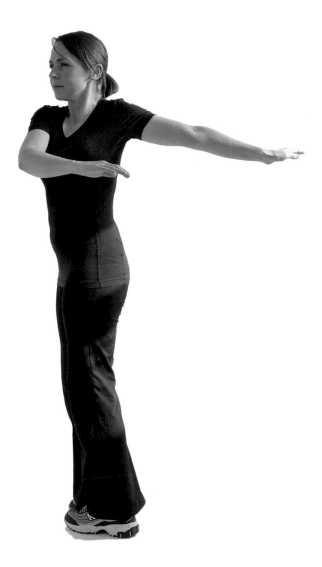

WEEK 9 TESTS

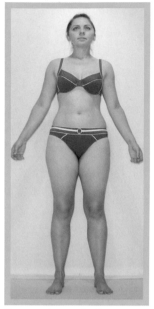 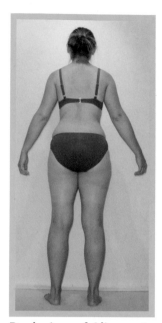

Front view of Alison at the end of week 9.

Back view of Alison at the end of week 9.

ALISON'S WEEKLY TESTS

Weight (kg)	53.5
Height (cm)	157.3
BMI	21.6
RHR	55
BP	110/58
Fat (%)	24.8

Measurements (cm)

Neck	29.84	
Chest	83.18	
Arms	R: 27.30	L: 27.30
Navel	73.66	
Hips	80.01	
Thighs	R: 55.24	L: 55.24
Calves	R: 35.56	L: 35.56

YOUR WEEKLY TESTS

Weight (kg)	
Height (cm)	
BMI	
RHR	
BP	
Fat (%)	

Measurements (cm)

Neck		
Chest		
Arms	R:	L:
Navel		
Hips		
Thighs	R:	L:
Calves	R:	L:

WEEK TEN NUTRITION PLAN WEEK 10

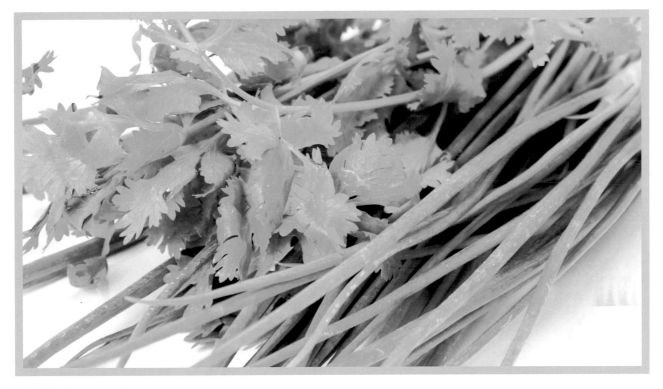

WEEK 10 OVERVIEW

Day	Breakfast	Lunch	Dinner
1	Fruit porridge	Butternut squash and coriander soup	Swordfish with courgette salad
2	Fruit salad	Beetroot salad	Baked lamb and vegetables
3	Muesli with fresh fruit	Beef salad pitta	Poached chicken
4	Wheat biscuits or muesli with fruit	Chicken wrap	Marlin steaks
5	Fresh fruit and seeds	Tuna and olive salad	Baked Mediterranean vegetables with ricotta and turkey
6	Omelette	Vegetable soup	Monkfish delight
7	Fruit smoothie 1	Tuna salad	Garlic lamb

SHOPPING LIST **WEEK 10**

CARBOHYDRATES
1 bag of brown rice
1 bag of couscous
240g of muesli
560g porridge oats
1 bag of sunflower seeds
1 bag of pumpkin seeds
4 sweet potatoes
4 organic tortilla wraps
4 wholemeal/brown pitta breads
1 bag of wild rice
Wheat biscuits

DAIRY AND NON-DAIRY ALTERNATIVES
8 eggs
200g ricotta cheese/goat's cheese
680ml skimmed/soya/rice/oat milk
1.5kg soya yoghurt

FISH
8 anchovy fillets
350g cod or haddock
4 marlin steaks
350g monkfish
16 large raw prawns
4 × 200g swordfish steaks
350g tuna steaks
4 small tins of tuna

MEAT
400g cooked roast beef
8 chicken breasts
400g lean ham
350g boneless lamb
800g rack of lamb
4 turkey breasts

FRUIT
6 apples
1 apricot
8 bananas
1 punnet of blackberries
4 lemons
2 limes
2 mangos
2 oranges
1 peach
1 large pineapple
1 punnet of raspberries
1 watermelon

VEGETABLES
2 aubergines
200g baby carrots
4 cooked beetroots
1kg butternut squash
24 black olives
4 carrots
8 celery sticks
8 courgettes
1 cucumber
175g French beans
200g green beans
1 green pepper
2 lettuces
50g mangetout
6 onions
200g peas
4 red onions
4 red peppers
22 red tomatoes
115g baby plum tomatoes
100g rocket salad
4 shallots
10 spring onions
2 yellow peppers

HERBS
Basil
Black pepper
Chilli powder
Chives
Cinnamon sticks
Cumin
Fresh ginger
1 garlic bulb
1 green chilli
Mint
Nutmeg
Oregano
Paprika
Parsley
Rosemary
Tarragon
4 thyme sprigs
Turmeric

OTHER
150g dried apricots
Balsamic vinegar
Chicken stock
Chinese rice wine
Cold-pressed extra virgin olive oil
Dijon mustard
Fish stock
Honey
Light soy sauce
Plain flour
Soy sauce
Brown sugar
Tabasco sauce
400g tinned tomatoes
Vegetable stock

SNACKS
Fruit
Wholegrain crispbread crackers
Flat breads
Small bowl of muesli
Yoghurt/soya yoghurt
Nuts (cashew, pine or occasionally mixed nuts)
Soya nuts
Seeds (pumpkin or sunflower)

FRUIT DRINKS
1 carton fruit juice

RECIPES **WEEK 10** DAY 1

BREAKFAST FRUIT PORRIDGE

See page 80

LUNCH BUTTERNUT SQUASH AND CORIANDER SOUP

See page 87

DINNER SWORDFISH WITH COURGETTE SALAD

4 × 200g swordfish steaks

1 tablespoon olive oil

Lemon wedges

2 tablespoons fresh parsley, chopped

Couscous

For the salad:

2 teaspoons olive oil

2 tablespoons lemon juice

½ red onion, finely sliced

12 olives (optional)

3 small courgettes

1 To make salad, combine the olive oil, lemon juice, onion and olives in a bowl.
2 Steam the courgettes until tender.
3 Transfer to salad mixture and toss to coat.
4 Boil and cook couscous.
5 Heat a non-stick frying pan over a medium heat, brush swordfish steaks with oil and pan fry for 2 minutes on each side.
6 Toss the parsley through courgette salad and spoon on to serving plates.
7 Place swordfish on top of salad and serve with couscous and lemon wedges to garnish.

RECIPES **WEEK 10** DAY 2

BREAKFAST FRUIT SALAD

See page 84

LUNCH BEETROOT SALAD

See page 96

DINNER BAKED LAMB AND VEGETABLES

1 tablespoon olive oil

4 thyme sprigs, chopped

1 tablespoon tarragon, chopped

1 tablespoon parsley, chopped

1 clove garlic

800g rack of lamb (200g per person), fat removed

1 lemon, zest finely grated

200g baby carrots

200g green beans

200g peas

1 Preheat oven to 200°C (400°F).
2 In a bowl mix half the oil with herbs, garlic and lemon zest.
3 Heat a large frying pan over a high heat.
4 Coat lamb in remaining oil and sear until golden on both sides.
5 Transfer to a baking dish, rub herb mixture into lamb rack and bake for 25 minutes.
6 Remove from oven, cover loosely with foil and set aside for 10 minutes.
7 Bring a large saucepan of water to the boil and cook carrots for 2 minutes, adding the beans and peas for a further 4 minutes.
8 Drain and serve with the lamb.

RECIPES **WEEK 10** DAY 3

BREAKFAST MUESLI WITH FRESH FRUIT

See page 79

LUNCH BEEF SALAD PITTA

See page 100

DINNER POACHED CHICKEN

2 tablespoons light soy sauce

1 tablespoon Chinese rice wine

2cm piece fresh ginger, sliced

1 tablespoon coriander

6 spring onions, finely sliced

1 litre of chicken stock

4 skinless chicken breasts

Brown rice and vegetables

1 In a large saucepan bring the soy sauce, Chinese rice wine, ginger, coriander, four of the spring onions and chicken stock to the boil.
2 Add the chicken, then reduce the heat and simmer for 12 minutes.
3 Remove from heat and allow chicken to rest in liquid for 5 minutes.
4 Slice chicken thickly and place on serving plate.
5 Pour liquid from saucepan over the chicken and sprinkle the rest of the spring onions over.
6 Serve with rice and vegetables.

RECIPES **WEEK 10** DAY 4

BREAKFAST WHEAT BISCUITS OR
MUESLI WITH FRUIT   *See page 82*

LUNCH CHICKEN WRAP   *See page 115*

DINNER MARLIN STEAKS

4 marlin steaks

For the dressing:

100ml olive oil

2 limes, juiced

1 clove of garlic, crushed

1 tablespoon parsley, of chopped

½ teaspoon dried oregano

1 tablespoon olive oil

Generous amounts of vegetables of
your choice

1. For the dressing, place the olive oil in a mixing bowl and slowly whisk in 70ml of hot water and lime juice.
2. Add the garlic, parsley and oregano and whisk until smooth.
3. Heat the olive oil in a large frying pan on high heat.
4. Add the marlin steaks and cook for 3 minutes on each side.
5. Serve with vegetables and drizzle the dressing over the top.

RECIPES **WEEK 10** DAY 5

BREAKFAST FRESH FRUIT
AND SEEDS   *See page 81*

LUNCH TUNA AND OLIVE SALAD   *See page 80*

DINNER BAKED MEDITERRANEAN VEGETABLES WITH RICOTTA AND TURKEY

1 red pepper, halved and deseeded

1 yellow pepper, halved and deseeded

4 courgettes, finely sliced lengthways

1 aubergine, finely sliced

1 tablespoon olive oil

1 clove garlic, crushed

2 small red onions, finely sliced

4 plum tomatoes, diced

115g fresh basil

200g low fat ricotta cheese or goat's cheese

4 turkey breasts

1 Preheat the oven to 180°C (350°F).
2 Place peppers, skin-side up, in a baking dish, drizzle with a little olive oil and roast for 20 minutes.
3 Remove from oven, cover with foil and allow to cool slightly.
4 Slice flesh into thick strips.
5 Preheat grill to high.
6 In a bowl toss the courgette and aubergine with half the oil. Grill vegetables until soft.
7 Heat the remaining oil in a large non-stick frying pan over a high heat. Add the garlic and onion and cook until soft.
8 Arrange vegetables, including tomatoes and basil, in layers in a non-stick baking dish.
9 Crumble ricotta cheese over the top and bake for 30 minutes.
10 Grill turkey breasts on medium heat for 8–12 minutes, or until cooked. Keep turning.
11 Serve the turkey with vegetables and ricotta cheese.

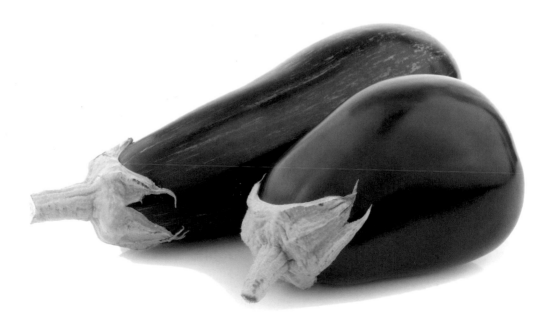

RECIPES **WEEK 10** DAY 6

BREAKFAST OMELETTE

See page 86

LUNCH VEGETABLE SOUP

See page 99

DINNER MONKFISH DELIGHT

16 large raw prawns, peeled

350g cod or haddock fillet, skinned and diced

350g monkfish, diced

2 onions, finely chopped

4 celery sticks, finely chopped

2 tablespoons plain flour

700ml fish stock

1 red pepper, deseeded and chopped

1 green pepper, deseeded and chopped

2 large tomatoes, chopped

1 tablespoon olive oil

1 garlic clove, crushed

½ teaspoon brown sugar

1 teaspoon ground cumin

4 tablespoons parsley, chopped

1 tablespoon fresh coriander, chopped

Dash Tabasco sauce

Brown or basmati rice

1. Heat the olive oil in a large saucepan. Add the onion and celery and cook for 5 minutes (stir occasionally).
2. Add the garlic and cook for 1 minute.
3. Next, stir in the flour, sugar and cumin and cook for 2 minutes – keep stirring.
4. Gradually stir in the fish stock and bring to the boil, stirring constantly.
5. Boil the rice.
6. Add the peppers and tomatoes to the saucepan and partially cover. Reduce the heat to very low and simmer gently for 10 minutes. Stir occasionally.
7. Add the parsley, coriander and Tabasco sauce and then gently stir in the fish and peeled prawns.
8. Cover and simmer gently for 5 minutes or until the fish is cooked through and the prawns have changed colour.
9. Gently mix and transfer to serving plates.
10. Serve with rice.

RECIPES **WEEK 10** DAY 7

BREAKFAST FRUIT SMOOTHIE 1   *See page 85*

LUNCH TUNA SALAD   *See page 134*

DINNER GARLIC LAMB

1 tablespoon olive oil

1 onion, chopped

350g lean boneless lamb, diced

600ml vegetable stock

1 orange, grated zest and juice

1 aubergine, halved lengthways and sliced thinly

4 tomatoes, chopped

115g no-soak dried apricots

1 garlic clove, finely chopped

1 teaspoon clear honey

1 cinnamon stick

1 cm piece ginger, finely chopped

2 tablespoons fresh coriander, chopped

Brown rice

1 Heat the olive oil in a large frying pan over a medium heat.
2 Add the onions and lamb cubes, stirring frequently, for 5 minutes, or until meat is slightly browned all over.
3 Add the garlic, vegetable stock, orange zest and juice, honey, cinnamon stick and ginger and bring to boil.
4 Reduce the heat, cover and simmer for 45 minutes.
5 Add the aubergine, tomatoes and apricots.
6 Cover and cook for a further 45 minutes, or until lamb is tender.
7 Stir in the coriander and season with black pepper.
8 Serve immediately with brown rice.

Lunch for tomorrow:
CHICKEN PITTA
Consider preparing the chicken in advance.

TRAINING DIARY **WEEK 10**

WEEK 10 OVERVIEW
Day 1: Weights – upper body
Day 2: CV – run
Day 3: Rest
Day 4: CV – cycle
Day 5: Weights – legs; myo cellulite massage
Day 6: Circuits
Day 7: Rest
Any day: Myo stretch

ALISON'S DIARY

Day 1 (Monday)
I was exhausted from yesterday's fun, but unfortunately had to go back to work. Gavin has surprised me and booked a holiday for after we finish the 12-week programme I now have another goal to aim for and that is to look even better for my holiday.
Tiredness 4
Stress 3
Sleep 5 hours 45 minutes

Day 2 (Tuesday)
I went and saw my family today, and on the way back I popped in to see a friend of mine. Also ran 5 miles.
Tiredness 3
Stress 1
Sleep 7 hours

Day 3 (Wednesday)
I'm really achy today after yesterday's run and Monday's weights session.
Tiredness 3
Stress 1
Sleep 6 hours

Day 4 (Thursday)
I cycled to Christchurch to see my sister and then back, but Gavin put in some detours so when I got home I was tired and my legs felt like jelly.
Tiredness 4
Stress 2
Sleep 8 hours

Day 5 (Friday)
I got up and had breakfast, but I didn't feel like it. I had my cellulite massage before I went into the leg workout. By the time I finished I only had another couple of hours before I had to go to work so I sat out in the sun.
Tiredness 3
Stress 2
Sleep 7 hours 30 minutes

Day 6 (Saturday)
I finished work early today so I could spend some more time with Gavin.
Tiredness 2
Stress 2
Sleep 8 hours 15 minutes

Day 7 (Sunday)
Test day and had lost a lot of weight. I only have two weeks to go and I can see the end now. I went out for a meal tonight to celebrate my test results.
Tiredness 3
Stress 2
Sleep 7 hours 45 minutes

TRAINING SESSION **WEEK 10** DAY 1

ALISON'S SESSION

AM Rest

PM Training session Weights – Upper body

Time trained 5.30–6.40 p.m.

Session time 1 hour 10 minutes

RPE 9/10

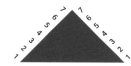

WORKOUT

This is a high-rep workout to help tone your muscles which you have developed by now.

Regular pull-ups
1–7 and 7–1
Total: 56

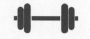

Note: This is quite a tough session due to the high reps to target each muscle group.

Dumbbell press
Set and Rep:	1. 30	2. 20	3. 20	4. 20	5. 20
Weight (lb):	5	12.5	12.5	12.5	12.5

Triceps kickbacks
Set and Rep:	1. 30	2. 20	3. 20	4. 20
Weight (lb):	10	10	10	10

¾ press-ups
Set and Rep:	1. 30	2. 20	3. 20	4. 20

Dumbbell arm curl
Set and Rep:	1. 30	2. 20	3. 20	4. 20
Weight (lb):	12.5	12.5	12.5	12.5

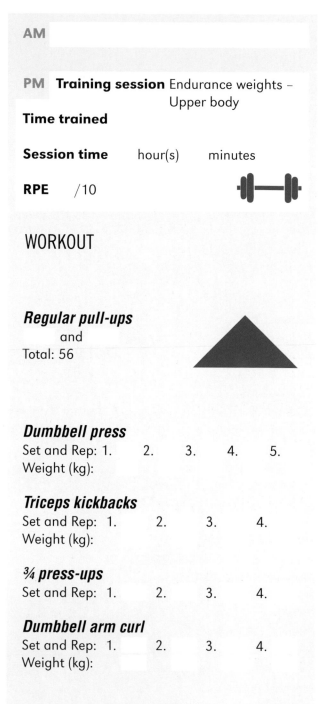

YOUR SESSION

AM

PM Training session Endurance weights – Upper body

Time trained

Session time   hour(s)   minutes

RPE   /10

WORKOUT

Regular pull-ups
          and
Total: 56

Dumbbell press
Set and Rep: 1.	2.	3.	4.	5.
Weight (kg):				

Triceps kickbacks
Set and Rep: 1.	2.	3.	4.
Weight (kg):			

¾ press-ups
Set and Rep: 1.	2.	3.	4.

Dumbbell arm curl
Set and Rep: 1.	2.	3.	4.
Weight (kg):			

¾ wide press-ups
Set and Rep: 1. 30   2. 20   3. 20   4. 20

Half sit-ups
4 × 20

Reverse curls
4 × 20

¾ wide press-ups
Set and Rep: 1.   2.   3.   4.

Half sit-ups
        ×

Reverse curls
        ×

Your notes:

TRAINING SESSION **WEEK 10** DAY 2

ALISON'S SESSION

AM Rest

PM Training session CV – Run

Time trained 7.00–7.55 p.m.

Session time 55 minutes

RPE 0/10

YOUR SESSION

AM

PM   Training session CV – Run

Time trained

Session time   hour(s)   minutes

RPE   /10

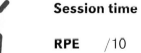

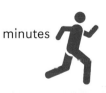

WORKOUT
Run: 5 miles
Actual distance: 5 miles
Time: 54.10 minutes
Average pace: 10.50 m/m

WORKOUT
Run: 5 miles
Actual distance: miles
Time: minutes
Average pace: m/m

Alison's notes: I really enjoyed this run. It was a beautiful day with a slight breeze, which was really refreshing. This was definitely a good running day for me.

Notes: On this run, we are trying to get the pace (minute/miles) down as much as possible by concentrating on putting maximum effort into how fast we can run the 5 miles.

Your notes:

TRAINING SESSION **WEEK 10** DAY 4

ALISON'S SESSION

AM Training session CV – Cycle

Time trained 10–11.55 a.m.

Session time 1 hour 55 minutes

RPE 9/10

PM Rest

WORKOUT

Cycle: 15 miles
Actual Distance: 16.0 miles

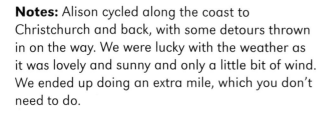

Notes: Alison cycled along the coast to Christchurch and back, with some detours thrown in on the way. We were lucky with the weather as it was lovely and sunny and only a little bit of wind. We ended up doing an extra mile, which you don't need to do.

YOUR SESSION

AM Training session CV – Cycle

Time trained

Session time   hour(s)   minutes

RPE   /10

PM

WORKOUT

Cycle: 15 miles
Actual Distance: miles

Your notes:

TRAINING SESSION **WEEK 10** DAY 5

ALISON'S SESSION

AM Training session Weights – Legs

Time trained 11.00–11.30 a.m.

Session time 30 minutes

RPE 6/10

PM Rest

WORKOUT

Bosu squats (bosu upside down)
1 × 20 warm-up with just Olympic bar
Set and Rep: 1. 16   2. 16   3. 16   4. 16   5. 16

Stiff leg deadlifts
Set and Rep: 1. 12   2. 12   3. 12   4. 12
Weight (lb):   15   15   15   15

Standing glute extensions
Set and Rep: 1. 10   2. 12   3. 14   4. 16

Standing hip abduction
Set and Rep: 1. 10   2. 12   3. 14   4. 16

Squats
As deep as you can go on the squats with no weight
Set and Rep: 1. 16   2. 16   3. 16

Calf raises
Set and Rep: 1. 20   2. 20   3. 20   4. 20

Leg levers
Set and Rep: 1. 20   2. 20   3. 20   4. 20

YOUR SESSION

AM Training session Weights – Legs

Time trained

Session time   hour(s)   minutes

RPE   /10

PM

WORKOUT

Bosu squats
1 × 20 warm-up with just Olympic bar
Set and Rep: 1.   2.   3.   4.   5.

Stiff leg deadlifts
Set and Rep: 1.   2.   3.   4.
Weight (kg):

Standing glute extensions
Set and Rep: 1.   2.   3.   4.

Standing hip abduction
Set and Rep: 1.   2.   3.   4.

Squats

Set and Rep: 1.   2.   3.

Calf raises
Set and Rep: 1.   2.   3.   4.

Leg levers
Set and Rep: 1.   2.   3.   4.

Superset

	Reverse crunch			Reverse curls		
Sets	1.	2.	3.	1.	2.	3.
Reps	25	25	25	25	25	25

Alison's notes: This was a really good leg and bum workout, I felt really good doing it and even better after I had finished as it all felt tighter.

Superset

	Reverse crunch			Reverse curls		
Sets	1.	2.	3.	1.	2.	3.
Reps						

Your notes:

TRAINING SESSION **WEEK 10** DAY 6

ALISON'S SESSION

AM Training session Circuits

Time trained 10.00–11.05 a.m.

Session time 1 hour 5 minutes

RPE 10/10

PM Rest

YOUR SESSION

AM Training session Circuits

Time trained

Session time   hour(s)   minutes

RPE   /10

PM

WORKOUT

Complete cycle 1 first, then move on to cycle 2, and finally cycle 3.

Follow the tables opposite by doing the exercises in the first set, then complete the exercises in the second set, third set and finally fourth set. You will notice as you go through the sets, the reps increase.

WORKOUT

CYCLE 1

Exercises	Set 1	Set 2	Set 3	Set 4
Half sit-ups	10	20	30	40
Step-ups	10	20	30	40
Skipping	30 secs	1 min	1 min 30	2 mins
Bosu squats	10	20	30	40
Arm haulers	10	20	30	40

CYCLE 2

Exercises	Set 1	Set 2	Set 3	Set 4
Oblique side crunch	10	20	30	40
Side lunge	10	20	30	40
Skipping	30 secs	1 min	1 min 30	2 mins
Wide squat thrusts	10	20	30	40
Pull-ups (regular)	3	6	9	12

CYCLE 3

Exercises	Set 1	Set 2	Set 3	Set 4
Reverse curls	10	20	30	40
Back lunges	10	20	30	40
Skipping	30 secs	1 min	1 min 30	2 mins
Alt squat thrusts	10	20	30	40
¾ press-ups	10	20	30	40

Alison's notes: Wow, what a workout, I don't think there was one muscle that wasn't worked in this one. You need to focus your mind on something else other than counting though – get someone else to count if possible.

CYCLE 1

Exercises	Set 1	Set 2	Set 3	Set 4
Half sit-ups				
Step-ups				
Skipping				
Bosu squats				
Arm haulers				

CYCLE 2

Exercises	Set 1	Set 2	Set 3	Set 4
Oblique side crunch				
Side lunge				
Skipping				
Wide squat thrusts				
Pull-ups (regular)				

CYCLE 3

Exercises	Set 1	Set 2	Set 3	Set 4
Reverse curls				
Back lunges				
Skipping				
Alt squat thrusts				
¾ press-ups				

Your notes:

WEEK 10 TESTS

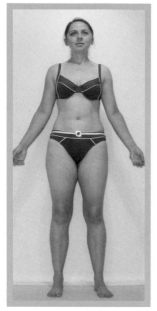

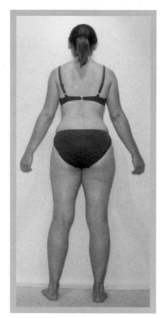

Front view of Alison at the end of week 10.

Back view of Alison at the end of week 10.

ALISON'S WEEKLY TESTS

Weight (kg)	53	
Height (cm)	157.3	
BMI	21.4	
RHR	57	
BP	115/60	
Fat (%)	23.8	
Measurements (cm)		
Neck	28.57	
Chest	83.18	
Arms	R: 26.67	L: 26.67
Navel	73.66	
Hips	80.01	
Thighs	R: 53.97	L: 53.97
Calves	R: 34.92	L: 34.92

YOUR WEEKLY TESTS

Weight (kg)		
Height (cm)		
BMI		
RHR		
BP		
Fat (%)		
Measurements (cm)		
Neck		
Chest		
Arms	R:	L:
Navel		
Hips		
Thighs	R:	L:
Calves	R:	L:

WEEK **ELEVEN** NUTRITION PLAN **WEEK 11**

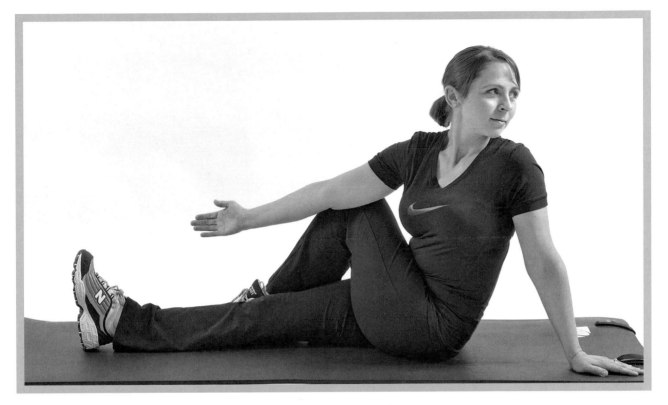

WEEK 11 OVERVIEW

Day	Breakfast	Lunch	Dinner
1	Fresh fruit and seeds	Chicken salad pitta	Fennel and halibut parcels
2	Scrambled eggs with wild mushrooms	Tuna salad	Mint chicken and lime
3	Muesli with fresh fruit	Yellow split pea soup	Mango and rum snapper
4	Fruit porridge	Salmon salad	Stuffed peppers
5	Fruit salad	Egg salad	Lamb curry with spinach
6	Omelette	Tomato and pepper soup	Hungarian goulash
7	Fruit smoothie 1	Chicken wrap	Chilli prawn salad

SHOPPING LIST **WEEK 11**

CARBOHYDRATES

1 bag of couscous
240g of muesli
560g porridge oats
1 bag of sunflower seeds
1 bag of pumpkin seeds
225g yellow split peas
5 sweet potatoes
4 organic tortilla wraps
4 wholemeal/brown pitta breads
1 bag of wild rice
Wheat biscuits

DAIRY AND NON-DAIRY ALTERNATIVES

13 eggs
40g feta/goats cheese
280g low fat fromage frais
680ml skimmed/soya/rice/oat milk
2kg soya yoghurt

FISH

8 anchovy fillets
4 halibut steaks
200g jumbo raw prawns
4 poached salmon fillets
500g red snapper
4 tins of tuna

MEAT

8 chicken breasts
8 boneless chicken thighs
800g lean braising streaks
400g lean ham
800g lean lamb leg

FRUIT

6 apples
2 apricot
10 bananas
1 punnet of blackberries
4 lemons
2 limes
3 mangos
1 melon
2 oranges
3 peaches
1 punnet of raspberries

VEGETABLES

1 avocado
1 baby gem lettuce
600g baby spinach
125g broccoli
12 button mushrooms
3 carrots
8 celery sticks
400g cherry tomatoes
2 cos lettuce
3 courgettes
1 cucumber
1 fennel bulb
2 green peppers
2 leeks
2 lettuces
50g mangetout
8 large wild mushrooms
335g mushrooms
8 onions
1 red onion
5 red peppers
18 red tomatoes
100g rocket salad
10 spring onions
750g tomatoes
10 yellow peppers

HERBS

Basil
1 bay leaf
Black pepper
Caraway seeds
Cardamon seeds
Chives
Ground cinnamon
Cumin
Garam masala
Fresh ginger
1 garlic bulb
Marjoram
Mint
Paprika
Parsley
2 red chillies
Thyme
Turmeric

OTHER

Balsamic vinegar
Cider vinegar
Cold-pressed extra virgin olive oil
Dijon mustard
Fish stock
Honey
Plain flour
Dark rum
800g tinned tomatoes
Tomato purée
Vegetable stock
75ml white wine

SNACKS

Fruit
Wholegrain crispbread crackers
Flat breads
Small bowl of muesli
Yoghurt/soya yoghurt
Nuts (cashew, pine or occasionally mixed nuts)
Soya nuts
Seeds (pumpkin or sunflower)

FRUIT DRINKS

1 carton fruit juice

RECIPES **WEEK 11** DAY 1

BREAKFAST FRESH FRUIT AND SEEDS

See page 81

LUNCH CHICKEN SALAD PITTA

See page 120

DINNER FENNEL AND HALIBUT PARCELS

4 halibut steaks (175g each)

2 leeks, cut into thin strips

2 courgettes, cut into thin slices

2 carrots, cut into thin slices

1 fennel bulb, halved and cut into thin strips

115g/4oz mushrooms, thinly sliced

4 teaspoons olive oil

4 tablespoons white wine

Vegetables of your choice

1 Preheat oven to 190°C (375°F).
2 Cut out four 30cm squares of baking paper and spread out on a work surface.
3 Divide the leeks, courgettes, carrots, fennel and mushroom equally between the paper squares.
4 Top each bed of vegetables with a halibut steak.
5 Fold up the edges of the paper, but do not seal.
6 Drizzle 1 teaspoon of olive oil and 1 tablespoon of white wine over each fish steak.
7 Fold over the edges of the paper to seal to make a loosely wrapped parcel.
8 Place the parcels on a large baking sheet and bake in the oven for 10–15 minutes or until parcels are puffed and fish is cooked.
9 Transfer to plates and serve with vegetables.

Lunch for tomorrow:
TUNA SALAD
See the following page and consider preparing the sweet potatoes in advance.

RECIPES **WEEK 11** DAY 2

BREAKFAST SCRAMBLED EGGS WITH WILD MUSHROOMS

See page 98

LUNCH TUNA SALAD

See page 134

DINNER MINT CHICKEN AND LIME

8 lean, boneless chicken thighs

Salad of your choice

For the marinade:

3 tablespoons fresh mint, finely chopped

4 tablespoons clear honey

2 tablespoons lime juice

For the sauce:

150g low fat natural soya/plain yoghurt

1 tablespoon fresh mint, finely chopped

2 teaspoons lime zest, finely grated

1 Mix the honey, mint and lime juice in a large bowl.
2 Add chicken to marinade and evenly coat both sides.
3 Cover with cling film and leave the chicken to refrigerate for at least 30 minutes, longer if possible.
4 Remove the chicken and reserve the marinade. Preheat the grill to medium.
5 Place the chicken on the grill tray and cook under a hot grill for 15–18 minutes, or until chicken is tender and cooked. Turn the chicken frequently and keep covering chicken with marinade.
6 Meanwhile, mix all the sauce ingredients together in a bowl.
7 Serve the chicken with the salad and use the remaining marinade for dipping.

Lunch for tomorrow:
YELLOW SPLIT PEA SOUP
Pre-soak the yellow split peas overnight in cold water.

RECIPES WEEK 11 DAY 3

BREAKFAST MUESLI WITH FRESH FRUIT

See page 79

LUNCH YELLOW SPLIT PEA SOUP

See page 151

DINNER MANGO AND RUM SNAPPER

2 tablespoons dark rum

50ml white wine

1 tablespoon ginger, finely chopped

1 clove garlic, finely chopped

1 Mix the rum, wine, ginger and garlic in a large, shallow, non-metallic dish and add the fish to the marinade.
2 Cover with cling film and leave in the refrigerator to marinate for 30 minutes.

500g red snapper fillets, cut into 4cm pieces

1 onion, cut into wedges

1 tablespoon olive oil

2 tablespoons plain flour

2 teaspoons tomato purée

500ml fish stock

2 large tomatoes, roughly chopped

1 mango, peeled, stoned and roughly chopped

1 red pepper, deseeded and roughly chopped

Basmati rice

Remove using a slotted spoon and reserve the marinade.

3 Boil the rice.
4 Heat the olive oil in a large saucepan, add the onion wedges and cook over a medium heat, stirring occasionally for 5 minutes.
5 Stir in the flour and add the tomato purée and red pepper.
6 Gradually stir in the fish stock and the reserved marinade and bring to boil, stirring continuously.
7 Reduce the heat and simmer for a further 3 minutes.
8 Add the fish, tomatoes and mango to the saucepan and cover.
9 Simmer for 8 minutes or until fish is cooked, then serve with rice.

RECIPES **WEEK 11** DAY 4

BREAKFAST FRUIT PORRIDGE

See page 80

LUNCH SALMON SALAD

See page 119

DINNER STUFFED PEPPERS

4 yellow peppers, halved lengthways and deseeded

150g baby spinach leaves

1 tablespoon olive oil

1 small onion, finely chopped

2 cloves garlic, crushed

3 tomatoes, chopped

12 button mushrooms, sliced

1 egg, lightly beaten

40g feta/goat's or mature cheese

2 tablespoons basil

Brown rice

1 Preheat oven to 180°C (350°F).
2 Heat the olive oil in a medium frying pan over a high heat and add the onions, garlic, tomatoes, mushrooms and spinach leaves and cook for 5 minutes, or until vegetables are soft.
3 Transfer to a large bowl and allow to cool slightly.
4 Add the egg and 1 tablespoon of water, and stir to combine.
5 Spoon the mixture into peppers and sprinkle the tops with cheese and basil.
6 Place peppers on baking tray and bake for 15–20 minutes, or until peppers are soft and cheese is slightly brown. Serve immediately with rice.

RECIPES **WEEK 11** DAY 5

BREAKFAST FRUIT SALAD   *See page 84*

LUNCH EGG SALAD   *See page 118*

DINNER LAMB CURRY WITH SPINACH

800g lean lamb leg, diced

2 tablespoons olive oil

2 onions, finely sliced

2 cloves garlic

115g soya/plain yoghurt

1 tin of chopped tomatoes

250g spinach

Fresh coriander, handful

Brown rice

Spices:

½ teaspoon cardamom seeds

1 teaspoon ground cinnamon

1 tablespoon garam masala

2 teaspoon turmeric

1 Heat olive oil in a large saucepan over a high heat and add the onion and garlic.
2 Cook for 5 minutes, or until onion is golden.
3 Add the spices and lamb, mix well and cook for 6–8 minutes, or until lamb begins to cook and change colour.
4 Stir through yoghurt and tomato.
5 Add spinach and 225ml of water, then reduce heat to medium and simmer for 40 minutes, or until meat is tender.
6 Stir through the coriander.
7 Serve with rice.

RECIPES **WEEK 11** DAY 6

BREAKFAST OMELETTE   *See page 86*

LUNCH TOMATO AND PEPPER SOUP   *See page 138*

DINNER HUNGARIAN GOULASH

800g lean braising steak

400g tinned chopped tomatoes

2 onions, finely chopped

220g mushrooms, sliced

2 green peppers, deseeded and diced

280g low fat fromage frais

Florets of broccoli

125g of peas

Brown rice

Herbs:

1 bay leaf

Marjoram, pinch

Thyme, pinch

2 level tablespoons paprika

¼ level teaspoon caraway seeds

1 Preheat oven to 150°C (300°F).
2 Place onions and tomatoes in pan and cook until onions are soft.
3 Add the mushrooms and peppers and cook for a further 5 minutes.
4 Cut the steak into strips and place in a casserole dish, adding the herbs and tomato mixture.
5 Cover and cook for about 1 hour 30 minutes.
6 Beat the fromage frais until smooth and pour over the casserole dish before serving.
7 Serve with the vegetables and brown rice.

RECIPES **WEEK 11** DAY 7

BREAKFAST FRUIT SMOOTHIE 1   *See page 85*

LUNCH CHICKEN WRAP   *See page 115*

DINNER CHILLI PRAWN SALAD

200g jumbo raw prawns

Handful fresh coriander

4 teaspoons lemon juice

1 yellow pepper

1 tablespoon olive oil

1cm ginger, peeled and finely chopped

2 cloves garlic, finely chopped

For the salad:

2 cos lettuces, torn into pieces

3–4 spring onions, finely sliced

2 fresh red chillies, deseeded and finely sliced

4 large tomatoes, sliced

1 Place the lettuce in a salad bowl, add the spring onions, tomatoes and yellow pepper and toss together.
2 Heat half of the olive oil in a large frying pan on a high heat.
3 Add the ginger, garlic, chillies and prawns.
4 Cook for 3 minutes, then reduce heat and squeeze the juice of a lemon over the frying pan.
5 Add the coriander, the rest of the olive oil and cook for a further minute.
6 Remove from the heat and season with black pepper.
7 Pour the prawn mixture over the salad and serve.

Lunch for tomorrow:
TUNA SALAD
Consider preparing the sweet potatoes in advance.

TRAINING DIARY **WEEK 11**

WEEK 11 OVERVIEW
Day 1: CV – run
Day 2: CV – cycle
Day 3: Rest; myo massage
Day 4: CV – run
Day 5: Weights – upper body
Day 6: CV – run PT
Day 7: CV – walk
Any day: Myo stretch

ALISON'S DIARY

Day 1 (Monday)
I had an amazing run today. I think training with someone else is much more motivating than training alone, especially when I'm running or cycling.
Tiredness 1
Stress 4
Sleep 6 hours 30 minutes

Day 2 (Tuesday)
I am putting more effort into my training, which is something I am really enjoying and it is helping to keep my stress levels down and keep my mind off the parts of my life that I am unhappy about.
Tiredness 3
Stress 3
Sleep 6 hours 45 minutes

Day 3 (Wednesday)
I have taken the next five days off, as Gavin said that I need to have some time out to relax and that we should spend some quality time together. I started my break with a myo massage.
Tiredness 2
Stress 1
Sleep 8 hours

Day 4 (Thursday)
I'm so glad I'm having time off as I can concentrate on my training sessions even more. I am now looking for a new job and starting to get my life back to normal instead of it revolving around work. I'm changing that back to work revolving around life.
Tiredness 2
Stress 2
Sleep 9 hours

Day 5 (Friday)
What can I say, after a few days off and time spent doing what I want to do, I have really been able to change myself and my views.
Tiredness 1
Stress 0
Sleep 9 hours

Day 6 (Saturday)
I didn't think I was going to get up today, and to be honest I didn't for ages. I had breakfast in bed and spent the day outside and seeing my family. What a lovely day.
Tiredness 0
Stress 0
Sleep 8 hours 45 minutes

Day 7 (Sunday)
Gavin did the tests this morning before we headed over to the Purbecks. I went with Gavin and his dogs again and we walked everywhere. I don't want to go back to work tomorrow, but I don't think I can get another day off.
Tiredness 1
Stress 1
Sleep 10 hours

TRAINING SESSION **WEEK 11** DAY 1

ALISON'S SESSION

AM Rest

PM Training session CV – Run

Time trained 6.00–6.44 p.m.

Session time 44 minutes

RPE 10/10

WORKOUT
Run: 4 miles
Actual distance: 4.25 miles
Time: 43 minutes 15 seconds
Average Pace: 10.15 m/m

Alison's notes: On this run we were trying to get the pace (minute/miles) down as much as possible by concentrating on putting maximum effort into how fast we could run the four miles. I got my minute mile down to 10m/m pace. This is a great average pace and a great start for my base fitness.

YOUR SESSION

AM

PM Training session Run

Time trained

Session time   hour(s)   minutes

RPE   /10

WORKOUT
Run: 4 miles
Actual distance: miles
Time: minutes
Average pace: m/m

Your notes:

TRAINING SESSION **WEEK 11** DAY 2

ALISON'S SESSION

AM Training session CV – Cycle

Time trained 9.00–11.25 a.m.

Session time 2 hours 25 minutes

RPE 10/10

PM Rest

WORKOUT
Cycle: 20 miles
Actual distance: 20.02 miles

Alison's notes: This cycle was only meant to be a short one, but we kept going and going until we reached Lymington and then I realised we had to go all the way back. This was a spectacular cycle as there were sections with flat paths to get up your speed, sections with big hills and sections that were off-road. We came back via the marshes, which were very flat and easy, but I found it really hard to get up speed and maintain it. I know Gavin found this frustrating, but for me this section was very boring – it went on and on. As soon as we were off-road though, on the coastal path, miraculously my speed came back.

YOUR SESSION

AM   Training session CV – Cycle

Time trained

Session time   hour(s)   minutes

RPE   /10

PM

WORKOUT
Cycle: 20 miles
Actual distance: miles

Your notes:

TRAINING SESSION **WEEK 11** DAY 4

ALISON'S SESSION

AM Training session CV – Run

Time trained 9.00–9.55 a.m.

Session time 55 minutes

RPE 8/10

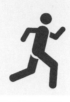

PM Rest

WORKOUT

Run: 5 miles
Actual distance: 4.95 miles
Time: 55 minutes
Average pace: 11 m/m

Alison's notes: I had a bit of a slower run today as my legs were aching (DOMS) from exercising this week. All I wanted to do was complete five miles in preparation for next week's 10km (6.2 mile) run.

YOUR SESSION

AM **Training session** CV – Run

Time trained

Session time   hour(s)   minutes

RPE   /10

PM

WORKOUT

Run: 5 miles
Actual distance: miles
Time: minutes
Average pace: m/m

Your notes:

TRAINING SESSION **WEEK 11** DAY 5

ALISON'S SESSION

AM **Training session** Weights – Upper body

Time trained 10.00–11.10 a.m.

Session time 1 hour 10 minutes

RPE 8/10

PM Rest

WORKOUT
Dumbbell press
Set and Rep: 1. 25 2. 25 3. 25 4. 25 5. 23
Weight (lb):   7.5   12.5 12.5 12.5 12.5

Dumbbell bench press
Set and Rep: 1. 25 2. 25 3. 25 4. 25
Weight (lb):   12.5   12.5 12.5 12.5

Lat pull-downs
Set and Rep: 1. 25 2. 25 3. 25 4. 25
Weight (kg):   12.5   12.5 12.5 12.5

Dumbbell arm curls
Set and Rep: 1. 25 2. 25 3. 25 4. 25
Weight (lb):   7.5   7.5   7.5   7.5

Triceps press-downs
Set and Rep: 1. 25 2. 25 3. 25 4. 25
Weight (kg):   10   10   10   10

Reverse shrug using a dumbbell
Set and Rep: 1. 25 2. 25 3. 25 4. 25
Weight (lb):   25   25   25   25

YOUR SESSION

AM **Training session** Weights – Upper body

Time trained

Session time   hour(s)   minutes

RPE   /10

PM

WORKOUT
Dumbbell press
Set and Rep: 1.   2.   3.   4.   5.
Weight (kg):

Dumbbell bench press
Set and Rep: 1.   2.   3.   4.
Weight (kg):

Lat pull-downs
Set and Rep: 1.   2.   3.   4.
Weight (kg):

Dumbbell arm curls
Set and Rep: 1.   2.   3.   4.
Weight (kg):

Triceps press-downs
Set and Rep: 1.   2.   3.   4.
Weight (kg):

Reverse shrug using a dumbbell
Set and Rep: 1.   2.   3.   4.
Weight (kg):

Bent-over lat raise
Set and Rep: 1. 25   2. 25   3. 25   4. 25
Weight (lb):   5   5   5   5

Abs
Complete 100 reps for each of the abs exercises below in any order, even if you manage to do it in one go.

Half sit-ups
100

Reverse curls
100

Heel taps
100

Notes: We are still keeping to an endurance and high-rep workout to finish toning the beautiful body Alison will now have.

Bent-over lat raise
Set and Rep: 1.   2.   3.   4.
Weight (kg):

Abs

Half sit-ups

Reverse curls

Heel taps

Your notes:

TRAINING SESSION **WEEK 11** DAY 6

ALISON'S SESSION

AM Training session CV – Run PT

Time trained 11.00 a.m.–12.10 p.m.

Session time 1 hour 10 minutes

RPE 8/10

PM Rest

WORKOUT
Run PT
Actual distance: 2 miles

Run for one mile, then move on to the exercises at station 1. Complete 100 reps for each of the exercises. Afterwards, move on to the next one-mile run before finishing at station 2.

Run 1 mile

Station 1
Alternate squat thrusts × 100
Wide squat thrusts × 100
Star jumps × 100
Spotty dogs × 100
Squat thrusts × 100
Jumping oblique twists × 100
Standing glute extension × 50 each side
Frog hops × 100
Heel to bum × 100

YOUR SESSION

AM Training session CV – Run PT

Time trained

Session time   hour(s)   minutes

RPE   /10

PM

WORKOUT
Run PT
Actual distance: miles

Run 1 mile

Station 1
Alternate squat thrusts ×
Wide squat thrusts ×
Star jumps ×
Spotty dogs ×
Squat thrusts ×
Jumping oblique twists ×
Standing glute extension ×   each side
Frog hops ×
Heel to bum ×

Run 1 mile

Station 2
¾ press-ups × 100
Dips × 100
Arm haulers × 100
Reverse shrug (no weight) × 100
Burpees × 30

Alison's notes: Good luck with this and keep going. I think the hardest exercise is left to last for a reason.

Run 1 mile

Station 2
¾ press-ups ×
Dips ×
Arm haulers ×
Reverse shrug (no weight) ×
Burpees ×

Your notes:

TRAINING SESSION **WEEK 11** DAY 7

ALISON'S SESSION

AM Rest

PM Training session CV – Walk

Time trained 10.00–2.00 p.m.

Session time 4 hours

RPE 7/10

YOUR SESSION

AM

PM Training session CV – Walk

Time trained

Session time   hour(s)   minutes

RPE   /10

WORKOUT

Walk: 15 miles
Actual distance: 15.02 miles
Time: 4 hours
Average pace: 16 m/m

Equipment

Food
2 bananas
1 apple
1 bag soya nuts
1 bag goji berries
1 turkey wrap
3 ltr water

Clothing
Walking boots
Walking trousers
Vest
Training t-shirt
Walking socks

Spare clothing
Sandals (in case feet hurt)
Warm jacket/top
Waterproof jacket

Other
First aid kit
First field dressing
Torch
Map and compass
Money
Mobile phone
Whistle

Alison's notes: What a walk, up and over towards Swanage and back again to Corfe Castle. This meant lots of hills and lots of walking, but we stopped twice. Both for five minutes each, one was to have a little bite to eat and the other to look at the beautiful view and have some water.

WORKOUT

Walk: 15 miles
Actual distance: miles
Time: minutes
Average pace: m/m

Equipment

Food

Clothing

Your clothing

Other

Your notes

WEEK 11 TESTS

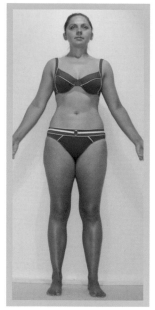

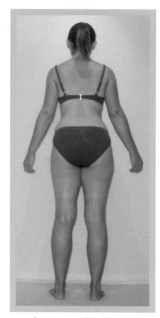

Front view of Alison at the end of week 11.

Back view of Alison at the end of week 11.

ALISON'S WEEKLY TESTS

Weight (kg)	53
Height (cm)	157.3
BMI	21.4
RHR	52
BP	111/59
Fat (%)	22.6

Measurements (cm)

Neck	28.57	
Chest	83.18	
Arms	R: 26.67	L: 26.67
Navel	73.02	
Hips	79.37	
Thighs	R: 53.97	L: 53.97
Calves	R: 34.29	L: 34.29

YOUR WEEKLY TESTS

Weight (kg)	
Height (cm)	
BMI	
RHR	
BP	
Fat (%)	

Measurements (cm)

Neck		
Chest		
Arms	R:	L:
Navel		
Hips		
Thighs	R:	L:
Calves	R:	L:

WEEK TWELVE NUTRITION PLAN WEEK 12

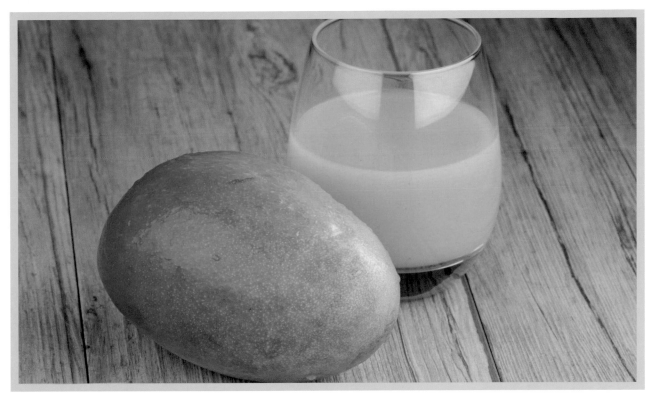

WEEK 12 OVERVIEW

Day	Breakfast	Lunch	Dinner
1	Fresh fruit and seeds	Tuna salad	Jambalaya
2	Fruit smoothie 2	Smoked salmon pitta	Grilled sea bass with fresh vegetables
3	Muesli with fresh fruit	Sweet potato and bean salad	Vegetable Thai curry
4	Fruit porridge	Chicken salad pitta	Monkfish salad
5	Wheat biscuits or muesli with fruit	Butternut squash and coriander soup	Baked rainbow trout
6	Fruit salad	Mackerel salad	Lamb shanks
7	Omelette	Tuna and olive salad	Butternut squash and lentil stew

SHOPPING LIST WEEK 12

CARBOHYDRATES
75g brown basmati rice
50g wholegrain brown barley
1 bag of brown rice
400g kidney beans
525g lentils
25g millet seeds
250g of muesli
125g new potatoes
1 bag of pine nuts
400g pinto beans
560g porridge oats
3 potatoes
1 bag of sunflower seeds
1 bag pumpkin seeds
12 sweet potatoes
8 wholemeal or brown
pitta breads
Wheat biscuits

DAIRY AND NON-DAIRY ALTERNATIVES
12 eggs
60g feta/goat's cheese
1880ml skimmed/soya/rice/
oat milk
1.7kg soya yoghurt

FISH
8 anchovy fillets
225g fresh mackerel
600g monkfish tail
8 king size prawns
4 rainbow trout
4 sea bass fillets
4 pack of smoked salmon
4 small tins tuna
350g tuna steaks

MEAT
4 chicken breasts
4 chicken thighs
100g raw chorizo
100g raw garlic sausage

2kg lamb shank
400g lean ham

FRUIT
8 apples
2 apricots
10 bananas
1 lime
3 lemons
1 mango
2 oranges
2 peaches
1 large pineapple
1 small packet of raisins
1 punnet of raspberries
1 watermelon

VEGETABLES
3 avocados
100g baby corn
3 bags of baby spinach
1.4kg butternut squash
25g black olives
250g cherry tomatoes
5 carrots
4 celery sticks
3 courgettes
½ cucumber
175g French beans
3 green peppers
2 lettuces
50g mangetout
1 marrow
4 onions
115g baby plum tomatoes
1 red onion
5 red peppers
8 red tomatoes
100g rocket salad
1 shallot
100g sugar snap peas
10 spring onions
2 yellow peppers

HERBS
Basil
2 bay leaves
Black pepper
Coriander
Ground coriander
Ground cumin
Dill
1 garlic bulb
Fresh ginger
1 lemongrass stalk
Nutmeg
Oregano
Paprika
Parsley
1 red chilli
Rosemary
Turmeric

OTHER
Balsamic vinegar
Chicken stock
400ml coconut milk
Cold-pressed extra virgin
olive oil
Dijon mustard
Plain flour
400g tinned plum tomatoes
Vegetable stock
115ml white wine
White wine vinegar

SNACKS
Fruit
Wholegrain crispbread crackers
Flat breads
Small bowl of muesli
Yoghurt/soya yoghurt
Nuts (cashew, pine or
occasionally mixed nuts)
Soya nuts
Seeds (pumpkin or sunflower)

FRUIT DRINKS
1 carton fruit juice

RECIPES **WEEK 12** DAY 1

BREAKFAST FRESH FRUIT AND SEEDS

See page 81

LUNCH TUNA SALAD

See page 134

DINNER JAMBALAYA

4 skinless, boneless chicken thighs, halved

1 tablespoon flour

1 onion, peeled and finely chopped

½ red pepper, deseeded and chopped

½ green pepper, deseeded and chopped

50g wholegrain brown barley, soaked in boiling water and drained

230g tinned chopped tomatoes

500ml chicken stock

75g brown basmati rice

1 tablespoon olive oil

8 king size prawns, peeled

100g raw garlic sausage, roughly chopped and lightly dry-fried

100g raw chorizo, roughly chopped and lightly dry-fried

1 clove garlic, peeled and finely chopped

1 teaspoon fresh thyme leaves

1 red chilli, deseeded and roughly chopped

25g millet seeds, dry-fried until they 'pop'

1 Dust the chicken in the flour.
2 Heat the olive oil in a large non-stick frying pan and add the onion, garlic, red and green pepper, thyme and chilli to the pan and cook over medium heat until onion is soft.
3 Add the barley, tomatoes, chicken stock and bring to boil.
4 Add the chicken and sausages, lower the heat and stir in the rice and millet.
5 Cover and cook for 20 minutes or until the rice is almost tender.
6 Remove the lid and simmer for a further 10 minutes.
7 Stir in the prawns and cook for a further 5 minutes.
8 Serve on warm plates.

RECIPES **WEEK 12** DAY 2

BREAKFAST FRUIT SMOOTHIE 2

See page 157

LUNCH SMOKED SALMON PITTA   *See page 79*

DINNER GRILLED SEA BASS WITH
FRESH VEGETABLES

4 fillets sea bass (150g each)

300g tinned lentils, drained and rinsed (try
and use fresh lentils if you have time)

Broccoli and other green vegetables

For the marinade:

3 garlic cloves, peeled and crushed

2 tablespoon fresh parsley, chopped

2 tablespoon water

Black pepper

3 teaspoons dried oregano

4 teaspoons olive oil

4 tablespoons lemon juice

1. To make the marinade, mix the oregano, garlic, olive oil, lemon juice, black pepper, water and parsley together.
2. Wash the fish fillet and pat dry with kitchen towel. Then place on plate and spoon over half the marinade. Cover and refrigerate for 1–2 hours.
3. Preheat the grill to high.
4. Grill the fillet skin-side down for 5–6 minutes until just cooked through – the flesh should be white.
5. Meanwhile, warm the lentils with the marinade.
6. Spoon on to warm plates and place the sea bass on top.
7. Serve with fresh vegetables.

Lunch for tomorrow:
SWEET POTATO AND BEAN SALAD
Consider preparing the eggs and sweet potatoes in advance.

RECIPES **WEEK 12 DAY 3**

BREAKFAST MUESLI WITH
FRESH FRUIT   *See page 79*

LUNCH SWEET POTATO AND
BEAN SALAD   *See page 202*

DINNER VEGETABLE THAI CURRY

400ml tin coconut milk

½ teaspoon ground coriander

½ teaspoon ground cumin

1. Heat coconut milk in a wok or large frying pan over a high heat.

2cm fresh ginger, peeled and sliced

1 stalk of lemon grass, cut into 2cm pieces

100g sugar snap peas

1 red pepper, deseeded and sliced

1 yellow pepper, deseeded and sliced

100g baby corn, halved lengthways

2 courgettes, trimmed and chopped

2 spring onions, trimmed and finely sliced

Basil leaves to garnish

Brown rice

2 Add ground coriander, ground cumin, ginger and lemon grass, and cook for 2–3 minutes.
3 Add the peas, peppers, baby corn and courgettes, and cook for a further 3–4 minutes or until vegetables are just cooked.
4 Garnish with spring onions and basil.
5 Serve with brown rice.

Lunch for tomorrow:
CHICKEN SALAD PITTA
See the following page and consider preparing the chicken in advance.

RECIPES **WEEK 12** DAY 4

BREAKFAST FRUIT PORRIDGE   *See page 80*

LUNCH CHICKEN SALAD PITTA   *See page 120*

DINNER MONKFISH SALAD

600g monkfish tail, washed with membrane removed

1 tablespoon olive oil

2 teaspoons rosemary, chopped

6 plum tomatoes

For the salad:

2 teaspoons olive oil

2 tablespoons pine nuts

1 garlic clove, peeled and sliced

450g baby spinach

2 tablespoons raisins

1 lemon, juice of

1 Preheat the oven to 220°C (425°F). Mix the olive oil and the rosemary in a small bowl, season with pepper and lightly coat the fish with this mixture.
2 Place the fish in a roasting tin with the tomatoes and bake in the oven for 20 minutes or until the fish is firm and white.
3 Meanwhile, heat the olive oil in a large frying pan, add the pine nuts and garlic, and cook until golden.
4 Add the spinach leaves, raisins and lemon juice a handful at a time.
5 Cut the fish from either side of the central bone.
6 Serve with the salad and cooking juices.

RECIPES **WEEK 12** DAY 5

BREAKFAST WHEAT BISCUITS OR
MUESLI WITH FRUIT

See page 82

LUNCH BUTTERNUT SQUASH AND
CORIANDER SOUP

See page 87

DINNER BAKED RAINBOW TROUT

4 rainbow trout, gutted

2 oranges, sliced with skin on

2.5cm fresh ginger, cut into slices

3 sweet potatoes, cut into small chunks

1 marrow, remove skin and cut into small chunks

2 garlic cloves, crushed

40g goat's/mature cheddar cheese

3 teaspoons dried basil

1 tablespoon olive oil

Salad leaves

For the dressing:

1 tablespoon fresh dill, finely chopped

250g plain soya/plain yoghurt

1 garlic clove, crushed

1 teaspoon balsamic vinegar

1 Preheat oven to 190°C (375°F).
2 Place the sweet potatoes, marrow, garlic and dried basil in a large baking dish and drizzle with olive oil.
3 Bake for 30–40 minutes or until cooked.
4 Add the cheese in the last 5–8 minutes.
5 Meanwhile, prepare the dressing by mixing all the dressing ingredients in a small bowl, then place in refrigerator.
6 Preheat the grill to medium.
7 Place two orange slices in each trout and sprinkle the ginger evenly between the fish.
8 Grill the fish for 12–14 minutes, turning occasionally.
9 Arrange the grilled trout on a bed of salad with the sweet potatoes and marrow.
10 Drizzle with the dressing and serve.

RECIPES **WEEK 12** DAY 6

BREAKFAST FRUIT SALAD

See page 84

LUNCH MACKEREL SALAD

See page 87

DINNER LAMB SHANKS

2 tablespoons olive oil

2kg lamb shanks on the bone

2 onions, chopped

1 celery stick

115ml white wine

675ml chicken stock

2 cloves garlic

2 bay leaves

2 tablespoons parsley

1 tablespoon lemon zest

Vegetables of your choice and new potatoes

1 Preheat oven to 160°C (325°F).
2 Heat a large heavy-based saucepan over a high heat.
3 Coat the lamb shanks with olive oil and cook in saucepan, turning occasionally, for 10 minutes or until well browned, then remove to a plate.
4 Add the garlic, onion and celery to the pan and cook for 5 minutes, or until soft.
5 Next add the wine, stock, lemon zest, parsley and bay leaves and bring to the boil.
6 Gently place the lamb shanks in a casserole dish and add the mixture from the pan.
7 Cover with foil and cook in oven for 1–2 hours, or until meat begins to fall off the bone.
8 Garnish with parsley and serve with steamed vegetables and new potatoes.

RECIPES **WEEK 12** DAY 7

BREAKFAST OMELETTE

See page 86

LUNCH TUNA AND OLIVE SALAD

See page 80

DINNER BUTTERNUT SQUASH AND LENTIL STEW

225g lentils

2 onions, peeled and finely chopped

750ml vegetable stock

3 carrots, peeled and chopped

½ butternut squash, peeled, deseeded and chopped

1 sweet potato, peeled and chopped

3 small white potatoes, peeled and chopped

1 celery stalk, trimmed and chopped

50g frozen or fresh peas

1 Soak the lentils in cold water for 20 minutes, rinse and drain.
2 Bring the vegetable stock to the boil in a large saucepan.
3 Next, add the onions, lentils, carrots, squash, sweet potato and white potatoes and bring back to boil.
4 Lower the heat and simmer for 10–20 minutes.
5 Add the celery and simmer for a further 5 minutes.
6 Add the peas and simmer for a couple more minutes.
7 Serve in bowls.

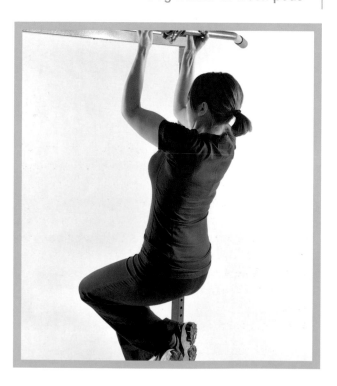

TRAINING DIARY **WEEK 12**

WEEK 12 OVERVIEW
Day 1: Rest
Day 2: CV – run
Day 3: CV – run PT
Day 4: Circuits
Day 5: CV – run; myo cellulite massage
Day 6: CV – walk; weights – upper body
Day 7: Tests

ALISON'S DIARY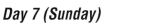

Day 1 (Monday)
Well I'm back to work this afternoon after yet another long sleep and lie in.
Tiredness 1
Stress 1
Sleep 6 hours 30 minutes

Day 2 (Tuesday)
It was so nice to have those days off, as I am ready for my biggest challenge so far, my 10km run. Trust me, I did not think I would do it but I did and I felt so good afterwards – no words can describe how I was feeling.
Tiredness 0
Stress 2
Sleep 6 hours 30 minutes

Day 3 (Wednesday)
After my euphoria from yesterday, and finishing the 10km run, all my colleagues have noticed how much weight I have lost and how my clothes seem to hang off me. I had a lymphatic massage after my run PT.
Tiredness 0
Stress 2
Sleep 7 hours

Day 4 (Thursday)
I'm not training as hard as I normally would, as Gavin doesn't want me to burn out now as the goal is in sight. I really enjoyed my last circuit training on this 12-week programme, and can't wait to get back into it after my holidays.
Tiredness 2
Stress 3
Sleep 5 hours 45 minutes

Day 5 (Friday)
I had a broken sleep last night, and I'm slightly nervous about this Sunday's tests. I'm worried I've not done myself proud, that the results aren't going to be that impressive, and that I'll decide not to have a book written about my training.
Tiredness 3
Stress 4
Sleep 8 hours

Day 6 (Saturday)
I'm feeling good with my thighs now, and I know I could always lose more weight and make them look even better, but I can finally say that I am happy with what I see.
Tiredness 2
Stress 3
Sleep 8 hours 45 minutes

Day 7 (Sunday)
Final test day is here. I was so happy with my end results, it was very emotional. The thing I'm most proud of is the way I look at myself and the way I feel. I have never been confident with my body, and I feel so good I can't wait to go on holiday, show it off and celebrate. I can't thank Gavin enough, and I hope when you read this you too can get to the stage that I've reached.
Tiredness 1
Stress 2
Sleep 7 hours

TRAINING SESSION **WEEK 12** DAY 2

ALISON'S SESSION

AM Training session CV – Run

Time trained 9.00–10.06 a.m.

Session time 1 hour 6 minutes

RPE 10/10

PM Rest

WORKOUT

Run: 10km (6.2 miles)
Actual distance: 6.2 miles
Time: 1 hour 6 minutes
Average pace: 11.05 m/m

Alison's notes: I can't believe I've done it. It was by far the best moment so far, as I never thought that I would ever be fit enough to run 10km.

Notes: On this run, don't worry at all about pace or time. You just want to run the full 10km without stopping and feel really good about it. A great tip for running your first 10km is to set little goals as you run and, if you can run with a running partner, you will both be able to push each other through your highs and lows.

YOUR SESSION

AM Training session CV – Run

Time trained

Session time   hour(s)   minutes

RPE   /10

PM Rest

WORKOUT

Run: 10km (6.2 miles)
Actual distance: miles
Time: minutes
Average pace: m/m

Your notes:

TRAINING SESSION **WEEK 12** DAY 3

ALISON'S SESSION

AM Training session CV – Run PT

Time trained 9.00–9.45 a.m.

Session time 45 minutes

RPE 7/10

PM Rest

YOUR SESSION

AM Training session CV – Run PT

Time trained

Session time   hour(s)   minutes

RPE   /10

PM

WORKOUT
Run PT
Actual distance: 2 miles

Run approximately 0.5 miles between the fitness stations.

During the run PT all the exercises were 1 × 100 reps. Alison broke the 100 reps into 5 × 20 reps, unless marked AIOH (all in one hit), which means that Alison completed all 100 reps without stopping.

Run 0.5 mile
Station 1
Dips × 100
Press-ups decline × 100

Run 0.5 mile
Station 2
Half sit-ups × 100
Crunch × 100

Run 0.5 mile
Station 3
Reverse curls × 100
Arm haulers × 100

WORKOUT
Run PT

Run 0.5 mile
Station 1
Dips ×
Press-ups decline ×

Run 0.5 mile
Station 2
Half sit-ups ×
Crunch ×

Run 0.5 mile
Station 3
Reverse curls ×
Arm haulers ×

Run 0.5 mile
Station 4
Calf raises × 100 AIOH
Squats × 100 AIOH
Pull-ups: 5 × 5 pull-ups and if needed negatives.

Notes: Alison didn't have too much time to do a workout before she had to go to work so I kept this workout as short as I could.

Run 0.5 mile
Station 4
Calf raises × ▢
Squats × ▢
Pull-ups: ▢ × ▢ pull-ups and if needed negatives.

Your notes:

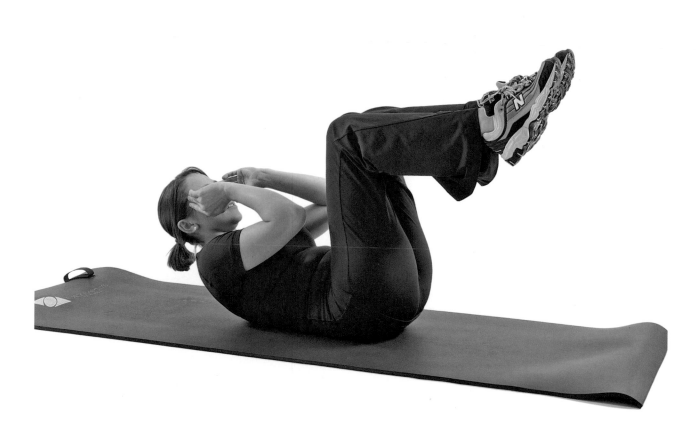

TRAINING SESSION **WEEK 12** DAY 4

ALISON'S SESSION

AM Training session Circuits

Time trained 8.00–8.45 a.m.

Session time 45 minutes

RPE 8/10

PM Rest

WORKOUT

As this is your final week, put as much effort into this as you can.

Two minutes for each exercise.

The weights used in this circuit were 3kg.

Again, don't count the reps as this can be mentally exhausting and demoralising. Go through each exercise in order, and in between each station you can have a break.

Station 1
Squats
Leg levers
Dumbbell press

Station 2
Lunges
Reverse curls
Bent-over rows

Station 3
Bosu squats (upside down)
Crunches
Dumbbell bench press

YOUR SESSION

AM   Training session Circuits

Time trained

Session time   hour(s)   minutes

RPE   /10

PM

WORKOUT

Station 1
Squats
Leg levers
Dumbbell press

Station 2
Lunges
Reverse curls
Bent-over rows

Station 3
Bosu squats (upside down)
Crunches
Dumbbell bench press

Station 4
Lunges
Reverse crunches
Lat pull-downs

Station 5
Standing glute extensions
Dorsal raise
Bent-over lat raise

Station 6
Standing hip abduction
Heel taps
Triceps press-downs

Station 7
Calf raises
Oblique side crunches
Supinated curl

Station 4
Lunges
Reverse crunches
Lat pull-downs

Station 5
Standing glute extensions
Dorsal raise
Bent-over lat raise

Station 6
Standing hip abduction
Heel taps
Triceps press-downs

Station 7
Calf raises
Oblique side crunches
Supinated curl

Your notes:

TRAINING SESSION **WEEK 12** DAY 5

ALISON'S SESSION

AM Training session CV – Run

Time trained 8.40–9.10 a.m.

Session time 30 minutes

RPE 10/10

PM Rest

WORKOUT

Run: 3 miles
Actual distance: 3.0 miles
Time: 28 minutes
Average pace: 9.20 m/m

Alison's notes: I thought I would be really pleased that this is the last run of the programme, but I think I'm actually beginning to enjoy them now. I'll continue running after I have finished the programme, but perhaps not quite as hard as Gavin has pushed me.

Notes: This was the the final run. Alison ran as fast as possible with the wind behind her all the way. Just look at the pace Alison set.

As this is the last run for the 12-week programme, just enjoy it and see what you can do.

YOUR SESSION

AM Training session CV – Run

Time trained

Session time   hour(s)   minutes

RPE   /10

PM

WORKOUT

Run: 3 miles
Actual distance: miles
Time: minutes
Average pace: m/m

Your notes:

TRAINING SESSION **WEEK 12** DAY 6

ALISON'S SESSION

AM Training session CV – Walk

Time trained 8.00–8.45 a.m.

Session time 45 minutes

RPE 4/10

WORKOUT
Walk: 4 miles
Actual distance: 4 miles

PM Training session Endurance weights – Upper body

Time trained 6.00–7.00 p.m.

Session time 1 hour

RPE 7/10

WORKOUT
Warm up on both exercises × 20 reps

Superset

	Dumbbell bench press			Pec fly		
Sets	1.	2.	3.	1.	2.	3.
Reps	30	30	30	20	20	20
Weight (kg)	15	15	15	10	10	10

YOUR SESSION

AM Training session CV – Walk

Time trained

Session time   hour(s)   minutes

RPE   /10

WORKOUT
Walk: 4 miles
Actual distance: miles

PM Training session Endurance weights – Upper body

Time trained

Session time   hour(s)   minutes

RPE   /10

WORKOUT

Superset

	Dumbbell bench press			Pec fly		
Sets	1.	2.	3.	1.	2.	3.
Reps						
Weight (kg)						

Superset

	Incline dumbbell press			Single arm cable row		
Sets	1.	2.	3.	1.	2.	3.
Reps	30	30	30	15	15	15
Weight (kg)	15	15	15	5	5	5

Superset

	Bent-over row			Dips		
Sets	1.	2.	3.	1.	2.	3.
Reps	30	30	30	30	30	30
Weight (kg)	15	15	15			

Superset

	Hammer curls			Lat raise		
Sets	1.	2.	3.	1.	2.	3.
Reps	30	30	30	30	30	30
Weight (kg)	7.5	7.5	7.5	7.5	7.5	7.5

Superset

	Incline dumbbell press			Single arm cable row		
Sets	1.	2.	3.	1.	2.	3.
Reps						
Weight (kg)						

Superset

	Bent-over row			Dips		
Sets	1.	2.	3.	1.	2.	3.
Reps						
Weight (kg)						

Superset

	Hammer curls			Lat raise		
Sets	1.	2.	3.	1.	2.	3.
Reps						
Weight (kg)						

Alison's notes: Well done. That's to me and to you. I think it is really important to carry on with the workouts and the nutrition plan. I'm going to have a week off first though, just to relax.

It's amazing just how anxious I became for test weeks, especially weeks 4, 8 and 12, but it has been totally worth it.

Your notes:

WEEK 12 TESTS

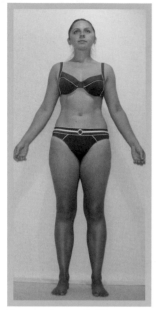

Front view of Alison at the end of week 12.

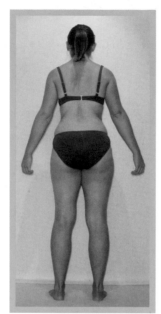

Back view of Alison at the end of week 12.

ALISON'S WEEKLY TESTS

Weight (kg)	52.5	
Height (cm)	157.3	
BMI	21.2	
RHR	50	
BP	110/61	
Fat (%)	21.3	
Measurements (cm)		
Neck	28.57	
Chest	83.18	
Arms	R: 26.67	L: 26.67
Navel	71.12	
Hips	78.74	
Thighs	R: 53.34	L: 53.34
Calves	R: 34.29	L: 34.29

YOUR WEEKLY TESTS

Weight (kg)		
Height (cm)		
BMI		
RHR		
BP		
Fat (%)		
Measurements (cm)		
Neck		
Chest		
Arms	R:	L:
Navel		
Hips		
Thighs	R:	L:
Calves	R:	L:

WEEK 12 HEALTH CHECK

ALISON'S RESULTS

Statistics

Weight (kg)	52.5
Height (cm)	157.3

Health tests

BMI	21.2
RHR	50
BP	110/61
Fat (%)	21.3
Glucose	3.8
Cholesterol	3.9
Lung function	450

Measurements (cm)

Neck	28.57	
Chest	83.18	
Arms	R: 26.67	L: 26.67
Navel	71.12	
Hips	78.74	
Thighs	R: 53.34	L: 53.34
Calves	R: 34.29	L: 34.29

Calliper test (mm)

Biceps	5
Triceps	8
Waist	7
Subscapularis	10
Total	30
Calliper fat (%)	23.3

Fitness tests

Bleep test (20m) level	8

Maximum reps in one minute

¾ push-ups	45
½ sit-ups	73
Squats	81
Dips	70
Max pull-ups	5

YOUR RESULTS

Statistics

Weight (kg)	
Height (cm)	

Health tests

BMI	
RHR	
BP	
Fat (%)	
Glucose	
Cholesterol	
Lung function	

Measurements (cm)

Neck		
Chest		
Arms	R:	L:
Navel		
Hips		
Thighs	R:	L:
Calves	R:	L:

Calliper test (mm)

Biceps	
Triceps	
Waist	
Subscapularis	
Total	
Calliper fat (%)	

Fitness tests

Bleep test (20m) level	

Maximum reps in one minute

¾ push-ups	
½ sit-ups	
Squats	
Dips	
Max pull-ups	

THE FINAL RESULTS

ALISON'S FINAL RESULTS

Overall statistics – increases and decreases	
Weight (kg)	–4.5
Height (cm)	157.3

Health tests	
BMI	–1.8
RHR	–27
BP	–2.7
Fat (%)	–10.8
Glucose	–2.4
Cholesterol	–1.3
Lung function	+80

Measurements (cm)		
Neck	–2.54	
Chest	–6.98	
Arms	R: –3.17	L: –2.54
Navel	–10.16	
Hips	–12.7	
Thighs	R: –6.98	L: –6.98
Calves	R: –1.27	L: –1.27

Calliper test (mm)	
Biceps	–3
Triceps	–10
Waist	–8
Subscapularis	–9
Total	–30
Calliper fat (%)	–8.6

Fitness tests	
Bleep test (20m) level	gained over 2.5 levels

Maximum reps in one minute	
Press-ups	+30
½ sit-ups	+30
Squats	+42
Dips	+47
Max pull-ups	+4.5

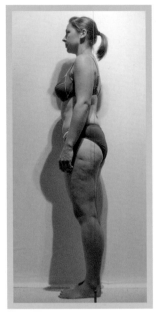

Alison's posture week 1.

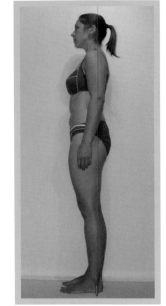

Alison's posture week 12.

YOUR FINAL RESULTS

Overall statistics – increases and decreases

Weight (kg)

Height (cm)

Health tests

BMI

RHR

BP

Fat (%)

Glucose

Cholesterol

Lung function

Measurements (cm)

Neck

Chest

Arms   R: L:

Navel

Hips

Thighs   R: L:

Calves   R: L:

Calliper test (mm)

Biceps

Triceps

Waist

Subscapularis

Total

Calliper fat (%)

Fitness tests

Bleep test (20m) level

Maximum reps in one minute

Press-ups

½ sit-ups

Squats

Dips

Max pull-ups

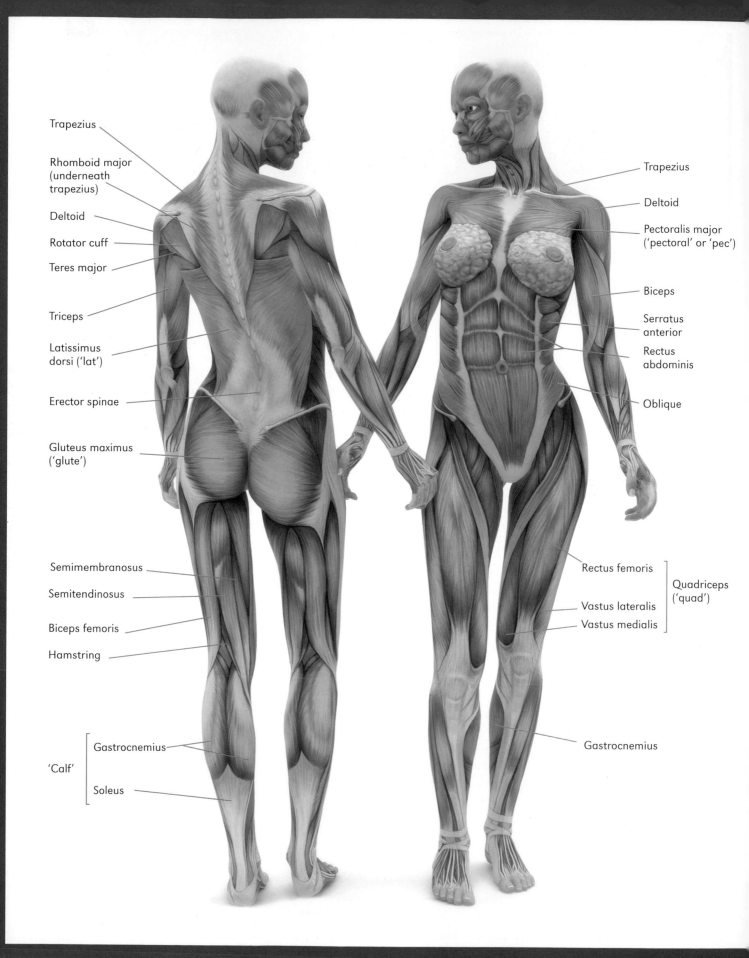

Trapezius

Rhomboid major
(underneath
trapezius)

Deltoid

Rotator cuff

Teres major

Triceps

Latissimus
dorsi ('lat')

Erector spinae

Gluteus maximus
('glute')

Semimembranosus

Semitendinosus

Biceps femoris

Hamstring

'Calf'

Gastrocnemius

Soleus

Trapezius

Deltoid

Pectoralis major
('pectoral' or 'pec')

Biceps

Serratus
anterior

Rectus
abdominis

Oblique

Rectus femoris

Quadriceps
('quad')

Vastus lateralis

Vastus medialis

Gastrocnemius

ANATOMY AND EXERCISES

07

CHEST MUSCLES

See the image opposite and take note of the muscles of the chest:

- *Pectoralis major*
- *Serratus anterior*

MIDDLE, OUTER AND INNER PECTORALS

Bench press (compound)

>>

Purpose

To build mass, strength and density in the pectorals, anterior deltoids and triceps.

Action

- Lie on the bench, with your feet flat on the bench, or on the floor.
- Your grip should be wider than shoulder width, with an overhand grip.
- Raise bar off rack.
- Lower the bar under control, until the bar comes in alignment with or slightly below your nipples.
- Press the bar back up until arms are almost locked out.

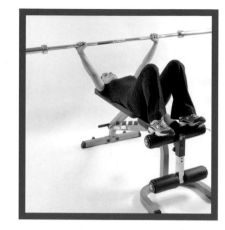

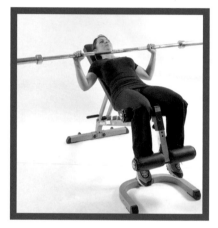

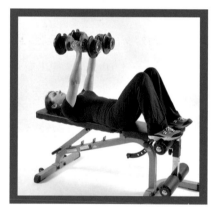

<< **Pec fly**

Purpose

To enhance the mass of the pectoralis major.

Action

- Lie on the bench, with your feet flat on the floor.
- Hold dumbbells above your chest, palms facing each other.
- Lower weights out and down, with your elbows slightly bent, until your pectorals are fully stretched.
- Return to the starting position following the same large arch, while squeezing your chest.
- Once at the top, keep a small gap between the weights and flex the pectorals to maximise full contraction.

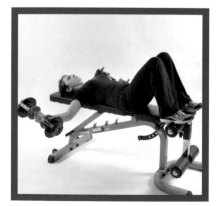

Dumbbell bench press

Purpose

Develops mass on the outer and middle pectorals.

Action

- Lie on the bench, with your feet flat on the floor.
- Grasp the dumbbells in your hands, and hold the weights above your chest, with your palms facing forwards
- Lower the dumbbells to your outer pectorals as far as you can go while feeling a stretch.
- Press the weight back up, squeezing your chest, until your arms are almost locked out and keeping a small gap between the weights.

>>

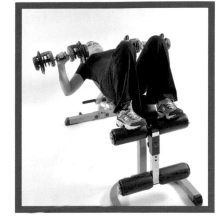

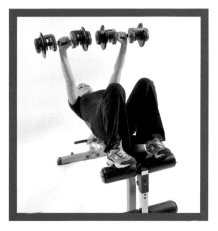

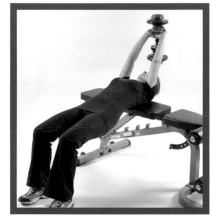

<< ## Straight arm pull-overs (dumbbells)

Purpose

This develops the pectoralis major, as well as expanding your ribcage.

Action

- Lie on the bench, with your feet flat on the floor.
- Hold dumbbell with both of your hands.
- Hold the weight above your chest with a small bend in your elbow.
- Lower the weight behind your head as far as you can go, until your pectorals and rib cage are fully stretched.
- Return to the starting position following the same large arch, while squeezing your chest.

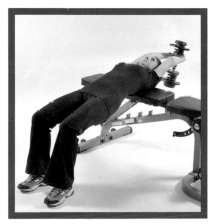

Cable cross-over

>>

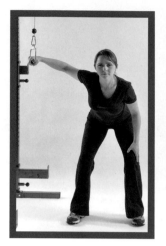
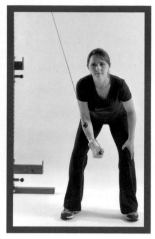

Purpose

To develop the inner portion of the pectoralis major and pectoralis minor.

Action

- While holding the pulley handles, step slightly forwards.
- Extend your arms to your sides and lean forwards from your waist.
- With your palms facing each other and your elbows slightly bent, bring your hands together following the same arch as pec fly.
- Contract the pectorals when your hands are in the centre, but keep going until your hands have crossed each other so that one hand is wrapped underneath the bar and the other is wrapped over the top of the bar. Alternate per repetition.

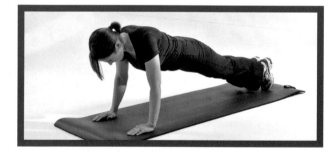

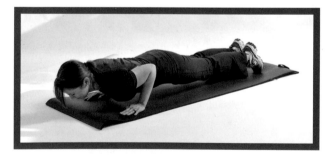

<< **Press-up**

Purpose

To develop the pectoralis major and triceps.

Action

- Lie flat on the floor face down.
- Place your hands on the floor slightly wider than your shoulders, pointing up towards your head and in line with your nipples.
- Place your toes on to the floor, and raise your legs and hips off of the floor.
- Keep your back nice and straight until you have finished your set.
- Extend your arms by pushing into the floor, without arching your back.
- Lower back down to the starting position, not allowing your knees or legs to come into contact with the floor.

¾ *press-up* >>

Use if you are unable to perform a regular press-up.

Action

- Lie flat on the floor face down.
- Place your hands on the floor slightly wider than your shoulders, pointing up towards your head and in line with your nipples.
- Place your toes and the tops of your knees on to the floor.
- Raise your hips and upper body off of the floor, keeping your back nice and straight.
- Extend your arms by pushing into the floor, without arching your back.
- Lower back down to the starting position.

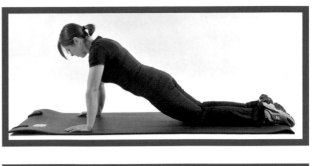

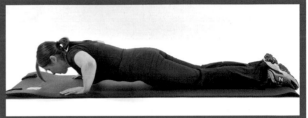

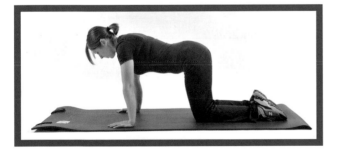

<< **Box press-ups**

Purpose

Another easier variation of the press-up.

Action

- Kneel with your shins on the floor
- Form yourself into the box position, with your hips above your knees, your back flat, your palms on the ground a little wider than your shoulders and your arms straight.
- Bending your elbows, lower yourself as close as your are able to the floor without touching it.
- Extend your arms by pushing into the floor and return to your starting position.

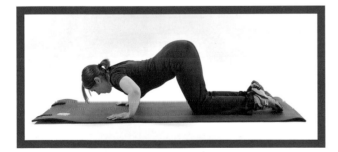

Wide press-ups

>>

Purpose
To develop the outer part of pectoralis major.

Action
- Lie flat on the floor face down.
- Place your hands on the floor wider than shoulder-width apart, pointing away from your body at 45° and in line with your nipples.
- Place your toes on to the floor and raise your legs and hips off of the floor.
- Extend your arms by pushing into the floor, without arching your back.
- Lower back down to the starting position, not allowing your knees or legs to come into contact with the floor.

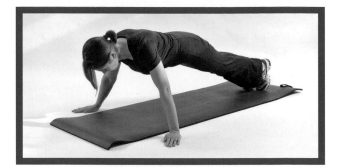

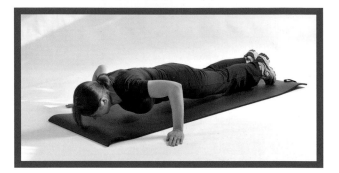

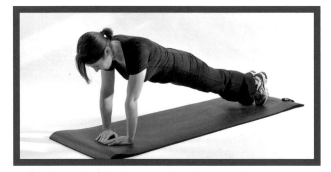

<< ## Diamond press-ups

Purpose
To develop the inner part of pectoralis major, and a lot of emphasis on your triceps.

Action
- Lie flat on the floor face down.
- Place your hands in a triangular shape, index fingers and thumbs touching, in front of your body in alignment with your lower pectorals.
- Place your toes on to the floor, and raise your legs and hips off the floor.
- Lean slightly over your hands and extend your arms by pushing into the floor, without arching your back.
- Squeeze your chest at the top to get the most out of your inner pectorals.
- Lower back down to the starting position, not allowing your knees or legs to come into contact with the floor.

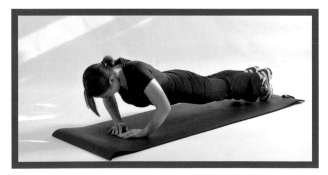

LOWER PECTORALS

Decline bench press

>>

Purpose
To develop mass, strength and density in the lower pectorals.

Action
- Place the bench at a decline angle of 30°.
- Lie on the bench, with your feet around the bench pads.
- Your grip should be wider than shoulder width, with an overhand grip.
- Raise bar off rack.
- Lower the bar under control until the bar comes into alignment with or slightly below your nipples.
- Press the bar back up until arms are almost locked out.

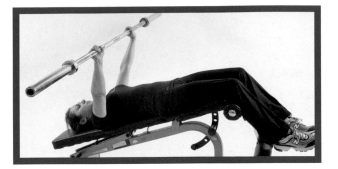

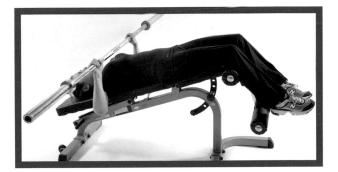

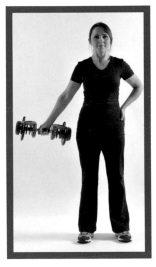

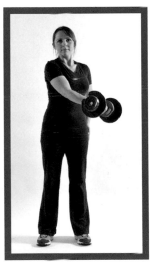

<< ### *Morey squeeze (lower)*

Purpose
To work the lower and middle pectorals.

Action
- Extend one arm to your side while supporting yourself with either a bench or weight.
- Draw your hands up and inwards until the weight is roughly in alignment with the opposite nipple, while keeping a slight bend in your elbow.
- Flex your lower pectoral to get the full benefit.
- Following the same arch bring the weight back down to your side.

UPPER PECTORALS

Incline press

>>

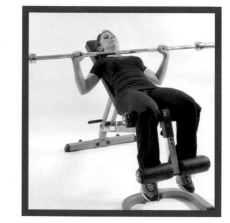

Purpose

To develop and build mass and strength of the upper pectorals, anterior deltoids and triceps.

Action

- Place the bench at an incline angle of 45°.
- Lie on the bench, with your feet flat on the floor.
- Your grip should be wider than shoulder width, with an overhand grip.
- Raise the bar off the rack.
- Lower the bar under control to your upper pectorals, just below your collarbone.
- Press the bar back up until arms are almost locked out.

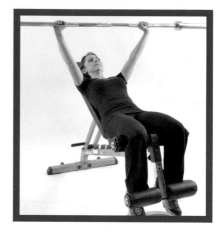

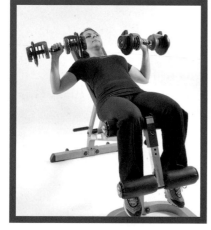

<< **Incline dumbbell press**

Purpose

To develop mass on the middle and upper pectorals.

Action

- Place the bench at an incline angle of 45°.
- Lie on the bench, with your feet flat on the floor.
- Grasp the dumbbells in your hands and hold the weights above your upper chest, with your palms facing forwards.
- Lower the dumbbells to your outer pectorals as far as you can go while feeling a stretch, in line with your upper pectorals, just below your collarbone.
- Press the weight back up until arms are almost locked out, while keeping a small gap between the weights.

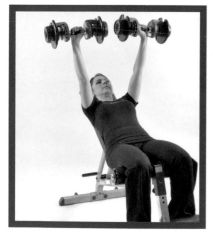

Incline fly

Purpose

To build mass on the upper pectorals.

Action

- Place bench at an incline angle of 45°.
- Lie on the bench, with your feet flat on the floor.
- Hold dumbbells above your chest, with palms facing each other.
- Lower weights out and down, with your elbows slightly bent, until your pectorals are fully stretched.
- Return to the starting position following the same large arch, while squeezing your chest muscles.
- Once at the top, keep a small gap between the weights and flex the pectorals to maximise full contraction.

>>

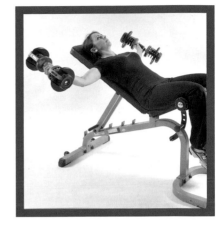

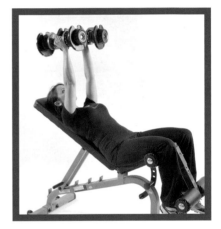

Morey squeeze (upper)

Purpose

To develop and define the upper and slight middle pectorals.

Action

- Extend one arm to your side while supporting yourself with either a bench or weight.
- Draw your hands up and inwards until the weight is roughly in alignment with the opposite shoulder, while keeping a slight bend in your elbow.
- Flex your upper pectoral to get the full benefit.
- Following the same arch, bring the weight back down to your side.

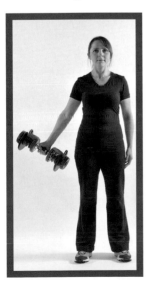
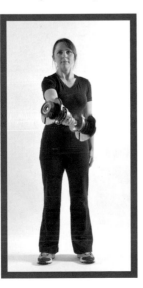
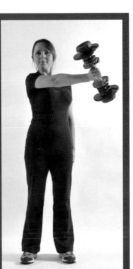

SERRATUS ANTERIOR

Rope pulls

Purpose
To work and develop the serratus anterior. Your abdominals and lats are also brought into use.

Action
- Hold on to the upper pulley and kneel on the floor.
- Keep your arms extended above your head, curl your body forwards and down, pulling with your lats.
- Keep pulling until your elbows have touched your sides, and curl your head towards your knees.
- Uncurl and come back up to the start, feeling a stretch in your lats.

>>

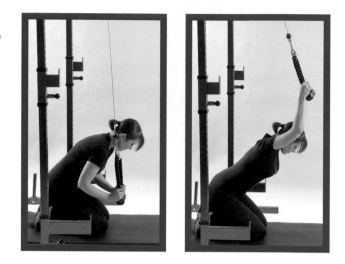

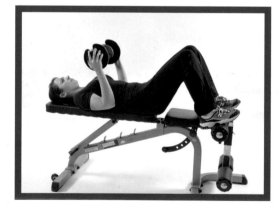

<< **Pull-overs**

Purpose
Works the lower lats and serratus anterior.

Action
- Lie on the bench with your arms bent and weight on your chest.
- Move the bar over your head slowly, while keeping your arms bent, until you feel your lats stretch (the weight should never touch the floor).
- You can also use the dumbbell instead of the bar.

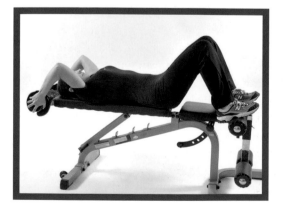

BACK MUSCLES

See the image on page 290 and take note of the muscles of the back:

- **Rotator cuff**
- **Teres major**
- **Rhomboids**
- **Latissimus dorsi**
- **Trapezius**
- **Erector spinae**

FULL SWEEP AND DEVELOPMENT OF THE BACK

Regular pull-ups

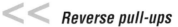

Purpose
To create the full sweep of the lats and develop the teres major.

Action
- Hold the chin bar, with your hands over a shoulder-width apart and with an overhand grip.
- Hang from the bar so that your feet are not touching the ground and your arms are straight.
- Pull your body up, trying to reach the top of your chest to the bar.
- At the top, hold yourself for a brief moment.
- Lower your body to the start, with your arms straight.

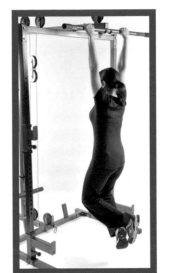

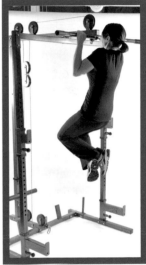

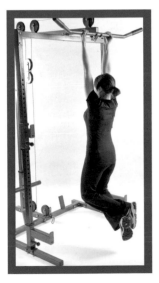

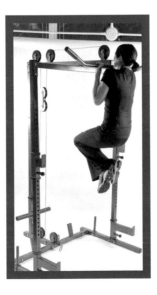

Reverse pull-ups

Purpose
To develop your lats, teres major and biceps.

Action
- Hold the chin bar, with your hands shoulder-width apart and with an underhand grip.
- Hang from the bar so your feet are not touching the ground and your arms are straight.
- Pull your body up, trying to reach the top of your chest to the bar.
- At the top, hold yourself for a brief moment.
- Lower your body to the start, with your arms straight.

Deadlifts (compound) Incline press >>

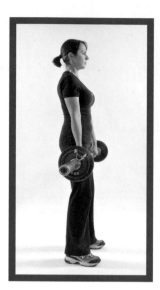
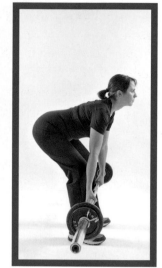

Purpose
An overall power exercise that involves more than one muscle group and works the lower back.

Action
- Place the barbell on the floor in front of you.
- With your legs hip-width apart, bend your knees and lean forwards from the hips to grasp the bar.
- Grasp the bar with a medium to wide grip, one hand in an overhand grip and the other in an underhand grip.
- Keep your abdominal muscles contracted and your back in a neutral position to protect from the strain.
- Lift by driving with your legs first, and then straighten up until you are standing upright.
- Push your chest out and shoulders back.
- Lower the weight by bending your knees and leaning forwards from the waist.
- Touch the weight just above the floor to begin your next rep.

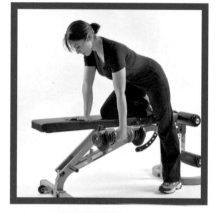

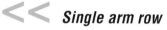

<< **Single arm row**

Purpose
Isolates the lats on one side, as well as developing and defining the centre of your back.

Action
- Grasp the dumbbell in one hand, with your palm facing inwards.
- Place the opposite knee and hand on the bench, keeping a neutral back.
- Begin with the weight hanging by your side at full stretch, allowing your body to tilt towards the weight.
- Raise your upper arm and elbow as high as possible, next to your body.
- Lower under control, and repeat until you have finished your reps, before repeating with the other arm.

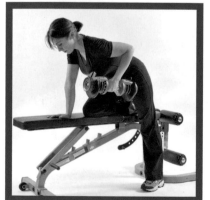

Low pull/seated row Incline press

>>

Purpose
To bulk and develop the thickness of the back and lower lats.

Action
- Sit facing the machine, with your feet on the pads and knees slightly bent.
- Extend your arms and lean slightly forwards, feeling a stretch in your lats, even when the weight stack is at the bottom.
- Pull the handle towards your upper abdominals, while squeezing your shoulder blades back and down.
- Your chest should stick out, sitting upright and not leaning back.
- Control the weight back to the start, again feeling the stretch in your lats.

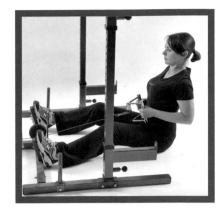

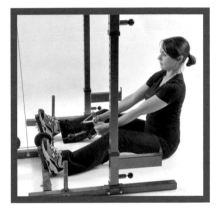

UPPER BACK DEVELOPMENT

<< **Bent-over rows**

Purpose
To develop and thicken the upper back.

Action
- Stand with your feet hip-width apart and your knees slightly bent.
- Grasp the bar with a wide and overhand grip.
- Bend forwards so your upper body is between 45° and parallel with the floor.
- Allow the bar to hang in front of your shin bones, with your head and back straight.
- Lift the bar up towards the upper abdominals/ diaphragm.
- Keep your elbows close to your body, and feel your back work.
- Lower the bar back down to the start.

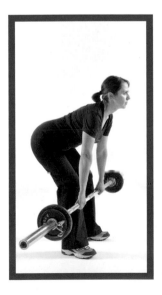

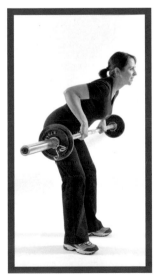

T-bar row (improvised)

>>

Purpose
Thickens your outer and upper back.

Action
- Straddle the bar, keeping your feet hip-width apart.
- Slightly bend your knees, bend forwards to 45° keeping a flat back, and take hold of the weight.
- Without changing position, lift the weight up to your lower pectoral before lowering it back down to get a full stretch.
- Remember, if you feel it in your lower back or legs you will need to take off some plates to isolate the upper back.

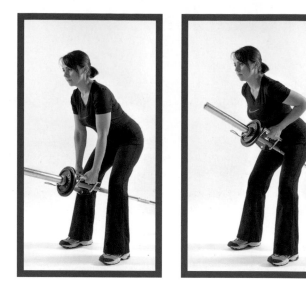

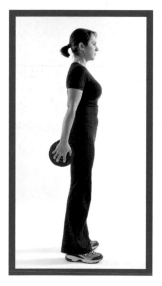 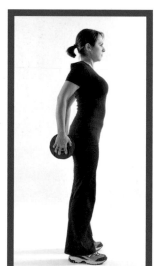

<< **Reverse shrug**

Purpose
To strengthen your lower trapezius. Excellent for office workers.

Action
- Place the weight on a squat rack.
- Face away from the bar, then back into and grasp the bar with your palms facing away (overhand grip).
- To begin, lift bar, rotate your shoulder blades back and down in one motion and squeeze, while sticking your chest out.
- Remember, the movement is very small and you should not feel anything in your upper traps.
- Return by allowing your arms to rotate forwards.

WIDEN YOUR BACK/LATS

Lat pull-downs

Purpose

To develop the bulk of your back and widen your upper lats.

Action

- Hold the bar with a wide overhand grip.
- Sit on the bench, with your knees/feet under the supports.
- While sticking out your chest and leaning backwards 5–10°, pull the bar down, squeezing your shoulder blades back and down while leading with your elbows until the bar is at the top of your chest in alignment with your collar bone.
- Allow your arms to extend back to the start under control before repeating.

\>\>

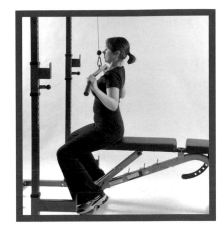

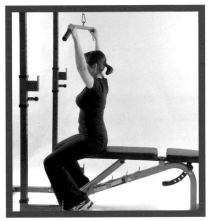

DEVELOPING LOWER LATS AND LOWER BACK

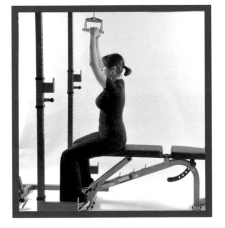

\<\< **Close grip pull-downs**

Purpose

To develop the lower lats.

Action

- Hold the bar with a close overhand grip.
- Sit on the bench, with your knees/feet under the supports.
- While puffing out your chest, pull the bar down with your elbows pulling back to the top of your chest.
- Allow your arms to extend back to the start under control.

Single arm cable row

Purpose

To develop your lower lats using the full range of motion.

Action

- Use a floor-level pulley.
- Take hold of the handle and stand in a balanced position with the opposite leg forwards.
- Begin with your arm fully outstretched in front of you, palm down.
- Pull the handle while twisting your hand to face up.
- Pull your elbow back as far as possible.
- Extend your arm back out in front while twisting your hand palm down to feel the stretch in your lats.

>>

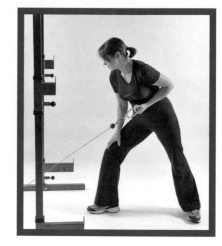

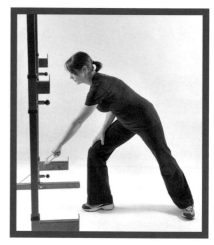

LOWER BACK

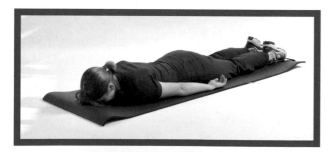

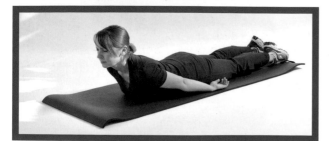

<< **Dorsal raise**

Purpose

To strengthen the spinae erector (lower back).

Action

- Lie face down, with your whole body touching the floor.
- Arm placement varies. Easy – arms by your side; medium – fingers on temples; hard – arms straight out in front.
- Raise your chest off the floor using your lower back.
- Remember to keep your hips and feet on the floor at all times.
- Lower yourself back down and repeat.

SHOULDER MUSCLES

See the image on page 290 and take note of the muscles of the shoulders:

- *Triceps*
- *Deltoid*

ANTERIOR AND MEDIAL DELTOIDS

Military press

Purpose
Bulks and thickens the anterior and medial deltoids.

Action
- Perform from a standing or seated position (seated is more challenging).
- Grasp the bar with an overhand grip, and hold it in alignment with your collar bone/shoulder with elbows tucked in.
- Press the bar straight up overhead, until your arms are straight but not locked out.
- Lower the weight under control to the start position.

>>

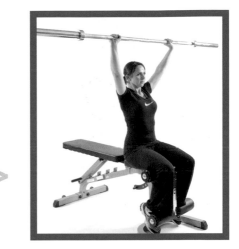

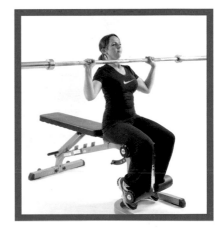

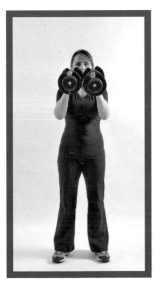

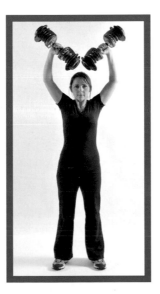

<< **Arnold press**

Purpose
Develops the anterior and medial deltoids.

Action
- From a standing or seated position, hold the dumbbells with your palms turned towards you.
- As you begin to press up, turn your arm and palms out in a smooth motion, while pushing your arms up until they are almost locked out.
- Once at the top pause for a second.
- Return by lowering the weight and rotating your palms back to the starting position.

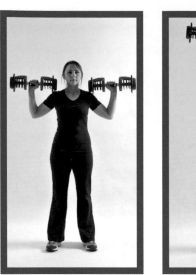

 Dumbbell press

Purpose
To develop anterior and medial deltoids, and give more range of motion than the military press.

Action
- Perform from a standing or seated position (seated is more challenging).
- Grasp the dumbbell, with palms facing forwards and in alignment with your collar bone/shoulder with elbows tucked in.
- Press the dumbbells straight up overhead until the weights almost touch at the top, and with your arms straight but not locked out.
- Lower the weight under control to the start position.

Upright rows

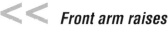

Purpose
Develops separation between deltoids and pectorals. Works the upper trapezius and anterior deltoids, while strengthening your shoulder girdle.

Action
- Stand with your legs hip-width apart and grasp the bar with an overhand grip, with a gap of 10–20cm between your hands.
- Lift the bar up towards your chin.
- Pause and then lower under control keeping the weight close to your body.

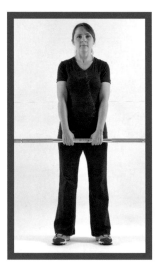
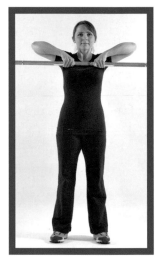

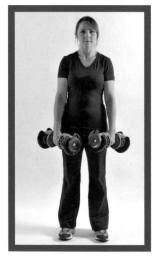
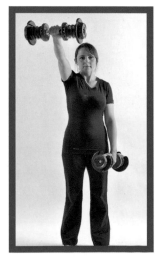

Front arm raises

Purpose
To develop the anterior deltoid.

Action
- Perform from a standing or seated position.
- Grasp the weight in your hand, and lift one hand up in a large arch until the weight is higher than your head.
- Make sure the weight passes in front of your face to maximise the anterior deltoid.
- Lower the weight smoothly and under control.

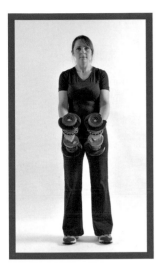
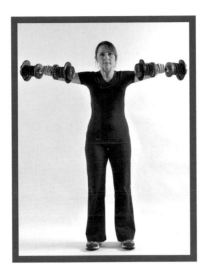
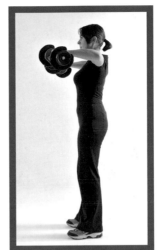

Lateral raise

Purpose

To develop the medial deltoids.

Action

- Hold the dumbbells in each hand, with the weights together and in front of you, and palms facing each other.
- Feet should be hip-width apart, and arms slightly bent and leaning partially forwards.

- Raise the weights up and out, leading with your elbow.
- Bring the weight slightly higher than your shoulder, while making sure the weight doesn't go higher than the elbow.
- Lower slowly and keeping control until the weight touches at the bottom, before the next repetition.

REAR DELTOID

Bent-over lat raise

>>

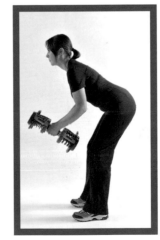
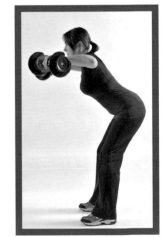

Purpose

To develop the rear deltoids.

Action

- Hold the dumbbells in each hand, with the weights together and to the front of you, and palms facing each other.
- Feet should be hip-width apart, and arms slightly bent.
- Lean forwards at the waist to about 45°, while keeping a straight back.
- Lift the weights to either side of your head, remembering not to allow them to go behind your shoulders.

- To accentuate the rear deltoids, twist your hands so the thumb ends up lower than your little finger.
- Lower the weight under control and repeat.

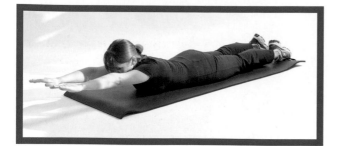

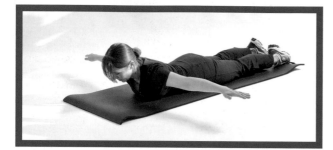

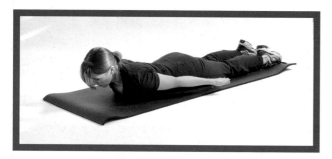

Arm haulers

Purpose

To work all of your deltoids, especially the rear deltoid.

Action

- Lie face down, with your back slightly arched.
- Start with your arm straight and above your head.
- Bring your arms directly down to your side.
- Remember, your arms or hands should not to touch the ground.
- Bring your arms back up to the top and repeat, always keeping your feet on the ground.

ALL-OVER SHOULDER

7-way kettle bell raises

Purpose
To work all of your deltoids.

Action
- Hold the kettle bell in one hand, palm facing you.
- Hold the weight to your side with a slight bend in your elbow.

1. Using the weight as a momentum, raise your arm diagonally to the front, across your body, so the weight comes into alignment with the opposing shoulder.
2. Front arm raise.
3. Arm raise to the front, which is 45° out to your side. Allow the weight to swing all the way through behind you.
4. Lat raise.
5. Arm raise behind you, 45° out to your side of the body. Raise as high as comfortable, with your palm facing diagonally forwards towards your body. Remember to swing the weight slightly in front of you.
6. Rear lat raise, palms facing forwards.
7. With your palm facing back and towards your body, raise the weight diagonally behind you, squeezing your shoulder blade, and trying to feel your rear deltoid.

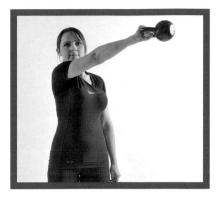

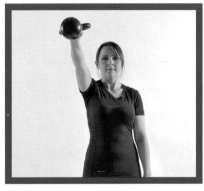

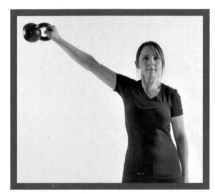

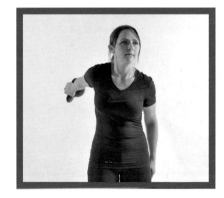

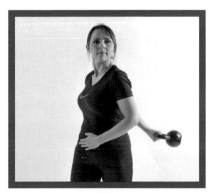

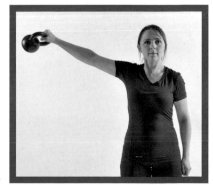

ARMS: BICEPS MUSCLES

See the image on page 290 and take note of the following arm muscles:

- *Biceps*
- *Deltoid*
- *Pectoralis major*
- *Triceps*

BICEPS SIZE AND SHAPE

Arm curl (Olympic bar)

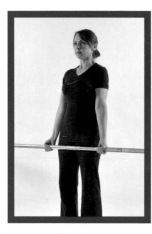 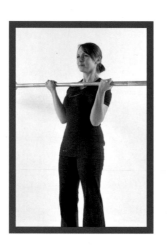

Purpose

To develop the mass and overall size of the biceps.

Action

- Stand with your back straight, and your feet hip-width apart.
- Grasp the bar with an underhand grip, with your hands shoulder-width apart.
- Let the bar hang in front of you with your arms straight.
- Curl the bar in an arch that goes up and out, bringing it as high as is comfortable.
- Keep your elbows close and pivoted to the side of your body.
- Contract the biceps at the top before lowering the weight back down under control to the start.
- A narrow grip mainly works the outer biceps (long head).
- A wide grip mainly works the inner biceps (short head).

Dumbbell arm curl

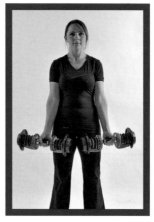 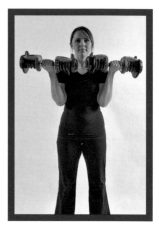

Purpose

Allows you to concentrate on the development of the individual biceps.

Action

- Stand with your back straight and your feet hip-width apart.
- Grasp the dumbbells with an underhand grip, with your hands shoulder-width apart facing away from the body.
- Let the dumbbells hang in front of you, with your arms straight.
- Curl the dumbbells in an arch that goes up and out, bringing it as high as is comfortable.
- Keep your elbows close and pivoted to the side of your body.
- Contract the biceps at the top before lowering the weight back down under control to the start.

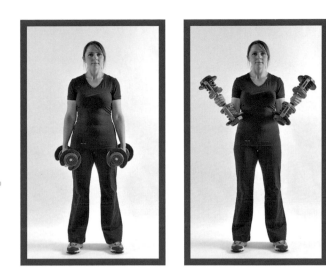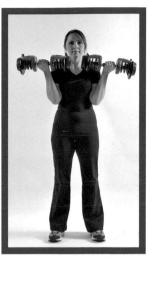

>>

Supinated curl

Purpose
Develops the size and shape of the biceps.

Action
- Stand with your back straight and your feet hip-width apart.
- Grasp the dumbbell with an underhand grip, with your hands facing your body shoulder-width apart.
- Curl one dumbbell in an arch, while twisting your wrist so your palm ends up facing you.
- Keep your elbows close and pivoted to the side of your body.
- Contract the biceps at the top before lowering and twisting the weight back down under control to the start.

HEIGHT OF BICEPS

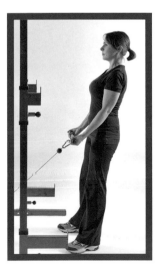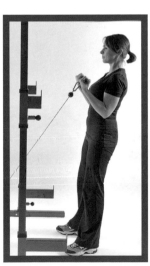

<< **Cable arm curl**

Purpose
Develops the shape and height of biceps.

Action
- Stand with your back straight and your feet hip-width apart.
- Grasp the bar from the lower pulley, with an underhand grip and your hands shoulder-width apart, facing away from the body.
- Allow your biceps to stretch, while being straight.
- Curl the bar in an arch that goes up and out, bringing it as high as is comfortable.
- Keep your elbows close and pivoted to the side of your body.
- Contract the biceps at the top before lowering the weight back down under control to the start.

Incline dumbbell curls

Purpose

Develops the mass of the biceps and gives you a greater range of motion.

Action

>>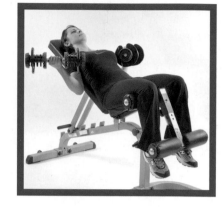

- Place the bench at an incline angle of 45°.
- Lie on the bench, with your feet flat on the floor.
- Grasp the dumbbells with an underhand grip, and your palms facing in towards your body.
- Keep your arms extended and your elbows forwards.
- Curl the weights up to your deltoid in an arch, while twisting your wrists so your palms end up facing you.
- Contract the biceps at the top before lowering the weights back down under control to the start.

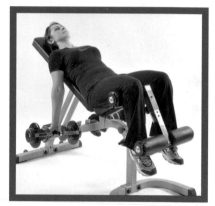

ARMS: TRICEPS AND FOREARM MUSCLES

See the image on page 290 and take note of the triceps and deltoid muscles of the upper arm and shoulder.

DEVELOP ALL THREE HEADS

Triceps press-downs

Purpose

To develop the whole triceps.

Action

>>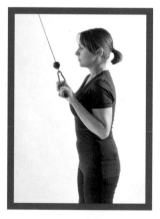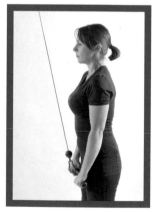

- Stand facing the machine, with your feet shoulder-width apart and back straight.
- Take hold of the bar from the upper pulley, with an overhand grip and your hands 10–20cm apart.
- Press the bar down towards your thighs as far as possible, while keeping your elbows tucked into your sides.
- Contract your triceps at the bottom, and then allow the bar to come back up to the top.
- Change the attachments and hand placements to work all the triceps heads.

- Medial head of triceps – reverse grip triceps press-down with bar.
- Lateral head of triceps – rope triceps press-down.
- Long head of triceps – overhead press with back to machine.

Triceps kickbacks

Purpose
To develop the whole triceps.

Action
- Hold one dumbbell with an overhand grip.
- Stand with one foot in front of the other.
- Place your free hand on your knee, or rest the free hand on a bench with the same hand and leg on the bench for stability.
- Keeping your back straight and leaning forwards from your waist, bend your elbow and raise it back to about shoulder height.
- Allow the weight to hang below your elbow.
- Keeping your elbow tucked into your side, raise the weight so your arm seems to be parallel with the floor.
- Squeeze at the top for the full benefits before allowing the weight to come back to the start.
- Make sure your upper arm doesn't move during the action.

>>

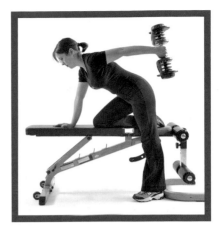

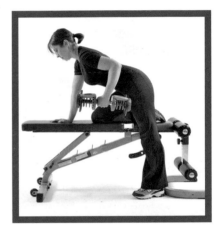

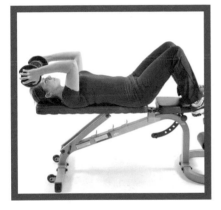

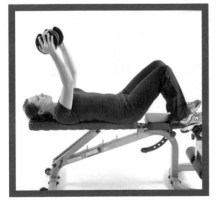

<< **Skull crusher**

Purpose
To develop the triceps.

Action
- Lie on the bench, with your head all the way down to the end.
- Grasp the bar with an overhand grip, approximately 12–24cm apart.
- Press the weight up above your pectorals until your arms are straight out in front of you.
- Keeping your elbows stationary, lower the bar past your forehead, and then pause before pressing it straight back up, but this time with the weight just above your head when fully extended. This keeps constant tension on your triceps.

Bench dips

>>

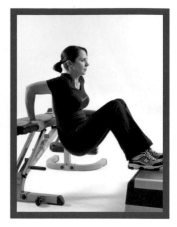

Purpose

To develop the thickness of the triceps.

Action

- Suspend yourself between two benches or chairs, with your feet on one and the heels of your hands on the other.
- Your hands should be shoulder-width apart and facing forwards.
- Keeping your arms straight, lower yourself to the floor while keeping upright and your back close to the bench.
- Once at the bottom press back up, and once at the top contract your triceps as much as possible to get the full benefits.

EMPHASIS ON LATERAL HEAD

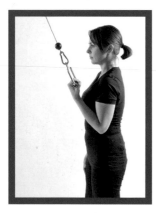
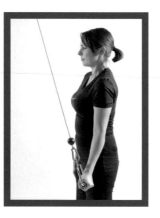
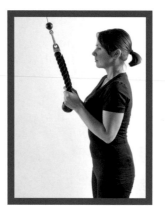
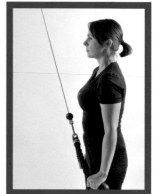

Rope triceps press-down

Purpose

To develop all three heads of the triceps, especially the lateral head.

Action

- Stand facing the machine, with your feet shoulder-width apart and back straight.
- Take hold of the rope from the upper pulley, with your hands in front of you and facing each other.
- Pull the rope down and out past your thighs as far as possible, while keeping your elbows tucked into your side.
- Squeeze your triceps at the bottom as hard as possible, and then allow the bar to come back up to the top, bringing your arms back to the front.

Single arm pull-downs

Purpose

Develops the horseshoe shape, and isolates the triceps (especially the lateral head).

Action

- Stand facing the machine, with your feet shoulder-width apart and back straight.
- Take hold of the handle from the upper pulley, holding the handle with a reverse underhand grip.
- Extend the handle down as far as possible towards your thigh, while keeping your elbows tucked into your side.
- Squeeze your triceps at the bottom as hard as possible, and then allow the bar to come back up to the top, bringing your arm back to the front.

LEG MUSCLES

See the image on page 290 and take note of the muscles of the legs and backside:

- *Glutus maximus*
- *Quadriceps*
- *Rectus femoris*
- *Vastus lateralis*
- *Vastus medialis*
- *Hamstring*
- *Biceps femoris*
- *Semimembranosus*
- *Semitendinosus*
- *Gastrocnemius*
- *Soleus*

QUADRICEPS

Squats (compound)

>>

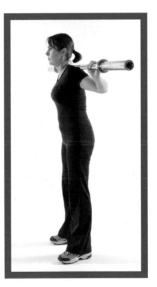
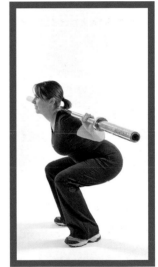

Purpose
To develop mass and strength in all four heads of the quadriceps, and strengthen your glutes.

Action
- With the barbell resting on a rack, stand under the bar and place it on to the trapezius.
- Hold on to the bar, with your hands at a comfortable width and in an overhand position.
- Lift the bar off the rack and step forwards, clear of the rack.
- Your feet should be shoulder-width apart, and toes naturally facing slightly outwards.
- Keeping your head up and back straight, bend at the knees and forwards from the hips.
- Try to remember to stick your glutes out on the way down, to help keep a straight back (as if you are about to sit down).
- When your thighs are horizontal with the floor or slightly below, push yourself back up to the starting position through your feet.
- Finish by walking the bar back on to the rack.
- Medial heads – feet facing out in squats.
- Lateral heads – narrow-stance squats.
- Medial heads and inner thighs – wide-stance squats.

Squat jumps >>

Purpose

To build muscular endurance and develop all four quadriceps and glutes.

Action

- Hold the dumbbells down by your side, with your hands in an overhand position.
- Your feet should be shoulder-width apart, and toes naturally facing slightly outwards.
- Keeping your head up and back straight, bend at the knees and forwards from the hips.
- Try to remember to stick your glutes out on the way down, to help keep a straight back.

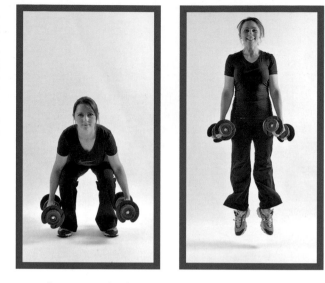

- When your thighs are horizontal with the floor or slightly below, push yourself back up and through into a jump, keeping the weights besides you.
- As soon as you land start the repetition.

Bosu squats >>

Purpose

To build muscular endurance, balance and develop all four quadriceps and glutes.

Action

- Hold the dumbbells down by your side, with your hands in an overhand position.
- Stand on the bosu (up or down), with your feet shoulder-width apart (or whatever the bosu allows), and your toes naturally facing slightly outwards.

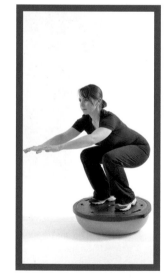
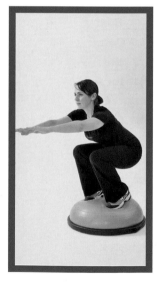

- Keeping your head up and back straight, bend at the knees and forwards from the hips.
- Try to remember to stick your glutes out on the way down, to help keep a straight back.
- When your thighs are horizontal with the floor or slightly below, push yourself back up to the starting position.

Single side squats >>

Purpose
To develop the quadriceps.

Action
- Hold the dumbbells down by your side, with your hands in an overhand position.
- Stand with one leg up on a step box and the other flat on the floor.
- Your feet should be slightly wider than shoulder-width apart, and your toes naturally facing slightly outwards.
- Keeping your head up and back straight, bend at the knees and forwards from the hips.
- Allow all your weight to be on the leg that is flat on the floor, while the other is for balance.
- Try to remember to stick your glutes out on the way down, to help keep a straight back.
- When your thigh is horizontal with the floor or slightly below, push yourself back up to the start.

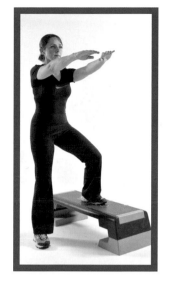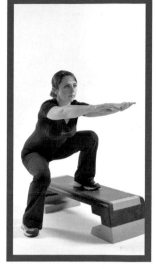

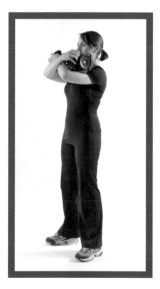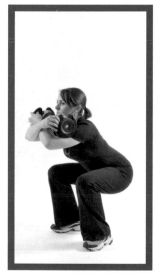

<< Front squats

Purpose
To develop the quadriceps and the lateral quadriceps.

Action
- With the barbell resting on a rack, face the barbell and keep the bar above your arms.
- With your arms in front, cross your arms and cross your elbows.
- Grasp the bar so it sits across the top of your shoulders and chest.
- Lift the bar off the rack and step backwards, clear of the rack.
- Stand with your feet shoulder-width apart, and toes naturally facing slightly outwards.
- Keeping your head up and back straight, bend at the knees and forwards from the hips.
- Try to remember to stick your glutes out on the way down, to help keep a straight back.
- When your thighs are horizontal with the floor or slightly below, push yourself back up to the starting position through your feet.
- Finish by walking the bar back on to the rack.

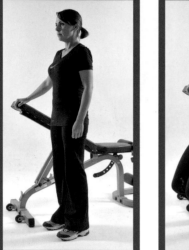
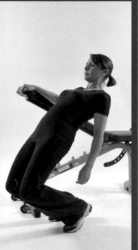

<< **Sissy squats**

Purpose

To isolate the lower quadriceps.

Action

- Stand upright, holding on to either a bench or rack.
- Keep your feet hip-width apart, bend your knees, and raise yourself on your toes.
- Allow your body to slowly drop towards the floor, pushing your hips and knees forwards.
- At the same time you should be tilting your head and shoulders back to keep balance.
- Go as low as is comfortable, before straightening your legs and coming back to the start.
- In the standing position, flex your quadriceps as hard as possible before doing your next repetition.

GLUTES AND QUADS

Lunges (static)

>>

Purpose

Develops the glutes and quadriceps.

Action

- With the barbell resting on a rack, stand under the bar and place it on to the trapezius.
- Hold on to the bar with your hands at a comfortable width and in an overhand position.
- Lift the bar off the rack and step forwards, clear of the rack.
- Keeping your trunk straight, head up and chest out, take a lunge forwards with your leading leg.
- The lunge should be long enough so that your trailing leg is almost straight.
- From this starting position bend your front knee, ensuring your front knee remains behind your toes and your trailing knee goes towards the ground.
- Push yourself back up with your leading leg.
- From this static position, repeat for the number of repetitions with this leg, and then swap to your other leg.

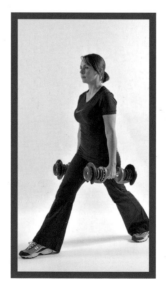
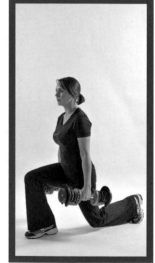

Bosu lunge (static)

Purpose

Develops the quadriceps and glutes, while improving balance.

Action

- Perform with or without a dumbbell (hold on to the dumbbells with palms facing your body).
- Keeping your trunk straight, head up and chest out, take a lunge forwards with your leading leg on the bosu, either way round.
- The lunge should be long enough so that your trailing leg is almost straight.
- From this starting position bend your front knee, ensuring your front knee remains behind your toes and your trailing knee goes towards the ground.
- Push yourself back up with your leading leg.

>>

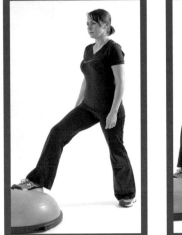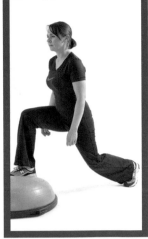

- From this static position, repeat for the number of repetitions with this one leg, and then swap to your other leg.

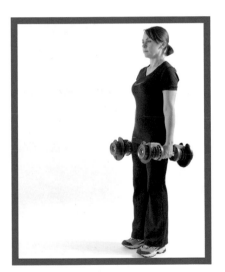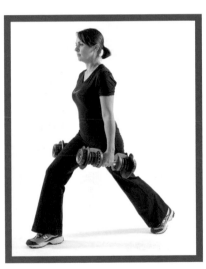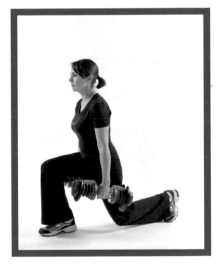

Lunges

Purpose

Develops the glutes and quadriceps.

Action

- With the barbell resting on a rack, stand under the bar and place it on to the trapezius. If using dumbbells, hold the weight next to your body, with palms facing in.
- Hold on to the bar with your hands at a comfortable width, and in an overhand position.
- Lift bar off the rack and step forwards, clear of the rack.

- Keeping your trunk straight, head up and chest out, take a lunge forwards with your leading leg.
- The lunge should be long enough so that your trailing leg is almost straight.
- Bend your front knee, ensuring your leading knee remains behind your toes and your trailing knee goes towards the ground.
- Push yourself back up to the standing position with your leading leg, so that your feet go hip-width apart
- Repeat for the number of repetitions with the same leg, and then swap to your other leg.

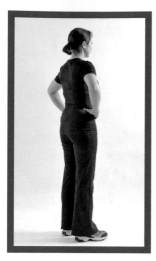
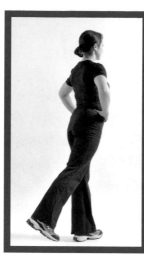

 ## *Standing glute extensions*

Purpose
To isolate and firm the glutes.

Action
- Stand facing a wall, with both arms on the wall for support.
- Keeping your pelvis forwards, extend your leg backwards from your hips with your knee slightly bent.
- Squeeze your gluteus muscle as hard as possible at the top of the movement, then return to the start.

Glute extensions

Purpose
To isolate and firm the glutes.

Action
- While on all fours, kneel on one leg and bring the other towards your chest, while leaning on your hands with your arms extended.
- Extend your leg backwards from your hips, leading with your foot.
- You can have your leg straight, but I prefer to keep my knee bent to hit the glutes even more.
- Squeeze at the top of the movement to get the most out of the glute extension, before returning your leg all the way through to your chest again.
- Repeat for the specific number of repetitions, before changing to your other leg.

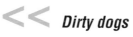

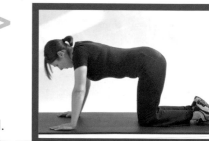

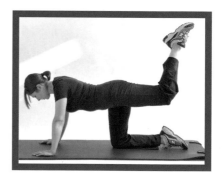

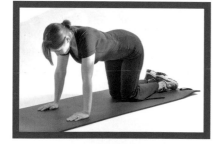

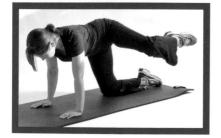

Dirty dogs

Purpose
To develop your gluteus medius and deeper gluteal muscles.

Action
- While on all fours, kneel on one leg and lean on your hands with your arms extended.
- Keep your leg in the bent position, and raise your leg up to your side from your hip.
- You should squeeze at the top and feel the burn on the side of your gluteals.
- Lower back down and repeat.

Standing hip abduction

>>

Purpose
To develop your gluteus medius and deeper gluteal muscles.

Action
- Stand facing a wall, with both arms on the wall for support, or if you have good balance stand as in the picture with your hands on your hips.
- Keeping your pelvis forwards, extend your leg backwards at a 45° angle from your hips, and with your knee slightly bent.
- Squeeze your gluteal muscles as hard as possible at the top of the movement, then return to the start.

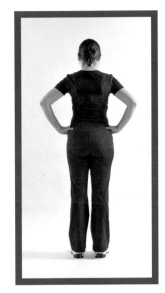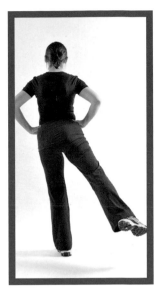

HAMSTRINGS

Stiff leg deadlifts

>>

Purpose
To develop the hamstrings.

Action
- Place the barbell on the floor in front of you.
- With legs hip-width apart, bend your knees and lean forwards from the hips to grasp the bar.
- Grasp the bar with a medium to wide grip, using an overhand grip with one hand and an underhand grip with the other.
- Keep your abdominal muscles contracted and back in a neutral position to protect from the strain.
- Lift by driving with your legs first, and then straighten up until you are standing upright.
- Push your chest out and shoulders back.
- Lower the weight by leaning forwards from the hips, keeping your legs as straight as comfortable, but making sure your knees are not locked out.
- At the bottom of the movement you should feel a stretch in your hamstrings before returning to the top. Repeat for the sets and reps specified.

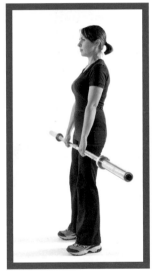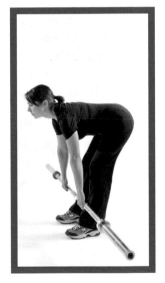

CALVES

Standing calf raises

Purpose

To develop the mass of the calves.

Action

- Stand either on the floor or on a block.
- With the barbell at knee height on the rack, take hold of it with an underhand grip for one hand and an overhand grip for the other.
- If on a block, lower your heels to the floor, stretching your calves.
- Keeping your knees slightly bent, raise up on to your tip-toes and flex as much as possible.
- Pause for a second, then return under control either to the floor or, if on a block, all the way down to a big stretch.

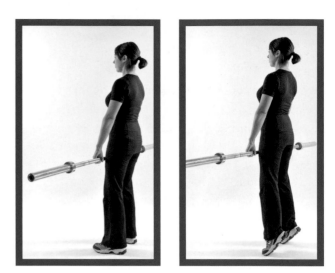

- Medial head of the gastrocnemius – toes turned out.
- Lateral head of the gastrocnemius – toes turned in.

ABDOMINAL MUSCLES

See the image on page 290 and take note of the abdominal muscles:
- *Rectus abdominis*
- *Obliques*

ABDOMINALS

Full sit-ups

Purpose

To work the rectus abdominis and hip flexors.

Action

- Lie on your back with your knees bent and together, and your feet, back and head flat on the floor.
- Hand position varies the difficulty: easy – arms across your body; intermediate – fingers by your temples; hard – arms straight and directly above your head.
- Curl your body off the ground with your head first, then shoulders, upper back, and finally your lower back.
- All the time you should be thinking of sucking your navel (belly button) into the ground.
- Once at the top pause, then return back to the start, but this time don't pause at the bottom.

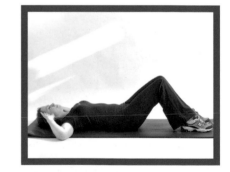

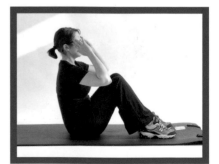

V sit-ups

Purpose

To work your upper and lower abdominals.

Action

- Lie on your back with your legs at a 35° angle, off the floor and together.
- Make sure your back and head are flat on the floor, and your arms straight out overhead.
- Simultaneously curl your upper body and lower body off the ground together.
- Upper body – raise your head first then shoulders, and finally your upper back and your arms following above your head.
- Lower body – raise your legs from 35° to approximately 80°, while keeping them straight and together.
- All the time you should be thinking of sucking your navel (belly button) into the ground.
- Once at the top pause, then return back to the start, but this time don't pause at the bottom.

>>

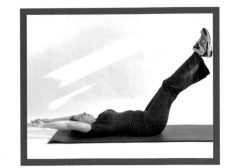

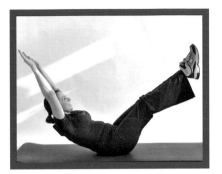

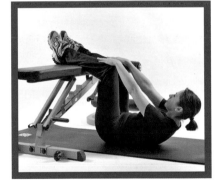

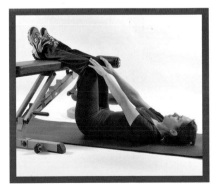

<< ## Incline sit-ups

Purpose

These put greater emphasis on your abdominals and hip flexors than a regular full sit-up.

Action

- Place the bench at a decline of approximately 45°.
- Hook your feet under the pads, and lie on your back with your knees bent and together if possible.
- Position your feet, back and head flat on the floor.
- Hand position varies the difficulty: easy – arms across your body; intermediate – fingers by your temples; hard – arms straight and directly above your head.
- Curl your body off the ground with your head first, then shoulders, upper back, and finally your lower back.
- All the time you should be thinking of sucking your navel (belly button) into the ground.
- Once at the top pause, then return back to the start, but this time don't pause at the bottom.

Plank

>>

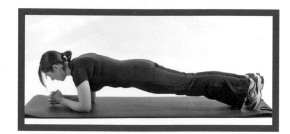

Purpose
To strengthen the core muscles.

Action
- Lie face down, supporting yourself on your forearms and toes.
- To start, raise your body off the ground so all your body weight is being placed on to your toes and forearms.
- Make sure your body is straight and flat and tighten your abdominals, obliques and lower back.
- Hold in this position for the time required, before returning back down.

UPPER ABDOMINALS

Half sit-ups

>>

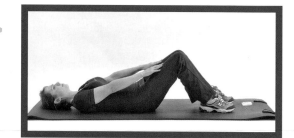

Purpose
To work the upper abdominals.

Action
- Lie on your back with your knees bent and together.
- Feet, back and head flat on the floor.
- Hand position varies the difficulty: easy – arms across your body; intermediate – fingers by your temples; hard – arms straight and directly above your head.
- Curl your body off the ground with your head first, then shoulders, and finally your upper back.
- All the time you should be thinking of sucking your navel (belly button) into the ground.
- Once at the top pause, then return back to the start, but this time don't pause at the bottom.

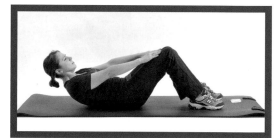

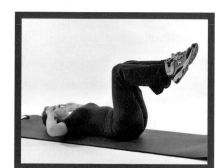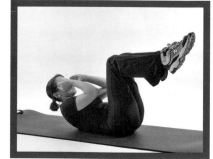

Crunches

>>

Purpose
Emphasises the upper abdominals.

Action
- Lie on your back, legs either in the air or resting on a bench.
- Keep your knees bent and together, with your back and head flat on the floor.
- Hand position varies the difficulty: easy – arms across your body; intermediate – fingers by your temples; hard – arms straight and directly above your head.

LOWER ABDOMINALS

Reverse crunch

>>

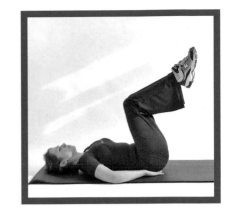

Purpose
To strengthen and develop your lower abdominals.

Action
- Lie on your back with your legs in the air.
- Keep your knees bent and together, with your back and head flat on the floor.
- Place your hands by your side.
- Curl your lower back and glutes off the ground. All the time you should be thinking of sucking your navel (belly button) into the ground.
- Once your knees are by your chest pause, then return back to the start, but this time don't pause at the start.

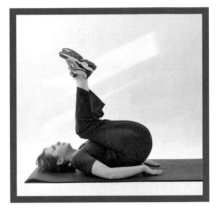

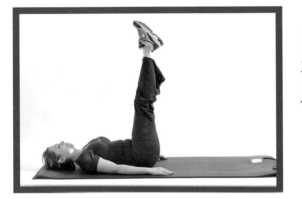

<< *Leg levers*

Purpose
To strengthen and develop your lower abdominals.

Action
- Lie on your back with your legs together and straight.
- Keeping your back and head flat on the floor, place your arms to your side for balance.
- Keeping your feet about 10cm off the floor, raise your legs up and out in a wide arch up to 80°.
- All the time you should be thinking of sucking your navel (belly button) into the ground.
- Once at the top pause, then return slowly back to the start, but this time don't pause at the bottom.
- Note that when you lower your legs and your lower back starts to arch off the floor, it is at this point you raise your legs back up to top. This stops any involvement with your lower back.

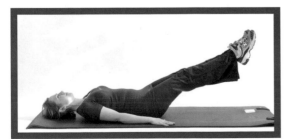

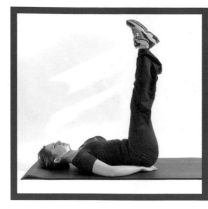
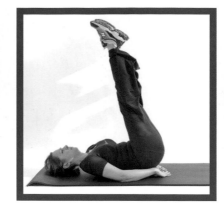
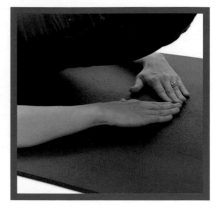

Reverse curls

Purpose

To strengthen your lower abdominals.

Action

- Lie on your back with your legs together and straight.
- Keeping your back and head flat on the floor, place your palms under your glutes/sacrum, face down making a triangular shape with your hands, with index fingers and thumbs touching.
- Raise your legs to start at a 90° angle in the air.

- Curl your lower abdominals, so your legs end up going up and towards you in a smooth diagonal motion.
- This is a small action – when you get it right you will feel a burning sensation from your navel (belly button) and below.
- All the time you should be thinking of sucking your navel (belly button) into the ground.
- Once at the top pause, then return slowly back to the start, but this time don't pause at the bottom.

OBLIQUES

Oblique side crunches

>>

Purpose

To strengthen the obliques.

Action

- Lie on one side, with your upper body resting on to the forearm and the lower body, hips, legs and feet in contact with the ground.
- Place your free hand either by your side or in front of you for balance.
- Raise your whole body off the ground, while supporting yourself on the side of your feet and forearm.
- Hold your body straight, almost like a side plank.
- Once in this position, raise your hip in the air by concentrating on contracting the oblique nearest the ground.

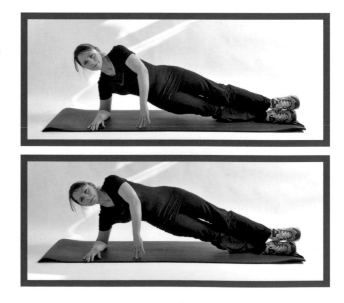

- Hold and flex, before lowering back down to the side plank position.

Heel taps

>>

Purpose
To work the obliques.

Action
- Lie on your back with your knees bent and together.
- Place your feet, back and head flat on the floor.
- Put your arms by your side and lift your head off the ground slightly.
- Crunch your body and arm towards one heel, squeezing your oblique.
- To complete a full repetition, move back to the centre, over to the other side, and back to the centre again.
- All the time you should be thinking of sucking your navel (belly button) into the ground.

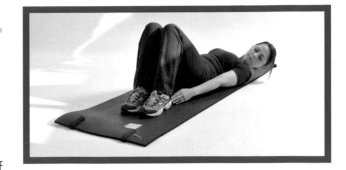

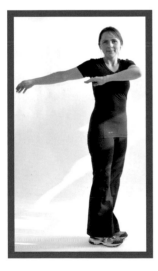 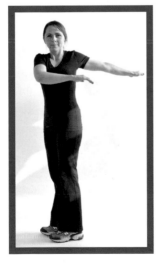

<< **Jumping oblique twists**

Purpose
Tighten and work obliques.

Action
- Start with your feet hip-width apart.
- Twist your lower torso to one side while trying to keep your upper body still.
- Twist your lower torso all the way round to the other side.

OTHER EXERCISES

Burpees

>>

Purpose

To condition and develop muscular endurance and strength in your whole body.

Action

- Start with your feet shoulder-width apart and ready to move into a squat position.
- Squat down and place your hands on the floor in front of you.
- Kick your feet back into a press-up position, while performing a regular press-up.
- On the way up from the press-up, immediately return to your feet in the squat position.
- Leap as high as possible, before returning back into the squat position for the next repetition.

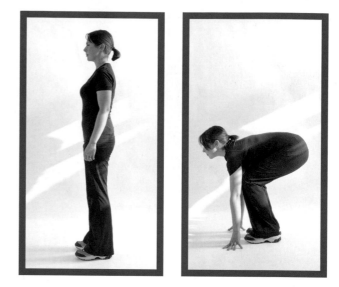

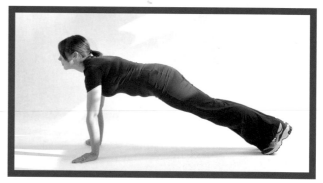

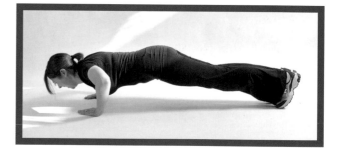

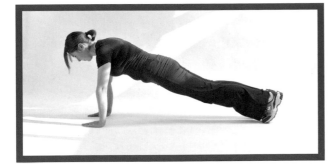

<< **Squat thrusts**

Purpose

To build muscular endurance in your legs.

Action

- Start with your feet shoulder-width apart, and ready to move into a squat position.
- Squat down, and place your hands on the floor in front of you.
- Kick your feet back into a press-up position.
- While in this position, bring your knees up as high as you can towards your chest.
- Return your feet back out straight to the press-up position. This is one repetition.
- Repeat for the specified number of repetitions, before returning to your feet.

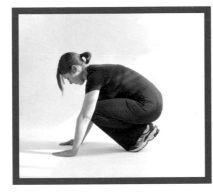

Alternate squat thrusts

Purpose

To build muscular endurance in your legs.

Action

- Start with your feet shoulder-width apart, and ready to move into a squat position.
- Squat down and place your hands on the floor in front of you.
- Kick your feet back into a press-up position.
- Stay in this position. Keep one leg out straight while you bring your other knee up as high as you can towards your chest.
- Then alternate your legs over, so the leg that was straight is now up by your chest and the other leg is out straight. Once both your knees have been up to your chest once, this counts as one repetition.
- Once you have finished the repetitions specified, return your feet out straight behind you and squat thrust up and on to your feet.

>>

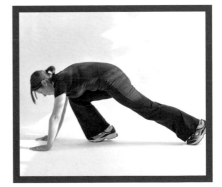

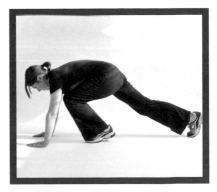

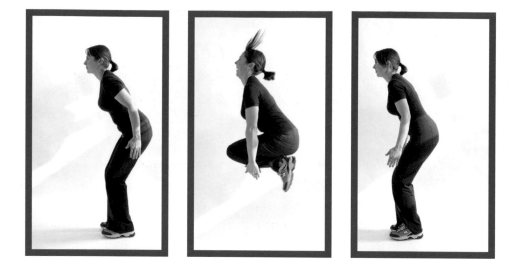

Frog hops

Purpose
To develop muscular strength and endurance in your lower legs.

Action
- Start from a squatting position, with your feet shoulder-width apart.
- Jump forwards as far and as high as you can, landing on both feet.
- Pause for a second, and then repeat for the specified number of repetitions.

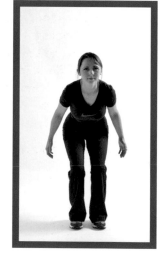
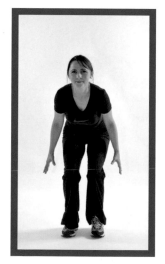
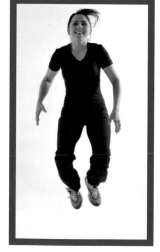

Jump overs >>

Purpose
To develop muscular strength and endurance in your lower legs.

Action
- Start with your feet hip-width apart, and next to a step box or an object approximately 45cm high.
- Jump over the object to the other side with your feet together and immediately back after touching the ground.
- Repeat for the specified number of repetitions.

Wide squat thrusts

Purpose

To build muscular endurance in your adductors and abductors.

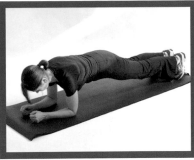

Action

- Start with your feet shoulder-width apart and ready to move into a squat position.
- Squat down and place your hands on the floor in front of you.
- Kick your feet back into a press-up position.
- While in this position, abduct your legs out to the side as far as possible, before adducting your feet together again.
- Repeat for the specified number of repetitions, before returning to your feet.

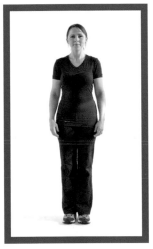 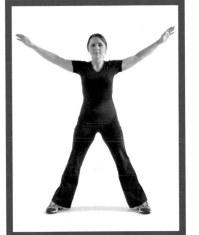

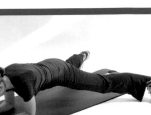 ## Star jumps

Purpose

Improves muscular endurance, fitness and coordination.

Action

- Stand with your feet shoulder-width apart, with your arms by your side.
- As you jump, raise your arms up to the side (shoulder height) and abduct your legs to the side as far as comfortable, then you will land in the position of a star.
- Jump back from that position to the start and repeat.

Spotty dogs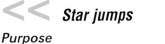

Purpose

Improves muscular endurance, fitness and coordination.

Action

- Stand with one foot forwards (leading leg), with the same-side arm out in front of you at shoulder height.
- Jump into the air so you swap your leading leg and arms over, so your opposite leg is now out in front.

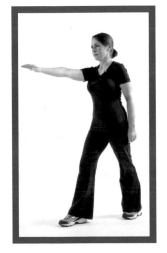 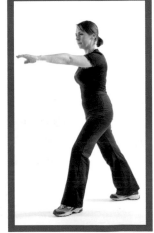

Skipping

>>

Purpose

Improves fitness, coordination and rhythm.

Action

- Hold on to the handles at waist height and slightly in front of you.
- As you jump, try to rotate the rope by making small rotations from your forearms, and with a little help from your wrists.
- One turn of the rope and one bounce counts as one repetition.

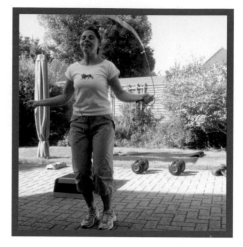

STEP BOX EXERCISES

STEP-UPS

Box Jumps

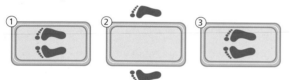

If you find this too much on your joints, do down, down, up, up instead.

Side Lunges

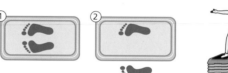

Down, Down, Up, Up

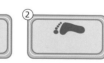

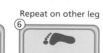

Repeat on other leg

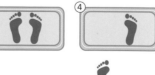

Back Lunges

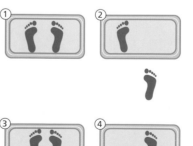

BOXING EXERCISES

Alternate punches

>>

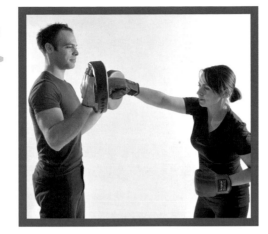
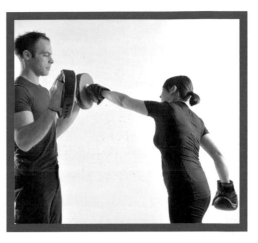

Straight punches

>>

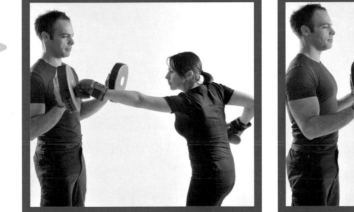
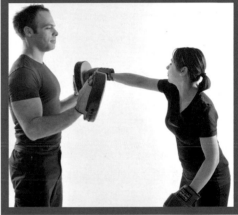

Upper cuts

>>

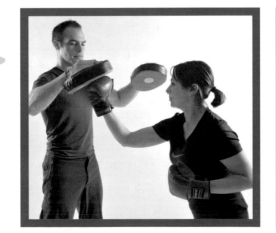
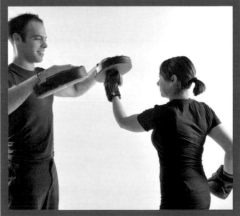

Wide punches

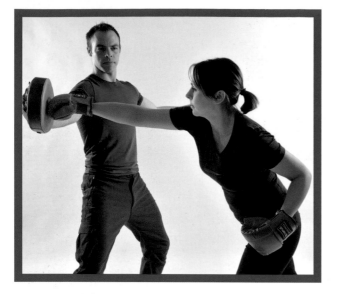 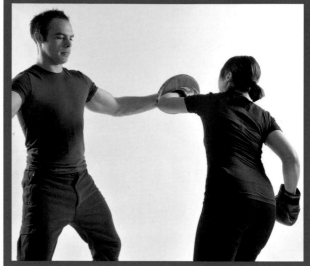

Reverse punches

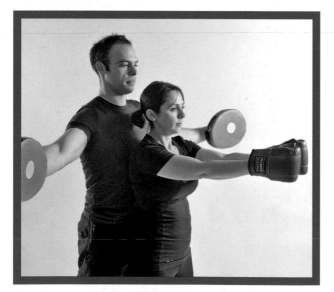 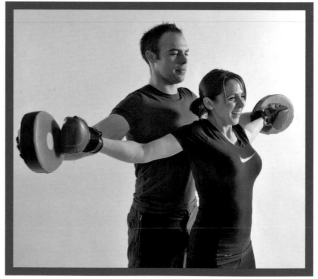

WEIGHT AND RUNNING CONVERSION CHARTS

WEIGHT CONVERSION CHART

Throughout the training sessions we have used kilograms and pounds. Use the weight conversion chart below to monitor and calculate the weight you have been lifting.

Kilograms (kg)	Pounds (lb)
1	2.2
5	11
10	22
15	33
20	44
25	55
30	66
40	88
50	110
60	132
70	154
80	176
90	198
100	220
110	242
120	264
130	286
140	308
150	330

MINUTE/MILE CONVERSION CHART

Use the following minute/mile conversation chart to see how long it takes you to run a certain distance. I have highlighted a good pace to be aiming for.

Miles	1	2	3	4	5	6	8	10
Minutes per mile	6	12	18	24	30	36	48	60
	7	14	21	28	35	42	56	70
	8	16	24	32	40	48	64	80
	9	18	27	36	45	54	72	90
	10	20	30	40	50	60	80	100
	12	24	36	48	60	72	96	120
	15	30	45	60	75	90	120	150

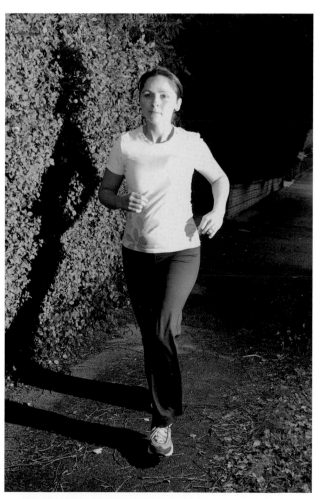

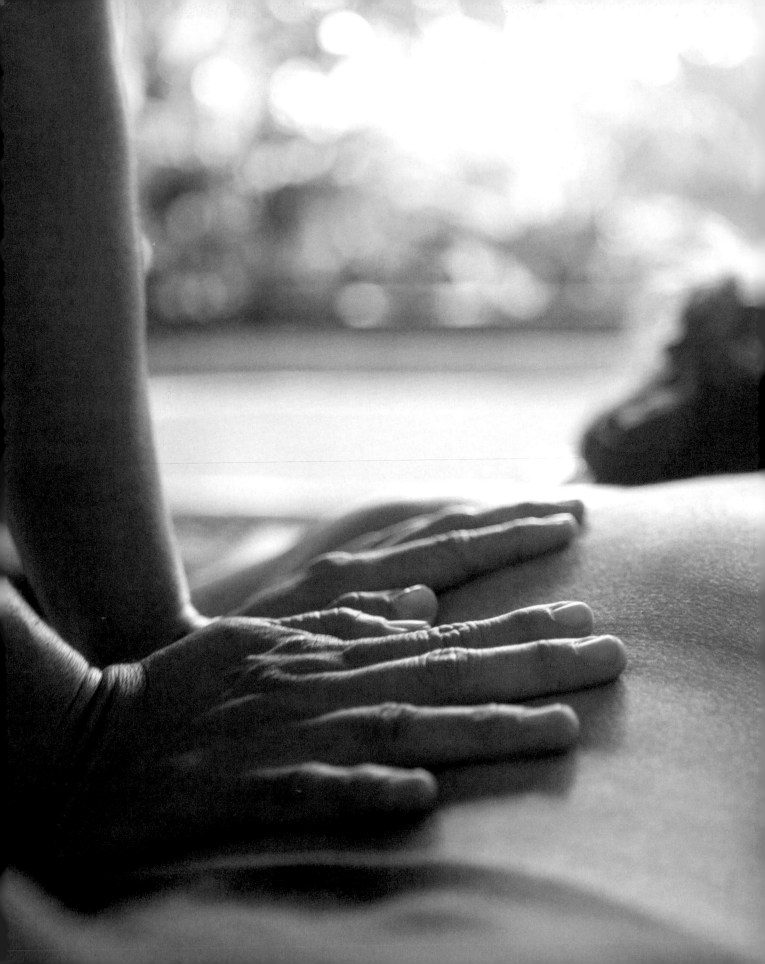

RELEASE THE PRESSURE

08

MASSAGE AND STRETCHING

MASSAGE

Massage is one of the oldest and simplest forms of medical care used to ease pain and anxiety, and to promote good health. Massage therapy and stretching provides relaxation and relief to muscle strain and fatigue, and this contributes to our overall health and well-being.

The benefits of massage therapy are almost endless, and include physical, emotional and physiological improvements to the body.

During the 12-week programme it is worth considering having massages to help relieve muscular spasms and tension, aid in the breaking down of cellulite, boost the immune system and stimulate the lymphatic system.

Muscular massage

Uses pressure or trigger points and essential oils to work with massage to eliminate pain patterns. This approach ultimately brings balance between the musculoskeletal system and the nervous system.

Lymphatic massage

Features special pumping strokes and vibrations to enhance the flow of the lymphatic system. Lymph is a whitish coloured liquid that flows throughout the body inside lymph vessels, which collect waste and toxins that cannot be absorbed through the capillary blood vessels. The combined movement and pressure encourages the movement of lymphatic fluid. This helps the immune and lymph systems, plus any other types of oedema, to return to full health and correct working order.

Cellulite massage

Uses a distinctive technique that picks up and rolls the connective tissue, skin, fascia and adipose tissue (fat) to separate them from each other. It helps release the build-up of cellulite which is then pushed to other specific areas with special strokes, to enable a fitness regime to take effect.

Alison used cellulite and lymphatic massages on a weekly basis, which along with the fitness programme and drinking plenty of water, helped to completely change the look of her skin around the thighs and on the stomach.

Myo stretching routine

Throughout the 12-week programme I used the myo stretch, which is an hour-long stretching routine. The myo stretch encompasses and works the majority of the muscles within your body to ensure an increase in muscle strength and resistance.

There are multiple benefits to stretching, and it should not be overlooked in your daily health routine. When we stretch properly we:

- Increase our range of motion (ROM)
- Increase performance in training and exercise (power and strength)
- Improve posture
- Reduce fatigue within muscles
- Reduce any delayed onset of muscle soreness after training or exercise (DOMS)
- Develop body awareness
- Promote circulation
- Improve relaxation within tense and tight muscles
- Aids stress relief

How to stretch correctly

There is no time limit to stretching, although do remember that less is best. The gentler you are with your stretching, the more you get out of the muscles.

When you find the first part of tension in your stretch, you should feel a really small amount, as if you are just about to stretch. It should be nice and simple, and isolate the muscle you are trying to focus on without involving any others. Allow the muscle adequate time to relax and elongate (there is no time limit).

If you are bouncing in stretches, feeling sharp pain in the muscle being stretched, feeling muscle spasm or shake, or feeling a burning sensation, then you are probably stretching the muscle too hard, and most likely incorrectly. Remember, less is best.

There are different types of stretching that can improve flexibility and strength, and are an important element when creating harmony within your body.

Static stretching

This means performing a certain stretch without movement. This is when you find the first tension within the muscle and hold, without moving from that position. Once it has released, you can either move on to the next stretch or gently repeat the action.

Developmental stretching

This works in the same way at the static stretch. You find the first point of tension and hold it until the muscle relaxes and elongates. Once you feel no stretch, go slightly further into the stretch until you feel tension for the second time. Repeat up to four times.

Proprioceptive neuromusular facilitation stretching (PNF)

An advanced stretching and flexibility technique that involves both the contraction and stretching of a muscle. This stretch is best performed with a professional or training partner, although some can be tried at home. Always remember to listen to your body and take note on how to perform the PNF correctly, and do not use the PNF stretch on muscles that are weak, elongated or overstretched.

To perform PNF stretching:
- Find the first bit of tension in the stretch and hold until the tension has elongated.
- Contract the same muscle that was being stretched for 20–40 per cent of your maximum effort.
- Hold the contraction of the muscle for 12 seconds.
- Release the contraction and allow the muscle to relax for a second.

- Now find the second stretch by going further until you find the tension again. You should have noticed a greater range before feeling the stretch.

MYO STRETCH

Developmental stretch for calf (gastrocnemius) muscles

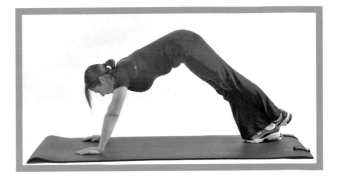

- From a press-up position, move your hand closer to your feet while raising your hips into the air.
- With your feet together, use one foot for support with the other foot flat on the floor and your legs extended straight, but not completely locked out.
- Bend the leg that is for support.
- Move your hands closer until you feel a small stretch in the calf of the foot that is flat to the ground.
- Once the stretch has elongated, move your hands closer again to your feet, or you can push your heel into the floor. You should now be feeling a stretch in the middle part of your calf muscle.
- Without dropping the position, allow your hands

- Again, allow the stretch to relax and elongate before repeating the process.
- You can repeat this process up to three times before coming out of the stretch.

to go back to the starting position and repeat for the other leg. You will also be working your upper body while in this position.
- Once you have completed the stretch on the other side, move your hands back to the start, keeping in the same position. You are now ready to perform the soleus stretch.

Developmental stretch for soleus muscles

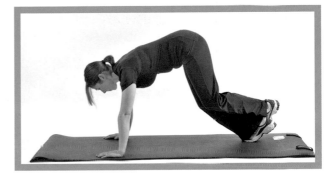

- Stay in the position of the calf stretch – with your hands out in front of you and your hips in the air.
- With your feet together, use one for support and the other almost flat on the floor, legs bent at the knee.
- Move your hands closer until you feel a small stretch in the lower calf.
- Once the stretch has elongated, move your hands closer to your feet, or you can push your heel into the floor. You should be feeling a stretch on the lower calf towards your Achilles tendon.
- Without dropping the position, allow your hands to go back to the starting position and repeat

for the other leg. You will also be working your upper body while in this position.
- Once you have completed the stretch on the other side, put both feet on the floor and go back down into the press-up position.
- Sit up and sit back on to your heels. You are now ready to move on to the lower back stretch.

Static stretch for the lower back

- While sitting on your heels, reach forwards from your hip with your hands out in front of you and let your head relax.
- You should be nice and relaxed, and you might be able to feel a stretch in your lower back and latissimus dorsi.

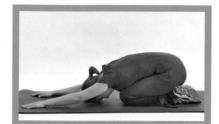

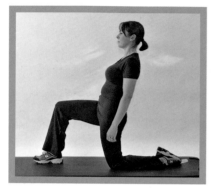

 ### Developmental stretch for hip flexor stretch

This is a good stretch for a lordotic posture:

- Kneel on one foot.
- If you need to, hold on to an object to help keep balance.
- Lean slightly forwards so your weight is on the front foot.
- Push your hip out forwards.
- To get more of a stretch, lean your torso slightly back in the opposite direction. You should feel a stretch in the front of your hip (iliacus, psoas major and rectus femoris).
- From this position go straight into the PNF stretch on the same leg.

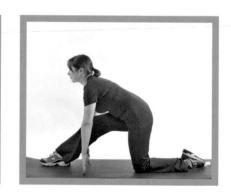

PNF stretch for hamstring muscles

This is a postural stretch for flat back/sway back:

- Kneel on one knee with your other leg out in front, so your foot is flat on the floor.
- Keep your back straight while leaning forwards to keep balance (you can either balance yourself with one or both arms down to the floor).
- Sit back on to your knee.
- Try to keep your leg out in front, with a small bend in your knee.
- Tilt your buttocks up in the air to feel more of a stretch. As long as you have the stretch in your hamstrings you can now perform a PNF stretch if your muscle requires it.
- Follow the rules for performing a PNF stretch (see page 340).
- While in the same position, and now that the first stretch has released, you can push your foot into the ground as if you were trying to curl your heel

up to your bum. You should now feel the same muscle contract that was just being stretched (if you can't feel the contraction in your hamstring, try moving until you do feel it).
- Hold the contraction at 20 per cent of your maximum effort for 12 seconds.
- Relax for one second, and then move into the stretch for a second time.
- Perform the PNF stretch two or three times. You should feel a stretch in the back of your thigh/ hamstring (semimembranosus, semitendinosus and biceps femoris).
- Sit back on to both of your heels.
- Now change legs and repeat these last two stretches.

Static stretch for the lower back
- Repeat exercise from opposite page.

>>

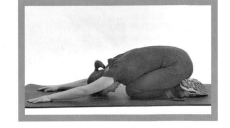

<< *Developmental stretch for quad with your knees bent*
- While sitting on your heels, place your legs under your buttocks.
- Lean back, keeping your body weight on your arms.
- You should then be able to feel a stretch in the middle part of your quads.
- To feel more of a stretch, or to develop the stretch, move your hands further behind you or squeeze your glute muscles/push out your hips. You should be able to feel a stretch within the middle part of your quads (rectus femoris, vastus medialis, vastus lateralis and vastus intermedius).
- Roll over on to your front and lie face down.

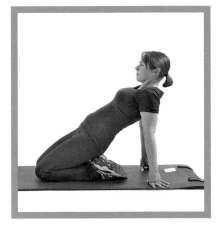

PNF stretch for quad lying face down
This is a posture stretch for lordotic postures:
- Lie face down.
- Bring one foot up towards your buttock while holding on to it with the same-side arm.
- Pull the foot to your buttock to feel the stretch within the middle/upper part of the quad.
- As long as you have the stretch in your quads you can now perform a PNF stretch if your muscle requires it. Follow the rules for performing a PNF stretch (see page 340).
- While in the same position, and when the first stretch has released, you can push your leg out as if you are trying to straighten it. You should now feel the same muscle contract. (If you can't, try to move slightly until you feel the muscle contract.)
- Hold the contraction at 20 per cent of your maximum effort for 12 seconds.

>>

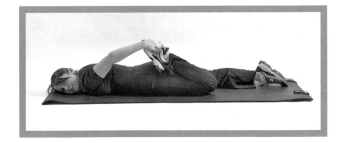

- Relax for one second, and then move into the stretch for a second time.
- Perform the PNF stretch two or three times.
- You should be able to feel a stretch within the middle to upper portion of the quads (rectus femoris, vastus medialis, vastus lateralis and vastus intermedius).
- Once you have stretched your quad, swap your hands over so your opposite hand is on the leg being stretched.
- From this position, go straight into the static stretch for the quads on the same leg.

>>

Static stretch for quad muscles lying down, opposite hand to opposite leg

- Lie face down.
- Bring one foot up towards your buttock, while holding on to it with the opposite arm.
- Pull the foot to your opposite buttock.
- Keep your hips on the ground. You should be able to feel a stretch on the outer part of the quad).
- Once you have finished stretching, move on to your other leg and repeat.

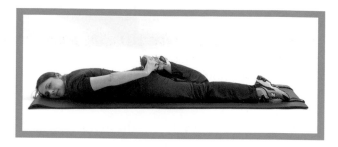

- Once you have finished your lying quad stretches you can relax for one or two minutes in this position.
- Roll on to your back and sit up for your hamstring stretch.
- Repeat these last two stretches on the other leg.

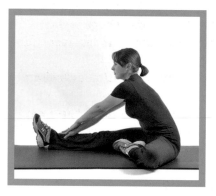

<< ## *Developmental stretch for sitting hamstring muscles*

This is a posture stretch for flat back or sway back.
- Place your arms on the ground beside you.
- Place both legs out in front of you.
- Sit with your back straight.
- Bend one knee enough so it falls to the side, while keeping your other leg straight.
- Lean forwards from the hip until you find a stretch in your hamstrings. You should now be able to feel a stretch within your hamstring muscles (semimembranosus, semitendinosus and biceps femoris).
- Once you have stretched one side, move on to the other side.
- When you have finished stretching your other leg, keep both legs out in front of you ready for the next stretch.

Developmental stretch for the wide leg adductor

>>

- Sit with your legs straight out and wide in front of you (make sure it is as wide as is comfortable so that you don't feel a stretch on your hamstring muscles).
- Sit with a straight back.
- Lean forwards until you feel a stretch on your adductors. You should be able to feel the inside of your thighs/adductors (adductor longus, adductor brevis, adductor magnus and gracilis).
- Bring both feet into your groin, if possible with your feet together, to stretch adductors.

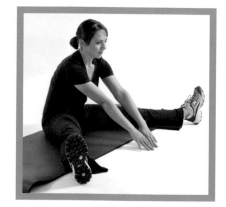

Developmental stretch for the sitting groin muscle >>

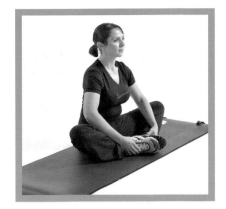

- Sit with your back straight.
- For support, hold on to your feet.
- Keep your feet together if possible, and allow your knees to drop out to the side.
- You should feel a stretch on the inside of your thighs. If not, bring your feet in towards your groin.
- You should be able to feel a stretch on the inside of your thighs/ adductors (adductor longus, adductor brevis , adductor magnus, gracilis and pectineus).
- Put both of your legs out in front of you and relax your body for one or two minutes.

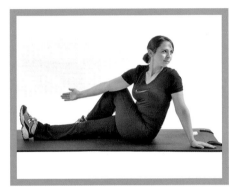

<< ## *Static stretch for sitting glute muscle extensions*

Perform this stretch if you feel pain in your lower back.

- Sit with one leg out straight, and cross the other leg over your knee.
- Turn your shoulders around so your torso is facing away from your body.
- Place one arm on to your raised knee to help you rotate even further, and your other arm out behind you to support yourself. You should be able to feel a stretch in your glute muscles (gluteus maximus, gluteus medius and gluteus minimus), as well as tensor fasciae latae and piriformis.
- Swap your legs over to stretch your other side.
- Keep your leg crossed but relaxed. Roll on to your back to stretch your deeper glute muscles.
- Change your legs over and repeat the same stretch.

Developmental stretch for glute muscles >>

Perform this postural stretch when suffering from sciatica (caused by your piriformis being too tight).

- Lie on your back on the floor, face up.
- Cross one leg over the other.
- Start to bring your foot down towards your buttock.
- Grasp on to the thigh (hamstrings) just under the knee.
- Pull the leg up and towards your chest. You should be able to feel a stretch in your glute muscles (piriformis, deep glute muscles and gluteus maximus).
- Stretch the other side, then relax with your feet on the ground and your knees in the air.
- Bring both knees into your chest to stretch your lower back.
- Change your legs over and repeat the stretch on the other side.

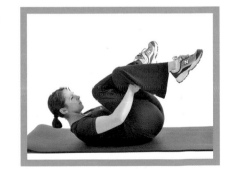

Developmental stretch for the lower back while lying down

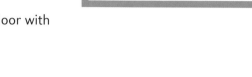

Perform this postural stretch if you have a lordotic posture.

* Lie on your back, face up.
* Hold on to the back of both of your thighs, just underneath the knees.
* Pull your knees towards your chest, allowing your buttocks to rise off the ground. You should be able to feel a stretch in your lower back and gluteus maximus.
* Once the stretch has released, drop your feet on to the floor with knees bent and relaxed.
* Drop legs flat to the floor for the next stretch.

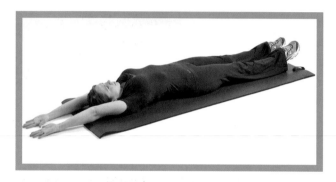

Static stretch for the whole body

* Lie on your back and extend your legs out straight in front of you, and your arms out straight overhead.
* Lengthen your body as much as possible by pointing your toes and pushing your arms overhead. You should be able to feel a stretch in different places of the body (including your abs, serratus anterior and lattisimus dorsi).
* Once the stretch has relaxed, bring your arms out to your side for the next stretch.

Static stretch for lying roll over

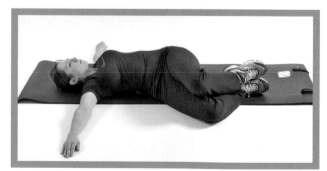

* Lie on your back.
* Keep your arms out to your side and bring your knees up, with your feet on the floor.
* Allow your knees to drop to one side and try to relax your back and hips to get the best stretch. You should be able to feel a stretch in your lower back muscles and glute muscles.
* Bring your knee back up to the centre and drop to the other side.
* Stay on your back in a relaxed position, and relax for 2–3 minutes.
* Roll on to your front for the abdominal stretch.

Static stretch for the abdominal muscles

>>

This is a postural stretch for a flat back.

- Lie face down on the floor.
- Keep your hands in front of you, about shoulder-width apart.
- Keep your hips, legs and feet flat on the ground.
- Raise your torso off the ground until your arms are almost straight, or you feel a stretch in your abdominals.
- Hold this stretch for no longer than 10 seconds.

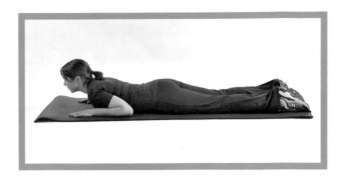

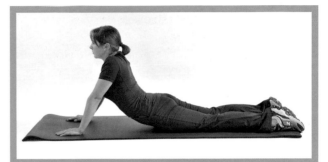

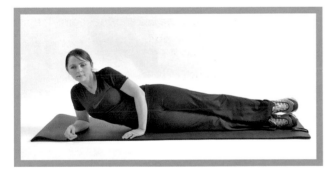

<< *Static stretch for the oblique muscles*

- Lie on your side, keeping your body straight.
- Make sure the leg you're resting is touching the floor.
- With your forearm resting on the floor and your other arm in front of you for support, extend your resting arm out straight so your body weight is resting on your hand instead.
- You should now feel a stretch on your side and in your oblique muscles.
- Roll onto your front, and then on to the other side, to stretch your other obliques.
- Once you have stretched your other side, roll back onto your front for the cat stretch.

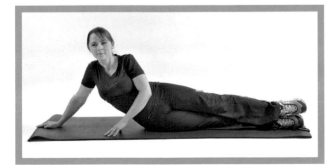

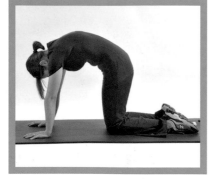

<< *Static cat stretch*

- Kneel on all fours.
- Let your head fall forwards and relax.
- Arch your back and draw in your belly button. You should be able to feel a stretch in your lower back.
- Relax from your stretch, and then sit back on your heels for another lower back stretch.

Static stretch for the lower back

- Repeat exercise from page 342.

>>

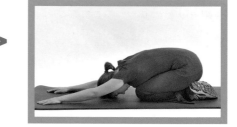

<< *Development lat stretch on the floor*

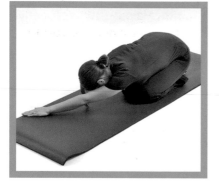

- Sitting on your heels, reach forwards with your hands.
- Place one arm across your body with it resting on the floor.
- Use your fingers to walk your arm diagonally away from your body to feel a stretch in your latissimus dorsi.
- Keep walking your fingers out to get a developmental stretch.
- Bring your arm back to the centre, and then swap over to the other side.

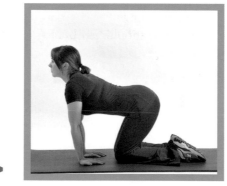 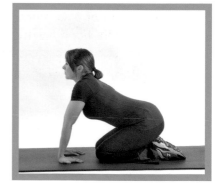

>>

Static stretch for the biceps muscles

- Kneel on all fours.
- Turn your arms so the insides of your forearms are facing away from you, and your fingers are pointing at you.
- Keep your arms straight, and sit back towards your heels.

- Try not to put too much body weight on to your arms. You should feel a stretch on the front of the top of your arms (the biceps, and possibly on your wrist flexors).
- Sit back up on to your heels, and relax for 2–3 minutes.

Static stretch for the triceps muscles

>>

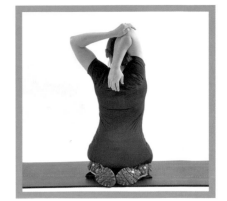

- Sit on your heels.
- Place one hand up and behind your head, with your elbow pointing upwards.
- With your other hand (depending on your flexibility), either pull the elbow down from the top, or you can push the elbow from the front. You should be able to feel a stretch on the back of your upper arm (triceps).
- Now stand up for the final stretches – you can move around to get the blood flowing around your muscles.
- Follow the next stretches one after the other while standing.

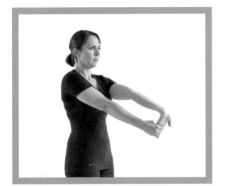

<< ## Static stretch for wrist flexor muscles

- With one hand, hold on to the fingers of your other hand and straighten your arm so your forearm is facing upwards.
- Pull your fingers/hand towards your body. You should be able to feel a stretch on the inside of your forearm.
- Repeat this stretch on your other hand.

Static stretch for the wrist extensor muscles

>>

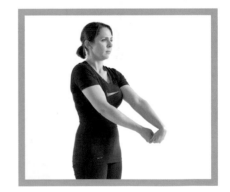

- With one hand, hold on to the opposite fingers/hand and straighten your arm so your forearm is facing down.
- Pull your fingers/hand towards your body. You should be able to feel a stretch on the back of your forearm.
- Repeat this stretch on your other hand.

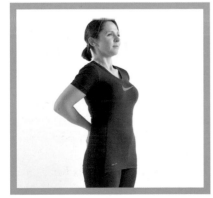

<< ## Static stretch for the anterior deltoid muscles

- Place your hands into the base of your back.
- Drop your shoulders forwards and raise up your chest, as if you're taking in a deep breath. You should be able to feel a stretch at the front of your shoulders (anterior deltoid).

Static stretch for the deltoid muscles

>>

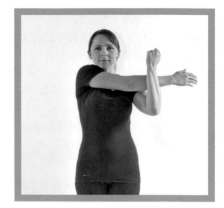

- Place one arm across the front of your body.
- You can either keep that arm straight or you can bend it to a 90° angle.
- Pull your arm in and towards the opposite arm until you feel a stretch. You should be able to feel a stretch in your shoulder, and slightly in the upper back (rear deltoid, rhomboids and trapezius).

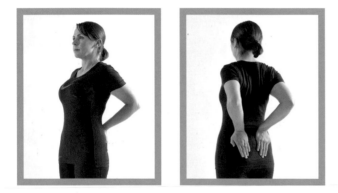

<<

Static stretch for the chest with hands behind the back

- Place your hands into the base of your spine.
- Bring your elbows as close together as possible and push your chest out. You should be able to feel a stretch in your chest (pectoral major, pectoral minor and anterior deltoid).

Static stretch for the chest on a wall

>>

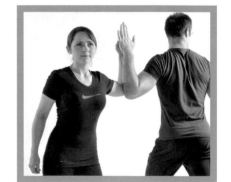

This is a postural stretch for the kyphotic posture:

- Stand beside a wall, with your feet shoulder-width apart.
- Bend your arm to a 90° angle at the elbow, and rest your forearm on to the wall or door frame.
- Place the same-side leg forwards.
- Turn your body and shoulders away from the bent arm until you feel a stretch in your chest (pectoral major, pectoral minor and anterior deltoid).

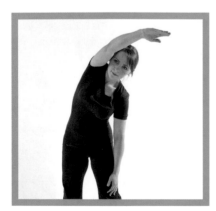

<< ### Static stretch for the lat muscle

- Place your feet shoulder-width apart, and extend one arm across your body in front of you.
- Reach across as far as possible with your hands, while leaning slightly forwards. The key is to try and arch the side of your back.
- You can vary this by holding on to an object or doorway (this will give you a deeper stretch into the lat muscle). You should be able to feel a stretch in the side of your back (latissimus dorsi).

Static stretch for the rhomboid muscles >>

- Place your hands together in front of you at about shoulder height.
- Reach forwards as far as comfortable with your hands, trying to round the middle/upper part of your back. You should be able to feel a stretch in the middle of your upper back between your shoulder blades (rhomboids).
- It's just like hugging a tree.

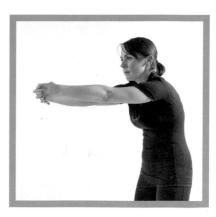

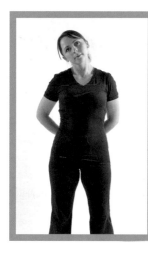
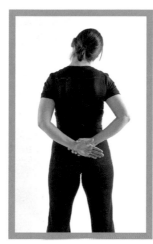

<<

Static stretch for the trapezius muscles

This can sometimes help kyphotic postures if you are feeling pain in the neck.

- While looking straight ahead, allow your head (ear) to drop towards the shoulder on the same side.
- Keep your hands behind your back to get the best stretch. You should be able to feel a stretch on the top of your shoulders into your neck (trapezius, levator scapulae).

Ending the myo stretch routine >>

To finish the routine, stand on your tip-toes and extend your arms overhead nice and straight. You should be able to feel a stretch throughout your body, and then release. Take a little walk around to get the blood moving throughout your whole body, including moving your arms.

You have now completed the myo stretch routine and should feel relaxed, with no tension in your body.

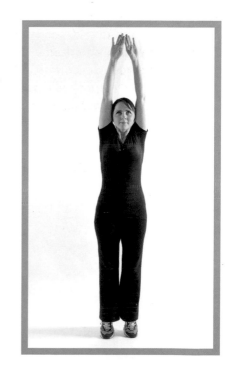

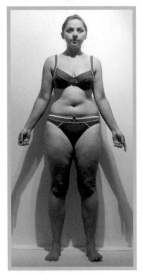

Week 1

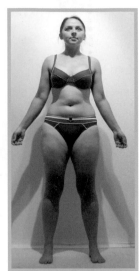

Week 2

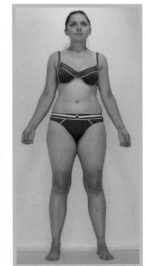

Week 3

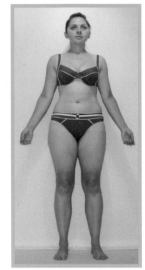

Week 4

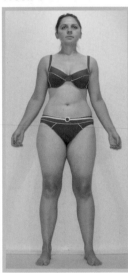

Week 5

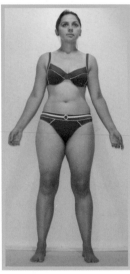

Week 6

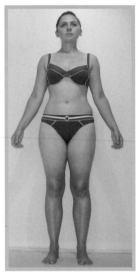

Week 7

Week 8

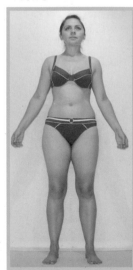

Week 9

Week 10

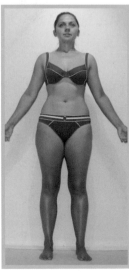

Week 11

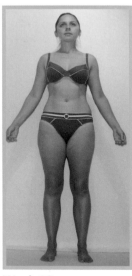

Week 12